Springer Series on Comparative Treatments for Psychological Disorders

Arthur Freeman, EdD, ABPP, Series Editor

Robert A. DiTomasso, PhD, ABPP, is professor, vice-chair, and director of clinical research in the Department of Psychology at the Philadelphia College of Osteopathic Medicine. He is a diplomate in clinical psychology from the American Board of Professional Psychology, a Fellow of the Academy of Clinical Psychology, and a Founding Fellow of the Academy of Cognitive Therapy. Dr. DiTomasso earned his doctoral degree in professional-scientific psychology at the University of Pennsylvania, where he received the William E. Arnold Award in recognition for outstanding leadership and scholarship. He completed a clinical psychology internship under the direction of the late Joseph Wolpe, MD, at the Behavior Therapy Unit at Eastern Pennsylvania Psychiatric Institute, Temple University School of Medicine, Department of Psychiatry. Dr. DiTomasso has had extensive teaching experience having served as adjunct associate professor at the University of Pennsylvania and as associate director of behavioral medicine at the West Jersey Health System Family Medicine Residency. His specialty is the cognitive-behavioral treatment of anxiety and anxiety-related medical disorders. He has published more than 32 chapters and articles.

Elizabeth A. Gosch, PhD, is assistant professor in psychology and director of the master of science program in clinical health psychology at the Philadelphia College of Osteopathic Medicine. She received her doctorate in clinical psychology from Temple University in Philadelphia. Dr. Gosch is a licensed psychologist who specializes in the treatment of anxiety disorders in her private practice. Her major research interests concern the process and effectiveness of psychotherapy with different populations. She is currently supervisor, therapist, and research consultant for an NIMH-funded clinical trial evaluating several forms of psychotherapy at the Child and Adolescent Anxiety Disorders Clinic at Temple University. As clinical instructor at the University of Pennsylvania, Dr. Gosch was assistant director of the Assessment Unit at the Center for Psychotherapy Research and involved in several NIMH-funded clinical psychotherapy trials. A member of the Publications Committee of the Association for the Advancement of Behavior Therapy, the Society for Psychotherapy Research, and the American Psychological Association, Dr. Gosch has published and lectured internationally on the cognitive-behavioral treatment of anxiety disorders in children.

ANXIETY DISORDERS

— A PRACTITIONER'S GUIDE TO —
COMPARATIVE TREATMENTS

ROBERT A. DiTOMASSO, PhD, ABPP
ELIZABETH A. GOSCH, PhD, Editors

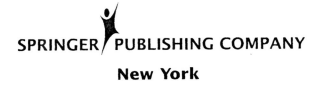

SPRINGER PUBLISHING COMPANY

New York

Springer Publishing Company, LLC
11 West 42nd Street
New York, NY 10036

Acquisitions Editor: Sheri W. Sussman
Production Editor: Janice G. Stangel
Cover design by Mimi Flow

06 07 08 09 / 5 4 3 2 1

New ISBN-13: 978-0-8261-2091-5 © 2006 by Springer Publishing Company, LLC

Library of Congress Cataloging-in-Publication Data

Comparative treatments for anxiety disorders / Robert A. DiTomasso,
    Elizabeth A. Gosch, editors.
            p. cm. — (Springer series on comparative treatments for
psychological disorders)
    Includes bibliographical references and index.
    ISBN 0-8261-4832-8
    1. Anxiety—Treatment. 2. Panic attacks—Treatment.
I. DiTomasso, Robert D. II. Gosch, Elizabeth A. III. Series
RC531 .C65 2002
616.85'223'06—dc21   2002019469
                                                                  CIP

Printed in the United States of America by Berryville Graphics

To Deborah, Natalie, and Alexis for their love, understanding, patience, and support. In memory of Lucy DiTomasso, William DiTomasso, and Robert DiGiovannantonio—RAD

To the many individuals with anxiety disorders who have shared their experiences with me in their search for answers. To my clinical mentors who have taught me to appreciate the contribution of differing theoretical orientations to treatment. And to Alan and Amelia for their unending support—EAG

Contents

Contributors

Katherine Crits-Cristoph, PhD
Clinical Assistant Professor
Center for Psychotherapy
  Research
Department of Psychiatry
University of Pennsylvania
Philadelphia, PA

Jay S. Efran, PhD
Professor
Temple University
Department of Psychology
Philadelphia, PA

Stephanie H. Felgoise, PhD
Assistant Professor
Department of Psychology
Philadelphia College of
  Osteopathic Medicine
Philadelphia, PA

Reed D. Goldstein, PhD
Clinical Assistant Professor
University of Pennsylvania School
  of Medicine
Dave Garroway
Laboratory for the Study of
  Depression
Pennsylvania Hospital
Philadelphia, PA

Jennifer Gregg, BA
Department of Psychology
University of Nevada, Reno
Reno, NV

Alan M. Gruenberg, MD
Professor of Psychiatry and
  Human Behavior
Jefferson Medical College;
President
Gruenberg & Summers, P.C.
Philadelphia, PA

Steven C. Hayes, PhD
Professor
Department of Psychology
University of Nevada, Reno
Reno, NV

Richard R. Kopp, PhD
Professor of Psychology
Alliant University
California School of Professional
  Psychology at Los Angeles
Encino, CA

Bruce Lackie, PhD
Licensed Psychologist
Affiliated Faculty
Walden University
Philadelphia, PA

Paul M. Lerner, EdD, ABPP
Licensed Psychologist in Private
   Practice
Camden, ME

Elizabeth A. Meadows, PhD
Associate Professor
Department of Psychology
Central Michigan University
Mount Pleasant, MI

Lynn Montgomery, MD, PhD
Clinical Associate Professor
Philadelphia College of
   Osteopathic Medicine
Philadelphia, PA

Arthur M. Nezu, PhD, ABPP
Professor
Department of Psychology
MCP Hahnemann University
Philadelphia, PA

**Christine Maguth Nezu, PhD,
   ABPP**
Professor
Department of Psychology
MCP Hahnemann University
Philadelphia, PA

Morrie Olson, RPh, MFT, CAAP
Executive Director
Behavioral Health Special
   Initiative
Philadelphia Behavioral Health
   System
Philadelphia, PA

Julieann Pankey, BA
Department of Psychology
University of Nevada
Reno, NV

Kelly A. Phipps, BA
Department of Psychology
Central Michigan University
Mount Pleasant, MI

Agnieszka Popiel, MD
Department of Psychiatry
Warsaw Medical University
Warsaw, Poland

Alan L. Schwartz, PsyD
Director of Psychology
Christiana Care Health Services
Department of Psychiatry
Wilmington, DE

Leonard C. Sitrin, PhD
Psychologist in Private Practice
Behavioral Medicine Consultants
Warren, NJ

**Major Stacey A. Williams, PhD,
   ABPP**
Chief, Pediatric Behavioral
   Health
Walter Reed Army Medical
   Center
Washington, DC

Preface

Anxiety disorders are costly, common, and debilitating. They often present challenging problems in the caseloads of practicing clinicians today. Thanks to the work of a myriad of dedicated clinicians and researchers, we know more about anxiety problems and their treatment than we ever have. The development of structured clinical interviews, new assessment tools, and treatment manuals attests to this fact. An enormous literature on the assessment and treatment of anxiety currently exists. Clinical case studies and empirical research in this area answer important questions, but in so doing often raise new and even more important questions. Real-world clinicians, practicing within the context of a given theoretical orientation, must often be innovative and creative in the applications of their models.

Clinicians are motivated to offer the very best services they possibly can by customizing and tailoring treatment to the individual. Theoretical models serve to drive and guide the thoughts and actions of therapists in assessing, conceptualizing, and planning treatment. Although commonalities exist across treatment paradigms, distinctions are often evident in how problems are assessed, formulated, and addressed. Coupled with the fact that no one theoretical orientation has accounted for all of the treatment outcome variance, we believe that understanding these different models will only serve to enhance our knowledge base about anxiety and its treatment.

The first chapter provides an overview of anxiety and its disorders including its prevalence, costs, associated problems, predisposing factors, and triggering factors. A brief description of each disorder, problems in assessment and diagnosis, and cultural factors are also included.

Chapter 2 introduces the case of Sandra, a composite portrait of a woman with an anxiety disorder whose history is informed by the scores of patients treated by the authors over the past 25 years. Sandra represents the history of an anxiety-disordered patient commonly seen in practice today. A standard list of questions for contributors is also included in this chapter.

Chapters 3 through 13 present the viewpoints of a variety of seasoned clinicians practicing from a single theoretical model. These clinicians were asked to elucidate how they would approach the case of Sandra from their own theoretical viewpoint. Each chapter provides a thorough description of the model, therapist skills and attributes, assessment plans, treatment goals, therapeutic relationship issues, common pitfalls, intervention strategies, and mechanisms of change. These chapters allow the reader to "sit in and observe" master clinicians at work—what they consider important and how they weigh various factors in the conceptualization and treatment of an anxious patient. Our hope is that clinicians, researchers, and graduate students will profit by a comparison of how each clinician approaches the same case from a different theoretical orientation. We are quite hopeful that this volume will prove extremely useful to clinicians of various theoretical persuasions who have an interest in comparing and contrasting differing approaches to the treatment of anxiety.

Acknowledgments

An edited volume of this nature would not have been possible without the assistance of a number of individuals. First and foremost, we extend our appreciation to Arthur Freeman, the series editor, for his expert guidance and assistance throughout the course of this project. Art was especially helpful in the development of the case presentation and in suggesting possible expert contributors. We also thank our colleagues in the Psychology Department at the Philadelphia College of Osteopathic Medicine for their support and encouragement.

Many thanks to our contributors who took time from their busy schedules and pressing responsibilities to participate in this project.

We thank Sandra Branche and Susan Hartman for their expertise in typing and word processing. They worked diligently in assisting us, especially with their timely turnaround of materials despite very busy schedules. We also appreciate the assistance of Sara O'Neal and Aaron Pollock, our graduate assistants. We thank Sheri Sussman and Janice Stangel for their patience and guidance through the editing process.

Finally, we would like to thank our families, Debbie, Natalie, and Alexis DiTomasso, and Alan and Amelia Schwartz for understanding the preoccupation and absences at times associated with the completion of this volume.

Series Editor's Note

> *Comparisons are odious . . .*
> —Cervantes, *Don Quixote*

The general view of comparisons is that they represent measurements against some standard or that they entail evaluating one experience or object against another. If one has had a sibling, one has likely come up against the parental statement, "Why can't you be like . . .?" Teachers also invariably compare students one with the other when they post grades or grade papers for all to see.

This view of comparisons is that they are somehow adversarial-one person, group, or effort "wins" and one "loses." In psychology we often use the construct of comparison as synonymous with the term "versus" (e.g., "The treatment of depression: Psychotherapy versus pharmacotherapy" or "A comparison of two treatments for Obsessive Compulsive disorder"). This implies that whenever there are two or more systems or objects available, one will be better than another. Yet not all comparisons are clear-cut. One choice may be appropriate for a certain sub-group, while another choice may work better in a different setting or with a different population. (This adversarial view seems to be very popular among mental health professionals. After all, we are a group that over the years when under attack have been known to circle our wagons and shoot at each other!)

Our goal in this series is to examine not who is better than whom, or what model works better than other models, but rather to examine and to compare, as cleanly as we can, the similarities and differences between different psychotherapeutic approaches. To do this most efficiently, we have used a standard patient. All contributors were asked to respond to the sample case prepared by the volume editors.

In this way the reader can compare the thinking, conceptualization, interventions, and questions that would be asked by the contributing authors. We have invited authors who are exemplars of a particular school, understanding that other therapists of the same school might see or do things differently. By aligning apparently diverse therapies side-by-side, we can look at what models share specific conceptual frameworks, philosophical biases, strategic foci, or technical interventions, as well as help us to make clearer distinctions between therapeutic models.

We have set as our goal the examination of those problems most frequently seen in clinical practice. We have not seen this need for cross-model comparison as an issue of professional discipline inasmuch as these clinical syndromes are seen by psychologists, psychiatrists, nurse practitioners, social workers, pastoral counselors, and counselors.

This series sprang from four roots. First, the powerful influence of the classic "Gloria" series produced by Dr. Everett Shostrum, when he arranged for Carl Rogers (Client-Centered Therapy), Albert Ellis (Rational Emotive Therapy), and Fritz Perls (Gestalt Therapy) to demonstrate their representative model of therapy with a standard patient, Gloria. He gave viewers the opportunity to compare and contrast the three models as practiced by the founders of the particular school of therapy.

The second influence on this series was the present state of affairs in psychotherapy. Between the models that are promoted for their purported science and efficacy and those models that are promoted for their purported humanism and eschewal of science, there are many treatment models. Without attempting to judge the value, efficacy, and importance of a model, we believe that it is important to offer mental health professionals the opportunity to make their own decisions about diverse treatment models.

The third impetus for this series was the availability of so many experts in the treatment of the broad range of psychological disorders. Both as editors and as contributing authors, it is their work that is being highlighted in this series.

Finally, this series was the result of encouragement and support from Bill Tucker, Acquisitions Editor of Springer Publishing Company, and Dr. Ursula Springer, the President of Springer Publishing Company. When I first approached Springer with the idea for the series, they were enthusiastic and eagerly agreed not to just produce one volume, but committed their resources to a series of several volumes. Given the publishing history of Springer, the breadth and quality of their book list, and the many professional groups that they reach, I can think of no better place for this series on comparative psychotherapy.

ARTHUR FREEMAN, EdD, ABPP
Department of Psychology
Philadelphia College of Osteopathic Medicine

1

Anxiety Disorders: An Overview

Robert A. DiTomasso and Elizabeth A. Gosch

Anxiety is a universal phenomenon experienced by all human beings at one time or another during the course of their lives. As a diffuse state of mood, anxiety has been considered to be an unpleasant affective experience marked by a significant degree of apprehensiveness about the potential appearance of future aversive or harmful events (Barlow & Cerny, 1988). The topic of anxiety has captured the attention of clinical psychologists, psychiatrists, and the lay public worldwide. Although anxiety was first recognized in the writings of Hippocrates (Reiger et al., 1988), it was only about 40 years ago that interest in this topic began to surge. Among many possible influences, Wolpe's classic book, *Psychotherapy by Reciprocal Inhibition*, may be partially credited with focusing attention on this important topic (Wolpe, 1958). Wolpe essentially challenged the professional community to develop and apply efficacious treatments for anxiety, based upon experimentally derived laboratory paradigms. Prior to that time, and perhaps related to the high prevalence of the experience of anxiety in the general population, considerably more professional attention was aimed at what appeared to be more serious, albeit rarer, and debilitating psychopathological states. Anxiety was naturally relegated to a secondary position in this regard.

In the ensuing years, however, what we have learned about anxiety has done much to accord this problem the attention it deserves.

Relative to other mental health difficulties, prevalence rates of anxiety are the highest (Dupont et al., 1996) making it not only common, affecting millions of people, but costly in terms of treatment expenditures and personal consequences for those who experience it. About 15% of the population are affected by an anxiety disorder at some time during the course of their lives (Brown & Barlow, 1992). Far fewer ever receive treatment for it. Those who have major anxiety problems may experience adverse consequences to their quality of life and their ability to function in the interpersonal arena (McLeod, 1994; Mendlowicz & Stein, 2000). Anxious, stress-related states are often associated with the precipitation and exacerbation of health problems and form a core component of psychophysiological or arousal disorders (Everly, 1989; Gatchel & Blanchard, 1994). Anxiety is one of the most common problems seen in the primary care setting (Marsland, Wood, & Mayo, 1976). It is among one of the most common precipitants motivating people to seek both medical care and mental health services (Brown & Barlow, 1992). Anxiety disorders impose a heavy economic burden on society with estimated annual costs at $42.3 billion in the 1990s (Greenberg et al., 1999). Patients with anxiety problems often experience coexisting mental health problem such as depression and substance abuse. Given the close association between danger and anxiety, perhaps no other emotion is so closely tied to the basic survival of an individual in the face of real threat. Yet when elicited in a chronic, maladaptive manner, anxiety may create a host of consequences that impair normal everyday functioning.

It is little wonder, then, that literally thousands of references appearing in the professional literature attest to the importance of this topic. In attempts to understand this phenomenon more fully, clinicians of varied theoretical persuasions have addressed issues of assessment, diagnosis, and treatment of this problem. Proponents of these diverse viewpoints promote notions that are theoretically consistent within their respective schools of thought. Not all schools are equal in the extent to which their constructs are subject to ongoing empirical validation. Of course, absence of evidence for a given theoretical construct does not necessarily translate into evidence of absence for that construct or its relevance to anxiety. It is possible and even likely, then, that hypotheses emanating from different theories, although untested, may add further to our existing knowledge of anxious traits and states. This possibility may stem, oddly enough, from empirical treatment validation studies themselves, which, though demonstrating the effectiveness of specific treatment protocols for anxiety disorders, fail to account for all of the variance in treatment outcome. Different theories may help to provide hypotheses and strategies to account for the unexplained residual outcomes. Barring any differences, however, these theorists appear to converge on one point: Anxiety and fear in the face of real, objective threat is adaptive.

As a mechanism of survival, anxiety motivates an individual to take some decisive action—to fight, to freeze, or to flee. Failure to do so would do little to promote the continuation of the species, or the individual in question for that matter. Understandably, then, exposure to real threat where there is a high risk of associated injury, or even death, warrants a relatively drastic adaptive reaction. Such an extreme reaction—or even a less intense apprehension or anticipation where no objective danger or minimal risk of threat exists—does little to promote the well-being of an individual.

BASIC CHARACTERISTICS OF ANXIETY

An understanding of the basic characteristics of anxiety facilitates the distinction between anxiety as a normal response and anxiety as a disordered response. Whatever theoretical differences exist between schools of thought about anxiety, issues in the study of this phenomenon abound. Although a major exposition of all of these issues is beyond the scope of this book, we now address several major issues.

Definition: Anxiety as a Disordered State

There are many more people who suffer from anxiety than from a disorder of anxiety. This distinction is critical in appreciating the impact of an anxiety condition on a person's functioning. Though everyone has likely experienced the state of anxiety at one time or another, many fewer individuals experience the pervasive, debilitating effects that accompany major anxious mental conditions. The defining characteristics of anxiety as a disorder necessitate a frequency, intensity, severity, breadth, and mix of symptoms powerful enough to adversely impact social, occupational, or other areas of functioning of an individual during the course of his or her life (American Psychiatric Association, *Diagnostic and Statistical Manual of Mental Disorder [DSM-IV]*, 1994). Of course, having an essential symptom of an anxiety disorder does not guarantee that a person is suffering from that disorder per se. As a case in point, while about 10% to 14% of the general population report having experienced a panic attack (*DSM-IV*, 1994), a much smaller proportion of individuals actually go on to develop a panic disorder. Many individuals appear to meet criteria for disorders not otherwise specified and thereby suffer from subthreshold clinical disorders. What differentiates those who do develop a full-blown major disorder from those who do not, then, is critical for understanding the factors that place a person at risk for an anxiety disorder, a topic to be addressed later.

Evocation of Anxiety

An important key to understanding the evocation of maladaptive anxiety appears to reside in the perceptions of the anxiety-prone individual. The manner in which an event is perceived has a determining influence on the type of reaction precipitated in an individual. The perception of an event or situation as a threat is sufficient but not necessary to elicit an anxiety response. Certain biogenic stressors (e.g., caffeine intoxication) may be enough to set a stress reaction in motion (Everly, 1989) even in the absence of the perception of an environmental event as a threat. Once the response is activated, however, perception may serve to exacerbate the reaction or diminish it. For example, a person who is over-caffeinated and attributes his discomforting arousal to an impending heart attack is likely to intensify his arousal symptoms. Unlike the person who perceives his arousal symptoms as a dangerous sign, the person who correctly attributes his arousal to too many cups of caffeinated coffee will not add to the existing symptom complex being experienced at the time.

The misperception of threat where there is none, and the misattribution of the cause of arousal to a malignant source when it is truly benign, clearly involves an overestimation of the likelihood of danger in a given circumstance confronting an individual. The exaggerated perception of the amount of danger believed to be inherent in a situation seems to be based upon the perceived catastrophic implications of imminent contact with an object. In either case, a mistaken perception of threat is often quite enough to precipitate an anxious reaction that is not warranted based on the actual amount of danger in the situation, which is usually none to minimal. A mistaken perception of the safety of a situation in which there is an objective but high likelihood of danger would be much more costly. From an evolutionary standpoint, erring in a more conservative direction makes the most sense. The fact that humans are prepared to acquire certain types of phobic reactions over others is also, then, more understandable (Seligman, 1971). In any case, without the perception, the anxiety response is not evoked.

If an individual's appraisal of a situation as dangerous is all that is necessary to set the anxiety process in motion, then the cognitive system must play a central and critical role in this regard. The appraisal, inaccurate as it may be, not only activates the response but promulgates it as well. The manner in which an individual actively processes information, and at a deeper level what the individual believes about an object or event, appears to be important. For example, take the case of a patient with irritable bowel who is extremely anxious about having a much needed sigmoidoscopy. He is so overwhelmed by the anticipation of the test that he fails to keep his appointment. Upon questioning to determine a cause for his active avoidance, he recounts that the liquid preparation he was instructed to ingest in order to clear his bowel for the exam precipitated intense cramping and pressure. His interpretation was that his condition was rapidly worsening.

To make matters worse, he recalled that his physician told him it would be necessary to pump some air into his bowel during the test. His interpretation of this information was that if air was put into his bowel it would explode and cause even more serious problems. The patient's appraisal (the test is dangerous) activated physiological (anxious tension), affective (panic), motivational (desire to avoid), and behavioral responses (active avoidance) in a congruent manner. In some clinical situations, such congruence may not be so matter of fact. There may be some discrepancy between what patients say, do, and feel. On the whole, however, the individual is usually prepared to meet threat and responds accordingly. The anxiety-prone individual may not only perceive relatively benign situations as dangerous, but may also underestimate his resources to cope with the situation, which in turn exacerbates his reaction. Once the judgement is made that danger is impending, the various systems may respond accordingly.

Anxiety patients tend to overestimate the probability of danger and negative events. This habit results in their characteristically predicting a threatening outcome across relevant situations. For example, patients with generalized anxiety disorder tend to expect the worst about a number of events or people in their lives. As a result they worry incessantly, which appears not only to dampen their emotional arousal but also to prevent their fully processing the situation in a realistic manner (Borkovec, Abel, & Newman, 1995). Estimates of the cost of a negative outcome or the probability of an aversive outcome do much to fuel the patient's maladaptive arousal. Evidence suggests (Bradley et al., 1995) that patients with generalized anxiety disorder may suffer from a preconscious inclination or bias for negative information toward which they guide their cognitive processing resources and efforts. The result may offer much in the way of not only precipitating anxiety states but also perpetuating them. Foa and colleagues (Foa et al., 1996) found a similar bias in those who are social phobics, which was eradicated after cognitive-behavioral treatment.

Onset of an Anxiety Problem

The onset of an anxiety problem is often preceded by a distressing life event, as per patient reports. Patients often become symptomatic after a life event that is emotionally upsetting. Patients with panic often have had distressing life experiences within the 6-month period preceding the development of the disorder (Barlow & Cerny, 1988), and those with obsessive compulsive disorder report a similar pattern (Steketee, 1993). Those with specific phobias appear more likely to acquire a phobic response during periods of high stress. It is likely, then, that such events may interact with some preexisting psychological or biological vulnerabilities to set the stage for the emergence of the condition.

Patients may also develop an anxiety disorder following a traumatic experience with an object or event. Although patients may not be able to recall a sensitizing event, this does not rule out the possibility that such an event did indeed occur and may be in part responsible for the onset of the disorder. On the other hand, the memory of a traumatic experience may simply be presumed by the patient to have been the sensitizing experience. In either case, some sensitizing experience may precede the onset of certain anxious conditions. In the simplest case, someone who is phobic about dogs may recall the onset of anxiety and fear associated with a ferocious attack by a pit bull. The patient with post-traumatic stress disorder (PTSD) may associate her condition with a date rape in college. In these two circumstances, the sensitizing events and the association between the event and the anxiety reaction are clear.

In other situations, however, the onset of the reaction may not be tied so closely in time to a particular event. Take the case of a dietician in her mid-40s who worked in the dietary department of a nursing home. One morning, another worker who was preparing breakfast accidentally cut her finger with a knife. The wound was bleeding so the dietician took her coworker by the hand and cleaned and dressed the wound. The dietician did not give the situation a second thought at that time. However, two years later when she accidentally discovered that the coworker had been HIV-positive for the past several years, she developed a phobic reaction of such intense proportions that she refused to counsel any patients with a history of drug abuse, sexually transmitted disease, blood transfusion, or HIV. She eventually was placed on disability and left her job. In the examples cited, the onset of the anxiety problem was closely tied to specific events in time. Yet with other disorders, such as generalized anxiety disorder, the worry and anxiety are more diffuse and may have persisted for many years and taken on a more characterological focus.

The onset of anxiety problems may be related to one or more possible mechanisms stemming from the experience of the patient. Three types of experiences seem possible and may solely or in combination account for the onset in some circumstances for certain disorders. These experiences are direct, informational, and vicarious (Craske & Barlow, 2001). The underlying process for their transmission is *learning*, a relatively permanent change in behavior as a result of the experience of the individual that is not attributable to other temporary causes including motivation, fatigue, drugs, or maturation. The *direct experience* of the individual undoubtedly plays an important role in the onset of anxiety problems and appears to be the most powerful source. For example, the actual experience of severe turbulence during a flight may be enough to sensitize an otherwise calm and experienced traveler and motivate him to seek alternative means for future travel. Otherwise, the apprehension in anticipation of a future flight as well as the raw panic response while in flight may both serve to ruin what would otherwise have been the joyful beginning of a much needed vacation.

Vicarious experience, acquired through what is observed or modeled, is another important source of information. In the wake of the terrorist attacks on the World Trade Center in New York, on September 11,

2001, the airline industry lost billions of dollars, secondary to active avoidance of air travel presumably due to fear. What an individual observes happening to another may sensitize the observer who may learn to associate anxiety with the situation and avoid it. Seeing a fellow student savagely beaten by the neighborhood bully over a seemingly benign remark may be all that is needed to evoke the observer's fear at the mere sight of the bully in the future. In this instance the observer may choose, albeit wisely, to avoid all contact with the bully, particularly idle conversation.

Extending our bully example even further, the reputation of the bully may be information that comes in quite handy to a new, otherwise uninformed adolescent boy on the block. In other words, the information itself may be enough to precipitate anxiety in the presence of the bully. The description of the experience by the observer to the new adolescent may serve to foster frighteningly vivid fantasies, providing not only information but also a sort of covert vicarious experience. Of course with anxious patients, what they learn and how they learn to respond is not nearly so adaptive. A related issue concerns whether anxiety is a truly distinct phenomenon. Even though we generally speak of anxiety as if it was a distinct entity, there is reason to question this notion.

Distinctiveness of Anxiety

Defining anxiety as a distinct emotional state has been a topic of considerable debate. Specifying the precise nature of anxiety is no simple task, as evidenced by its overlap with depression. The relationship between anxiety and depression has not only caused confusion but has presented a significant challenge to those attempting to understand and define it more precisely. Nowhere is this problem more clear than in the observed correlation between measures of anxiety and depression. The moderately positive correlations observed between measures of these two constructs have cast doubt upon the distinctiveness of either (Burns & Eidelson, 1998). Such relationships between measures of the same construct are commonly used to support the construct validity of the measures in question. Scores on one measure of anxiety are expected to correlate with those of another measure of anxiety. After all, if two measures are presumably measuring the same construct, people would be expected to respond to the item contents of each instrument in a similar fashion, a phenomenon referred to as convergent validity. On the other hand, a measure of a given construct should not correlate with a measure of a different construct, commonly called divergent validity. How then might one account for the observed correlations between measures of anxiety and depression? Attempts to do so have taken many forms.

At the most basic level, one must question the distinguishing features of the actual definitions of each construct and the items selected to measure each one. Item overlap and redundancy could easily account for the correlations between them. The *DSM-IV* (1994) criteria for generalized anxiety disorder (GAD) are a case in point. The diagnostic criteria for GAD contain six symptoms: restlessness, fatigue, difficulty concentrating, irritability, muscle tension, and sleep disturbance. The criteria for diagnosing a major depressive episode include psychomotor agitation, fatigue, diminished ability to think and concentrate, and sleep disturbance. The symptom overlap is somewhat striking.

Another way of accounting for the anxiety and depression overlap may be the mere coexistence of two distinct phenomena. The association between Down's syndrome and malignancies is a good case in point (Burns & Eidelson, 1998). Despite this association, each condition reserves its distinctiveness. The existence of one of these conditions is not considered pathognomonic of the other. Likewise, anxiety and depression may be considered two separate conditions, which frequently co-occur. Beck, Emery, and Greenberg (1985) postulate that anxiety and depression derive from two distinct cognitive states. The thinking of the anxious individual is characterized by themes of threat; the depressed individual, themes of loss. These distinct themes lead to particular affective states. The experience of a given life event could easily lead to the elicitation of both states. For example, the sudden death of a significant other could conceivably precipitate thoughts of both loss and threat in a simultaneous and synergistic manner, with one fueling the other.

Take the case of an older woman in a traditional marriage who has recently lost her spouse of 50 years. Her husband had handled all business and financial affairs. His sudden loss may not only precipitate thoughts of loss ("I've lost my best friend") but also thoughts of threat ("I'll never be able to handle my financial matters without him").

An alternative explanation focuses upon what is common between anxiety and depression and what is specific to each state. Clark, Steer, and Beck (1994) have proposed that the correlation between anxiety and depression may be explained by a general distress factor. This nonspecific factor comprises items that are common on both anxiety and depression measures and straddles both constructs. Clark et al. point to several lines of evidence to support their view. As noted previously, anxiety and depressive disorders share diagnostic criteria. Also, patients who have anxiety problems are frequently diagnosed with depressive disorders as well. Both conditions may share a common hereditary basis. Finally, patients with anxiety disorder are often treated successfully with antidepressant medication. Later, Clark et al. (1994) argued that although general distress may be common to both conditions, loss of pleasure is unique to depression while physical arousal is unique to anxiety. These findings may help to distinguish between individuals who have an anxiety disorder and those who have a depressive disorder. However, the co-occurrence of both disorders in the same individual is likely.

Comorbidity

Brown and Barlow (1992) have defined comorbidity as the simultaneous occurrence of two separate disorders within the same person at a given point in time or all of the diagnoses for which a person has ever met diagnostic criteria over a given period of time. A key question then is the determination of which disorder is primary and which is secondary. Clinically, the existence of this primary versus secondary distinction may have important implications for treatment. Targeting treatment at the primary disorder may cause improvement in the secondary diagnosis. For instance, what one may learn about effectively coping with anxiety may generalize to depression.

Years ago, Klerman (1990) proposed three definitions of primary versus secondary diagnoses. One way of conceptualizing a primary versus secondary diagnosis has to do with the time dimension related to problem onset. The differentiation is made on the basis of when the problems manifested in relation to each other. In this sense, the primary diagnosis is simply that which appeared first. A second approach to this problem is to consider how one problem may be causally linked to the development of another problem. For example, a patient who has initially begun to experience debilitating panic attacks may become secondarily depressed about the impact and interference the attacks are producing. One might expect that focused treatment of the panic attacks may also relieve the depression in this instance. The final approach is to consider the degree of impairment caused by a problem. Primary disorders would then be defined as those that cause the greatest problem or functional impairment for the patients.

Individuals with anxiety disorders tend to have high rates of coexisting problems with other anxiety disorders, depression, substance abuse, and personality disorders. This comorbidity among these disorders may be explained in a number of ways. Anxious patients with panic disorder may high levels of generalized anxiety between attacks. This generalized anxiety may lower the threshold for the onset of future panic attacks, as the patient worries persistently not only about the implications of these attacks but the probability of future attacks occurring. Problems in controlling attacks may create hopelessness and feelings of depression. In an effort to quell the effects of anxiety and possibly improve mood, anxious individuals may learn to rely on alcohol and other substances known to reduce arousal. Habitual reliance on such methods, prescribed or nonprescribed, may result in substance abuse or dependence. Long-standing patterns of thinking, feeling, and behaving in ways that promote anxiousness and fearfulness may set the stage for the occurrence of anxiety problems. Such personality disorders may exert their influence in a negative fashion by not only complicating treatment but also by producing a greater likelihood of negative outcome. To address this problem, clinical researchers (Brown & Barlow, 1992) have called for a dimensional approach to the assessment of specific symptoms or features of a disorder, as opposed to a categorical diagnostic approach to identify those factors that are more predictive of outcome.

Cultural and Individual Diversity Factors

The valid and reliable assessment and diagnosis of anxiety disorders presupposes a careful consideration of factors related to cultural and individual diversity (Friedman, 1997). In general, there are a host of variables that may affect the accuracy of information obtained from patients in different cultures. Sue and Sue (1990) provide a thorough treatise on the topic in the context of providing mental health services to those who are culturally different. Failure to attend carefully to such factors undermines the assessment process. Given the high prevalence of anxiety disorders in the general populations as well as the ever increasing cultural mix of the population in this country, cultural sensitivity is likely to assume even more importance in the future. Cultural factors contribute to problems in obtaining useful information on issues related to self-disclosure, language barriers, patterns of communication, and even what it means to have a mental health problem for a given individual in a certain culture. Cultural mores against disclosing personal information about self and family may operate and result in an inaccurate or incomplete picture of a problem. Difficulties in comprehending important subtle meanings of words may drastically alter the interpretation of questions. Deference to authority figures may prevent an individual from correcting a misconception held by a clinician (Sue & Sue, 1990).

Although found across all cultures, anxiety, more specifically panic disorder, may actually relate to a variety of culture-bound syndromes (*DSM-IV*, 1994). The specific presentation and nature of phobic reactions may depend considerably upon specific cultural beliefs that may alter the presentation of the phobia. The number of Italian immigrants who fear the evil eye is a case in point. Certain cultures may prescribe rituals that to the naïve observer may mistakenly signal an OCD problem. Finally, certain cultural groups may have fled countries where they witnessed or experienced horrifying events and fear disclosing these experiences.

Gender differences are also important to consider in diagnosing anxiety disorders. The base rates for certain disorders are higher for women than men. Panic disorders and agoraphobia are two examples. The types of specific phobia as reported by men and women also differ. The evidence of social phobia across the sexes may depend upon the types of samples studied (*DSM-IV*, 1994).

Finally, age differences are an important consideration in anxiety disorders. Knowledge about the differences in how anxiety disorders present across the age range should be carefully considered, especially when working with children.

Diagnosis of an Anxiety Problem

The reliable diagnosis of an anxiety disorder is a critical task for the practicing clinician. The failure to create an accurate diagnostic picture of the anxious patient may create significant problems for the clinician and patient alike. For the clinician faced with the responsibility of diagnosing the anxious patient, this task may be fraught with several possible pitfalls. First and foremost is the failure to rule out organic causes for the patient's complaints, which is a dangerous practice. The patient with an unsuspected adrenal-secreting tumor who is misdiagnosed as having panic attacks may receive an ill-conceived treatment plan. This plan may fail to address the actual problem and possibly place the patient at undue physical risk. Second, lack of knowledge, poor understanding, and misunderstanding of diagnostic criteria may not only unnecessarily complicate the clinical picture, but also lead to serious inaccuracies in diagnosis. Current knowledge of the diagnostic criteria for anxiety and other disorders will serve the clinician well in helping the patient. Third, the quality of the information obtained from the patient may be flawed unless the clinician is able to frame questions in ways that are understandable to the patient and accurately reflect the diagnostic criteria. Individual differences in the manner in which clinicians may ask questions related to the diagnostic criteria may also account for some of the unreliability. All of the factors described may present serious challenges that undermine the diagnostic process and create potentially serious professional, ethical and even legal risks for the clinician. For example, in view of existing empirically supported treatments for anxiety disorders (Barlow, 2000; Foa & Olasov Rothbaum, 1998; Hope et al., 2000; Steketee, 1993), misdiagnosed patients may simply fail to receive adequate care. They may also be saddled with an inaccurate label that is difficult to shed in the future.

Further issues of a diagnostic nature emanate from the structural nature of the *DSM-IV* (1994) classification system. Critics of this approach to diagnosis (Scotti et al., 1996) have argued that this system overlooks and grossly fails to account for information that is essential for the effective treatment of psychological conditions including anxiety disorders. The core issue with the structural classification system stems from the fact that specific target behaviors comprising the diagnostic criteria may evolve from very different sources and experiences that are evident only from knowledge of the patient's learning history. These historical events may be functionally related to the onset and maintenance of ongoing patterns of maladaptive behavior and, therefore, necessitate a specific set of interventions. For example, in the cases of two social phobics seen by one of the authors (RAD), the first patient was a college professor of mathematics who was extremely anxious in the classroom setting. He had a long history of teasing and rejection by his peers during his teenage years and not unexpectedly anticipated rejection from others in situations where he was the focus of attention. Unable to avoid his classroom duties, he endured the situation repeatedly under considerable duress. The second patient was a 41 year-old librarian and bachelor who lived a rather sheltered life, never learned the social skills necessary to sustain comfortable interpersonal interactions, and had significant difficulty in forming relationships. Although their treatment shared some similarities, specific differences were required. The first patient responded to a hierarchical exposure-based treatment protocol and showed no need for social skills training. The second responded to training in social skills and assertion. Though each met the criteria for social phobia, a functional analysis of their symptoms revealed the need for different treatments, not otherwise evident from their diagnostic classification. So even when reliable diagnoses of anxiety problems are made with *DSM-IV*, little may be offered in the way of informing useful treatment decisions. It is the formulation (Needleman, 1999; Persons, 1989) of the patient's anxiety problem and not the diagnosis per se that should drive the treatment process.

As discussed previously, unreliable diagnoses only further undermine attempts to provide effective treatments. For this reason, in an attempt to overcome this problem, clinical researchers have developed standardized semistructured interviews such as the Anxiety Disorders Interview Schedule (ADIS). As Chorpita, Brown, and Barlow (1998) have reported, "the collective evidence suggests that structured interviews posses acceptable reliability for the diagnosis of most anxiety disorders" (p. 1).

The question of what specific factors may contribute to diagnostic unreliability of the *DSM-III-R* (1987) anxiety disorders using the ADIS-R was addressed by David Barlow and his associates (Chorpita et al., 1998). These researchers tested the effects of several variables on diagnostic reliability including the existence of a comorbid diagnosis, the severity of the disorder being assessed, the patient's level of education, and the presence of behavioral indices (e.g., compulsions) of a disorder. These findings shed light on factors that attenuate reliability in diagnosing anxiety problems and will be discussed in depth. First, comorbidity appears to adversely impact diagnostic reliability of social phobia. Clinicians demonstrate better agreement when this condition is the sole diagnosis; reliability suffers when one or more comorbid diagnoses are made along with this disorder. Further analyses across all of the anxiety disorders demonstrated a significant overall improvement in agreement statistics when comorbid diagnoses were absent. The implications, then, are clear. The reliability of a diagnosis for anxiety may be attenuated when more than one anxiety disorder is present and such circumstances therefore warrant careful consideration by the clinician.

The effects of clinical severity were such that when clinical severity of an anxiety disorder was rated high, diagnostic agreement between the interviewers was high. This finding points to the potential difficulty of differentiating subclinical from clinical manifestations of anxiety in the treatment setting, especially when dealing with panic disorder, social phobia, and generalized anxiety disorder. Simply put, more severe problems may be more easily identified and delineated by a clinician. Surprisingly, a patient's level of education does not appear to exert an influence on diagnostic reliability.

Clinicians diagnosing anxiety disorders would also do well to be aware of other potential reliability problems in diagnosing anxiety disorders without noted behavioral indices. The presence of behavioral markers such as avoidance and compulsions may enhance reliability of diagnosis.

In differentially diagnosing anxiety disorders, the clinician must pay particular attention to the specific manner in which the disorder is manifesting. Though increased arousal is one hallmark of the anxiety disorders, the specific situation or event with which the anxiety is associated must be carefully determined. Identification of this factor will have a determining influence on the diagnosis obtained. However, the situation is not as simple as it may seem. For example, a clinician seeing a patient with a complaint of fear of driving may be tempted to assign a diagnosis of specific phobia. Further probing may uncover that this individual is fearful in many situations, happened to have had a panic attack while driving her car, and is remarkably fearful of the anxiety symptoms themselves. A diagnosis of panic disorder would be more indicated in this situation. In sum, the reliability of the diagnosis of anxiety disorders may be impacted by a number of variables. In diagnosing such disorders clinicians must be aware of possible situations under which their diagnostic reliability may be adversely affected.

DSM-IV ANXIETY DISORDERS: A BRIEF REVIEW

The *DSM-IV* classification scheme for anxiety disorders comprises several conditions. These problems include panic disorder, panic disorder with agoraphobia, specific phobia, social phobia, generalized anxiety disorder, posttraumatic stress disorder, acute stress disorder, and anxiety disorder NOS. The key characteristic across all of the anxiety disorders is what Barlow and Cerny (1988) have called anxious apprehension, a mood state that is oriented toward the future in which a person becomes prepared to deal with an anticipated negative event. Anxious apprehension is a state associated with three core characteristics: negative affect, chronic overarousal, and a sense of uncontrollability (Fong & Silien, 1999). The focus of the anxiety varies across the disorders and is specific to each disorder. For example, while the specific phobic is fearful of a circumscribed object or situation, the social phobic is overly concerned with evaluation by other individuals and being the focus of others' attention.

Other common features across the anxiety disorders include the marked, persistent, excessive, and unreasonable nature of the symptoms. In other words, regardless of the anxiety diagnosis, these patients have intense responses to feared events, responses that are ongoing over time, are extreme and disproportionate to the circumstance, and make little sense when viewed objectively regarding what the circumstances warrant. To qualify as disorders, by definition they cause distress that is clinically significant or that interferes significantly with the person's social, occupational, or recreational functioning. Of course, the means by which these disorders affect these consequences depends on the nature of the disorder. The symptoms must not be due to the effects of a substance, general medical condition, or another psychological problem. Active and more subtle forms of avoidance are usually present as well. A brief review of each anxiety disorder will suffice to illustrate this point (For a full discussion, see *DSM-IV*, 1994).

Panic Disorder

The critical feature of panic disorder (*DSM-IV*, 1994) is the presence of repeated, unexpected anxiety attacks accompanied by the subjective, frightening experience of panic. These attacks are typically experienced "out of the blue," are not precipitated by a situational trigger, but as a result of experience may become associated with certain situations. The patient with panic disorder who has a panic attack while driving a car, for example, may come to associate the two and begin to fear driving. Although the frequency, intensity, duration, pattern, number, and type of symptoms may vary between panic suffers, these patients display a fear of the symptoms of anxiety itself. This "fear of fear" has the effect of creating a hypervigilance for anxiety symptoms, which only serves to foster their appearance. The patient then gets caught in a vicious cycle of creating and exacerbating the very symptoms that are feared. Hypervigilance for future attacks appears to be fueled by anticipation about having attacks and worriment about what the attacks signify or the catastrophic outcomes that may ensue. Some patients with panic exhibit a fear of losing control and going insane; others, a fear of having a cardiac event or stroke. Not surprisingly, then, the patient's generalized anxiety is heightened between attacks, which only serves to lower the threshold for precipitating a panic reaction. The earliest sign of anxiety may become a signal for a full-blown panic attack and may seriously and adversely impact the patient's functioning (Barlow, Brown, & Craske, 1994).

Agoraphobia

Agoraphobia, "fear of open spaces," is a condition that may result as a complication of panic disorders (*DSM-IV*, 1994). It may also be associated with a more limited form of panic called limited symptom attacks, which does not meet diagnostic criteria for panic disorder. The defining characteristic of agoraphobia is the experience of anxiety about being present in circumstances from which it would be difficult to escape in the event that it became necessary to do so. These patients may also fear being in situations in which assistance would be unavailable to them in case they experience a full-blown panic attack or symptoms related to panic. Whatever the case, a person with agoraphobia may exhibit fear about a variety of situations. At its most extreme, some patients may restrict their travel to the point of becoming housebound. Others will travel only with another individual who has been designated as their safe person. When placed in fearful circumstances such as a church or a movie theater they may choose to sit in the back in an aisle seat close to an exit.

An agoraphobic person may avoid specific situations or experience significant distress if avoidance is not possible. Typical agoraphobic situations include traveling alone outside of the home. Some of these patients may have a safe distance they are willing to travel. Other situations include being in a crowded situation, which precludes their going to places like shopping malls and events like concerts. These patients may also report inability to stand in grocery store lines and may have escaped such situations leaving shopping carts filled with groceries. Not unexpectedly, they may fear riding in elevators, cars, buses, or trains, or traveling through tunnels or over bridges.

Social Phobia

The person who is a social phobic exhibits a marked and persistent fear in situations in which he or she is the focus of scrutiny or attention by others. These patients are overconcerned that they will do or say something that causes embarrassment and makes a fool out of them (*DSM-IV*, 1994). Not surprisingly, they are typically self-conscious in social situations, are preoccupied with fears of negative evaluation and rejection, and are overly focused on their performance. This negative self-presumption increases the anxiety level, makes them more removed from the social interactions, and disrupts their performance, which only serves to heighten anxiety. As a result they avoid situations that require social interaction or endure the situations with great distress. Those who are social phobics typically fear situations such as public speaking, answering a phone, eating in the presence of others, and even sitting in the presence of others. They may also avoid jobs that require interpersonal interaction. Failure to make effective contact with people may place them at risk for depression.

Generalized Anxiety Disorder (GAD)

The essential symptom of a patient with GAD is excessive unreasonable worries about a number of people or events in life (*DSM-IV*, 1994). These patients exhibit chronic worriment over a number of matters including, for example family, children, and their homes. When compared to normal controls, GAD patients tend to worry about the same things. However, a distinguishing feature is difficulty controlling the worry. Episodes of worry are accompanied by a variety of arousal symptoms, and the worry and anxiety cause clinical distress. There is evidence that worry behavior may actually preclude a patient's fully processing his or her worst fear, which is unrealistic, and may dampen the anxiety. They may also engage in a variety of safety behaviors. For example, the patient with GAD who worries about some tragedy befalling her spouse while he is driving home from work may engage in repeated attempts to reach the loved one on a cell phone or may call area hospitals to be certain the spouse has not been admitted to the emergency room. These patients may benefit form learning to confront their worst fears, abandoning their safety behaviors, and learning to use problem-solving and time-management strategies.

Acute Stress Disorder (ASD) and Posttraumatic Stress Disorder (PTSD)

The defining characteristic of ASD and PTSD is that the patient has experienced or witnessed a traumatic event in which the patient or others have been exposed to life-threatening circumstances or danger to their well-being (*DSM-IV*, 1994). During this event the patient has experienced a sense of horror or helplessness; what distinguishes ASD from PTSD is the duration of the problem. Traumatized patients typically experience a multitude of symptoms including efforts to avoid recollections of the trauma, a general numbing of sensitivity and reexperiencing of the trauma, and arousal problems. Events that may precipitate trauma may include war, natural disasters, rape, and accidents.

Typically these patients prefer to avoid talking and thinking about the trauma because of the associated distress in doing so. They may recall the event in an intrusive sense, experience nightmares, and have dissociative experiences during which they may feel or behave as if the traumatic events were reoccurring. Exposure to events or situations that are similar to the event causes psychological distress and physiological reactivity. These patients may also report a general numbing of sensitivity, including inability to have feelings and a sense of a shortened life. Heightened arousal symptoms often include a variety of problems including exaggerated startle and hypervigilance.

Obsessive-Compulsive Disorder (OCD)

Patients with OCD are characterized by the experience of obsessions, repeated involuntary thoughts, images, or impulses, that are associated with increased anxiety or compulsions, ritualistic behaviors or thoughts, which serve to neutralize the anxiety (*DSM-IV*, 1994). Obsessions are experienced as being out of the control of the individual, being a product of their own mind, and as excessive or unreasonable. Compulsions may be elaborate ritualized behaviors, which result in a decrease in anxiety. For example, the patient obsessed with fear of contamination usually experiences not only a fear of exposure to germs and dirt but also may spend hours on end engaging in handwashing or taking showers. Another variant of OCD is the checker who may repeatedly have an irresistible urge to check doors, locks, and the kitchen range to offset the likelihood of an otherwise impending disaster.

SUBSTRATE, TRIGGERING, AND MAINTENANCE FACTORS IN ANXIETY

The onset, duration, and persistence of anxiety and anxiety-related problems may stem from multiple sources. We have divided these sources into three major categories: the mental and physical substrate factors, triggering factors, and maintenance factors. Substrate factors include those influences that appear to set the stage for the eventual onset of an anxiety problem. They may be viewed as distal risk factors, which alone or in combination create the predisposition for an anxiety problem. These mental and physical events make a person vulnerable and susceptible to the experience of anxiety. Triggering factors include those experiences that alone or in combination have the potential for activating an already existing vulnerability. In this sense, life experiences or a series of stressful events may lower the threshold for precipitating an already existing predisposition to react with anxious affect. Finally, maintenance factors are those features that serve to fuel the anxiety in an enduring manner and preclude its resolution. These variables may contribute to continuation of the problem, despite an individual's motivation to do otherwise. These factors, while circumventing or reducing the unpleasant emotion in the short term, actually contribute to strengthening the anxiety response in the long run.

In the following sections, we discuss each of the specific factors within each category that are likely to influence the onset, development, and persistence of anxiety and anxiety-related problems. We posit that individual differences in proneness, onset, duration, and recalcitrance of anxiety problems within an individual may be explained by the unique combination and interaction of variables within and between each of the categories discussed above. For instance, an individual with a strong anxious predisposition who is undergoing multiple and fairly intense triggering events at a given point in time and who engages in dysfunctional behavioral patterns to deal with the anxiety is more likely to suffer an anxiety reaction than a person with an opposing profile.

Physical and Mental Substrate Factors

These are several factors that may predispose an individual to anxiety: genetic inhabitability, disease states, traumatizing mental events, locus of control, overprotectiveness, maternal sensitization, dysfunctional coping patterns, dysfunctional cognitive patterns, distressing vicarious experiences, classically conditioned events, chronic hyperventilation, and acquired misinformation.

Genetic Inhabitability

The role of a genetic loading for anxious arousal appears to be an important factor manifesting its influence by creating a potential for an individual to react with stress-related responses. In this sense, some individuals inherit nervous systems that are more easily aroused. Studies of the influence of anxiety disorders in twins and first-degree biological relatives of anxious disordered patients support this contention. Recently, in a study of monozygotic and dizygotic twins, anxiety sensitivity—the fear of anxiety symptoms themselves—was found to have a strong hereditary component (Stein, Lang, & Livesley, 1999). Hereditability was found to account for 50% of the variability in anxiety sensitivity scores.

Of course, the remaining 50% of the variability in anxiety sensitivity may be accounted for by other factors. The role of heredity can not be fully appreciated in the absence of environmental, psychological, and social factors (Barlow & Cerny, 1988).

Disease States

Physical disorders also have the capacity to place an individual at risk for anxiety problems. Certain disease states, of course, may imitate anxiety and may be mistakenly identified as an anxiety disorder. Anxiety problems may also occur simultaneously and interact with a disease state, rendering an individual vulnerable to the sequellae of both conditions. In certain instances, the sympathetic symptoms associated with disease states (e.g., hyperthyroidism) may lower the threshold for responding with anxiety to stressful events. In other instances, the symptoms of disease states themselves may become the focus of selective attention and fear, which in turn may exacerbate the symptoms.

Traumatizing Mental Events

The occurrence of mental trauma during the course of an individual's development may render an individual more prone to experience anxiety in situations similar to the traumatic event (Beck et al., 1985). The nature, number, duration, timing, and intensity of these events may play a significant role in creating a psychological vulnerability. An anxious vulnerability may be stored in a network of fear memories containing themes of threat, which are activated by special triggering events (Foa & Kozak, 1986). Under the appropriate set of triggering circumstances, this vulnerability may manifest itself in overt anxiety. In a manner somewhat akin to physical vulnerability factors, these psychological factors provide a sort of mental latent substrate. When activated by precipitating events, this mental substrate provides the vehicle through which experiences are filtered which, in turn, may set off an anxiety reaction. How an individual perceives the control of events, that is, from within oneself or outside of oneself may also be important.

Locus of Control

Early experience with lack of control has been posited to create a psychological vulnerability for anxiety (Barlow, 2000). In more recent research (Bennett & Sterling, 1998) comparing an anxiety-disordered group with nonclinical high-anxiety and nonclinical low-anxiety control groups, the anxiety disordered group and the high-anxious control group exhibited a more external locus of control. Those individuals with an external locus of control may have never learned the appropriate coping skills to foster a sense of self-reliance or internality. In the face of stressors, these same individuals may become more dependent on others and without help from outside themselves have difficulty coping with stressful events. One can speculate that perhaps such factors may account for the higher incidence of dependency traits and need for reassurance commonly seen in clinical situations with anxious patients.

Overprotectiveness

The role of parental overprotectiveness of an offspring may also create a risk for anxiety problems. In the same study (Bennett & Sterling, 1998), anxiety disordered individuals and high-trait-anxious nonpatients reported more maternal overprotection than low-trait-anxious individuals. In fact, the anxious patients reported more maternal overprotection than the high-trait-anxious group. The anxious patients also reported higher paternal overprotection than the other two comparison groups. These variables may be important in setting the stage for anxiety. The manner in which these recalled early experiences may affect an individual and create a vulnerability risk for anxiety problems is interesting. Overprotection may rob an individual of the opportunity for valuable learning experiences including perhaps the development of efficacy beliefs and coping behaviors.

Maternal Sensitization

Comparing anxious patients with high-anxious controls and low-anxious controls, Bennett and Sterling (1998) found that the patients reported more maternal sensitization than either of the control groups. Individuals who have become sensitized to fear certain things such as insects or disapproval by other individuals may be at more risk to develop certain types of anxiety problems.

Dysfunctional Coping Patterns

The absence of effective and adaptive coping strategies may place a person at considerable disadvantage when confronting overwhelming events in life. Individuals who have not learned useful means of coping through direct or vicarious experiences may be placed at risk. Repeated exposure to stressors in the environment with no coping strategies, or ineffective ones at best, may serve to sensitize an individual to react with heightened autonomic arousal under similar circumstances in the future. Under extreme circumstances, one could conceivably learn to become overwhelmed and helpless in the face of such stressors. Role-modeling of failure to cope or maladaptive strategies for coping by significant figures in a child's environment, coupled with exposure to repeatedly highly stressful events, may be important factors in setting the stage for this predisposition. The individual then may learn to rely on negative, overlearned strategies that may serve to preclude effective coping and only worsen the individual's anxiety.

Dysfunctional Cognitive Patterns

Anxiety-prone individuals are more likely to perceive threats to themselves in the absence of objectively threatening situations. The tendency to perceive threat in its absence appears to be related to the anxious individual's dysfunctional attitudes, beliefs, and assumptions, which in turn fuel a biased cognitive set for organizing, processing, integrating, and interpreting internal and external events. These maladaptive cognitive patterns appear to create a systematic pattern of selective attention, stimulus extraction, cue interpretation, and assimilation of threat-related material. In other words, the anxious individual tends to pay particular attention to certain aspects of situations to the exclusion of others, makes a faulty interpretation based on this limited data, and fits this information to a preexisting belief system that supports the risk of threat. As a result, anxious individuals may be primed to react with threat under what would otherwise be perceived as innocuous circumstances by nonanxious responders. Beck et al. (1985) and Barlow (2000) view the anxiety-prone person as making probability estimates that are not congruent with the real probability of threat occurring in their present and future experiences. These patterns are so overlearned that the validity of the appraisals and associated predictions are never really questioned.

Distressing Vicarious Experiences

Proneness to react with anxiety and panic to certain external and internal stimuli may also be rooted in the vicarious experiences of the individual. The mere act of observing the occurrence of an intensely threatening situation to another person (model) may be enough to promote vicarious learning, which in turn sets the stage for the expectation of threat to the observer under similar circumstances in the future. An individual may react in a similar manner to the presentation of a similar situation.

Take the case of a frightened young boy who watched his grandfather gasping for air in the front seat of his father's car as the grandfather was dying from a heart attack. Several years later, this same boy, now in late adolescence and physically fit, experienced a severe panic attack following a 5-mile jog, feeling out of breath with a racing heart. His interpretation as he raced in his own car to the local emergency room was that he was dying from a heart attack, as his grandfather had several years earlier. It is quite likely that without this priming frightening experience he would probably have realized that his heart was quite strong, that it was racing for good cause, and that being short of breath after a 5-mile run seemed reasonable under the circumstances.

Acquired Misinformation

During the course of their lives individuals acquire all sorts of information, some accurate and useful and some not so accurate or even useful for that matter. What a person believes to be true about a situation will determine how this person responds to this situation. Inaccurate information or lack of information may fuel a phobic reaction in this regard. For example, take the person whose belief that there is a 99% chance of dying in a plane crash is based on lack of knowledge about aerodynamics and how planes stay up in the air. She may be helped, in part, by learning about this subject. Although it is unlikely that such information alone will cure her phobia, it may help to get her on the plane to test her ominous prediction. In the absence of corrective or even new information, anxiety may be further and unnecessarily perpetuated.

Classically Conditioned Events

Experiences during which a person is exposed to a repeated, previously neutral stimulus paired with an unconditioned stimulus (which reliably elicits an unconditioned response) may also create a vulnerability. Under these circumstances the person may learn to respond to certain stimuli or classes in an anxious manner. In this sense, even internal events—such as the early signs of an anxiety symptom that has repeatedly signaled the onset of a full-blown panic attack—may acquire the capacity to do so, a process called interoceptive conditioning.

Chronic Hyperventilation

Individuals suffering from chronic hyperventilation, a type of breathing whereby a person blows off too much carbon dioxide, are at risk for the development of panic attacks. This condition may create the frightening symptoms the panic patient fears the most. In summary, there are a variety of factors, which may predispose an individual to reliably respond with anxious affect in the face of certain stressful events. Alone or in combination, these factors may create and reinforce an anxiety-prone vulnerability awaiting manifestation. What converts a predisposition into a sustained anxiety response is the right precipitants or combination of such, the topic of our next section.

Triggering Factors

A number of triggering events are likely to exert their influences by creating the occasion for responses or episodes of anxiety to occur (Beck et al., 1985). These factors include physical disease states, ingestion of psychoactive substances, exposure to toxic substances, an acute insurmountable stressor, ongoing long-term stressors, and stressors striking at a particular vulnerability of the person. The effects of each of these factors are discussed below.

Physical Disease States

The development of a physical disease state may precipitate anxiety and may not be an uncommon reaction during an individual's attempt to adjust. Some physical disease states may even imitate anxiety and be mistaken for an anxiety disorder. Physical problems appear to trigger anxiety in a number of possible ways. Physical disease may create a state in a person that overtaxes and compromises a person's ability to tolerate even normal everyday stressors at times. This state may then lower the threshold for triggering an anxiety reaction. Even when a physical problem mimics an anxiety problem, some patients may become threatened by the symptoms and unwittingly set a vicious cycle in motion. In this case, the person's catastrophic interpretation of real, organically-based symptoms may precipitate an anxiety reaction.

Exposure to Toxic Substances

An anxiety reaction may be triggered by exposure to a toxin, which creates one or more physical symptoms (for example, dizziness). Accidental ingestion of a toxic substance or inhalation of toxic fumes may create symptoms interpreted in a threatening manner by an individual. In the absence of an obvious reason to account for the aversive symptoms, catastrophic interpretations of the symptoms may trigger a panic reaction and worsen the very symptoms the person is motivated to escape. These substances have been termed biogenic stressors as evidenced by their ability to elicit a stress response in the absence of a triggering threat appraisal (Everly, 1989).

Ingestion of Stimulants and Other Psychoactive Substances

Taking an over-the-counter medication or an illegal street drug that produces sympathomimetic effects may create physical symptoms that reflect a change in physical state. If the person perceives these changes as threatening in some manner, an anxiety state is likely to ensue.

Hyperventilation

Under stressful circumstances breathing patterns may change. Rapid shallow breathing may disrupt the optimal level of oxygen and carbon dioxide in a person's blood. As a result a variety of physical symptoms may occur that may be perceived as threatening.

Overwhelming Life Stressor

The occurrence of major life events may be perceived as insurmountable and as a result precipitate a major anxiety state. The impact of the event itself is mediated by the manner in which the event is interpreted.

Long-Term Stressor

The occurrence of a stressor or a series of stressors over a protracted period of time may serve to overwhelm a person's resources. The threshold for responding with anxious affect may then be significantly lowered.

Events Activating Specific Vulnerabilities

The occurrence of an event that taps a particular vulnerability in a person may be expected to precipitate anxiety. A person who has already been primed for threat by a past event may be expected to respond in a similar manner to a similar event.

Maintenance of Anxiety

Once an anxiety reaction has been precipitated in an anxiety-prone individual, an interesting question has to do with what factors actually maintain the anxiety and associated responses. In the face of anxiety, an aversive condition, most individuals who proceed to develop an anxiety disorder actually engage in one or more behaviors that help to sustain the reaction. While effective for lowering the anxiety in the short-term in the long run these overlearned patterns of behavior tend to solidify the response.

The result is that a patient is caught in an unending vicious cycle that perpetuates the response. Three factors appear to be implicated here; namely escape, avoidance, and safety behaviors.

Escape and Avoidance Behaviors

Escape tendencies are those responses that remove a person from a threatening situation. In this sense these responses have the capacity for becoming overlearned because the person is usually quite motivated to remove himself from a frightening circumstance. Typically, these action tendencies are set into motion at the first sign of a perceived threat. Not surprisingly, they are quickly reinforced by the reduction of anxiety and removal from the aversive stimulus situation. In the case of a patient with panic, at the first sign of palpitation this individual might leave a situation that has previously been associated with a full-blown panic attack. The person never remains in the situation long enough to discover that there is no real danger.

As a short-term solution, avoidance patterns serve to reduce or prevent anxiety by precluding contact with a feared object or situation. Some patients engage in more subtle forms of avoidance by using safety behaviors that alter the nature of the contact with a feared object. The panic patient who never leaves home without a bottle of anti-panic medication is a good example.

Whether using escape or avoidance the result is the same: The patient never learns that the feared object or situation is truly not dangerous. The consequence is that the anxiety disorder is maintained and resistant to becoming extinguished.

CONCLUSION

Anxiety disorders are common, costly, and often debilitating problems that impair functioning in everyday life. In the next chapter, we present the case of Sandra, a young woman plagued by anxiety problems. In many ways, Sandra demonstrates the unique thinking, feeling, and behavior patterns so often characteristic of anxiety patients discussed in this chapter. Her history provides a thorough overview of the predisposing, triggering, and maintenance factors commonly seen in this population of patients as well as the challenges these patients present to clinicians.

REFERENCES

American Psychiatric Association (1994). *Diagnostic and statistical manual of mental disorders* (4th ed.). Washington, DC: Author.

Barlow, D. H. (2001). Unraveling the mysteries of anxiety and its disorders from the perspective of emotion theory. *American Psychologist, 55,* 1245–1263.

Barlow, D. H., & Cerny, J. A. (1988). *Psychological treatment of panic.* New York: Guilford.

Beck, A. T., Emery, G., & Greenberg, R. (1985). *Anxiety disorders and phobias: A cognitive perspective.* New York: Basic Books.

Bennett, A., & Sterling, J. (1998). Vulnerability factors in anxiety disorders. *British Journal of Medical Psychology, 71,* 311–319.

Borkovec, T. D., Abel, J. L., & Newman, H. (1995). Effects of psychotherapy on control conditions in generalized anxiety disorders. *Journal of Consulting and Clinical Psychology, 63,* 479–483.

Bradley, B. P., Mogg, K., Millard, N., & White, J. (1995). Selective processing of negative information: Effects of clinical anxiety, concurrent depression, and awareness. *Journal of Abnormal Psychology, 104,* 532–536.

Brown, T. A., & Barlow, D. H. (1992). Comorbidity among anxiety disorders: Implications for treatment and DSM-IV. *Journal of Consulting and Clinical Psychology, 60,* 835–844.

Burns, D. D., & Eidelson, R. J. (1998). Why are depression and anxiety correlated? A test of the tripartite model. *Journal of Consulting and Clinical Psychology, 66,* 461–473.

Clark, D. A., Steer, R. A., & Beck, A. T. (1994). Common and specific dimensions of self-reported anxiety and depression: Implications for the cognitive and tripartite models. *Journal of Abnormal Psychology, 103,* 645–654.

Craske, M. G., & Barlow, D. H. (2001). Panic disorder and agoraphobia. In D. H. Barlow (Ed.), *Clinical handbook of psychological disorders* (pp. 1–59). New York: Guilford

Chorpita, B. F., Brown, T. A., & Barlow, D. H. (1998). Diagnostic reliability of the DSM-III-R anxiety disorders. *Behaviors Modification, 22,* 307–315.

Dupont, R. L., Rice, D. P., Miller, L. S., Shiraki, S. S., Rowland, C. R., & Harwood, H. J. (1996). Economic costs of anxiety disorders. *Anxiety, 2,* 167–172.

Everly, G. (1989). *A clinical guide to the treatment of the human stress response.* New York: Plenum.

Foa, E. B., Franklin, M. E., Perry, K. J., & Herbert, J. D. (1996). Cognitive bases in generalized social phobia. *Journal of Abnormal Psychology, 105,* 433–439.

Foa, E. B., & Kozak, M. J. (1986). Emotional processing of fear: Exposure to corrective information. *Psychological Bulletin, 99,* 20–35.

Foa, E. B., & Oslasov Rothbaum, B. (1998). *Treating the trauma of rape: Cognitive behavioral therapy for PTSD.* New York: Guilford.

Fong, M. L., & Silien, K. A. (1999). Assessment and diagnosis of DSM-IV anxiety disorders. *Journal of Counseling and Development, 77,* 209–217.

Friedman, S. (1997). *Cultural issues in the treatment of anxiety.* New York: Guilford.

Gatchel, R. J., & Blanchard, E. B. (1994). *Psychophysiological disorders: Research and clinical applications.* Washington, DC: American Psychological Association.

Greenberg, P. E., Sisitsky, T., Kessler, R. C., Finkelstein, S. N., Berndt, E. R., Davidson, J. R., Ballenger, J. C., & Fryer, A. J. (1999). The economic burden of anxiety disorders in the 1990's. *The Journal of Clinical Psychiatry, 60,* 427–435.

Hope, D. H., Heimberg, R. G., Juster, H. R., & Turk, C. L. (2000). *Managing social anxiety: A cognitive-behavioral therapy approach.* New York: The Psychological Corporation.

Klerman, G. (1990). Approaches to the phenomena of comorbidity. In J. D. Maser & C. R. Cloniger (Eds.), *Comorbidty of mood and anxiety disorders* (pp. 13–37). Washington, DC: American Psychiatric Press.

Marsland, D. W., Wood, M., & Mayo, F. (1976). Content of family practice: A data bank for patient care, curriculum and research in family practice. *Journal of Family Practice, 3,* 25–68.

McLeod, J. D. (1994). Anxiety disorders and marital quality. *Journal of Abnormal Psychology, 103,* 767–776.

Mendlowicz, M. V., & Stein, M. B. (2000). Quality of life in individuals with anxiety disorders. *The American Journal of Psychiatry, 157,* 669–682.

Needleman, L. D. (1999). *Cognitive case conceptualization.* Mawah, NJ: Laurence Erlbaum.

Persons, J. (1989). *Cognitive therapy in practice: A case formulation approach.* New York: Norton.

Reiger, D. A., Boyd, J. H., Burke, J. D., Rae, D. S., Myers, J. K., Kramer, M., Robins, L. N., George, L. K., Karno, M., & Locke, B. Z. (1988). One-month prevalence of mental disorders in the United States: Based on five epidemiologic catchment area sites. *Archives of General Psychiatry, 45,* 977–986.

Scotti, J. R., Morris, T. L., McNeil, C. B., & Hawkins, R. P. (1996). DSM-IV and disorders of childhood and adolescence: Can structural criteria be functional? *Journal of Consulting and Clinical Psychology, 64,* 1177–1191.

Seligman, M. E. P. (1971). Phobias and preparedness. *Behavior Therapy, 2,* 307–320.

Stein, M. B., Lang, K. L., & Livisly, J. W. (1999). Heritability of anxiety sensitivity: A twin study. *The American Journal of Psychiatry, 156,* 246–251.

Steketee, G. S. (1993). *Treatment of obsessive-compulsive disorder.* New York: Guilford.

Sue, D. W., & Sue, D. (1990). *Counseling the culturally different: Theory and practice.* New York: Wiley and Sons.

Wolpe, J. (1958). *Psychotherapy by reciprocal inhibition.* Stanford, CA: Stanford University Press.

2

Clinical Case Presentation: The Case of Sandra

Elizabeth A. Gosch and Robert A. DiTomasso

Sandra came to my office (EG) at the Clinical Psychology Clinic of a medical school in the Midwest early one Saturday morning. She presented as a capable, tall, slender, and attractive 26-year-old professional. Beneath her calm façade, Sandra lived her life in a constant state of apprehension and fear. She had struggled with this anxiety for as long as she could remember. It was only now, at the behest of Ted, her boyfriend of 5 years, that she sought psychological help. Ted, an accountant for the IRS, encouraged her to seek help because he could see the heavy toll her fears were taking on her life. Trapped in her phobic world and paralyzed by avoidances, her everyday existence conformed to a rigid set of rules designed to allay her anxieties. When she awakened, where she went to sleep, when she showered, how long she worked each day, where she parked her sport utility vehicle—all these activities were governed by her unrelenting fear that she would be physically harmed by an assailant.

Each day Sandra wakens hours earlier than necessary in order to shower, iron her clothes, and eat breakfast, when her parents or her boyfriend are still in the house. She routinely leaves the house early to avoid any chance of being alone in the house. She arrives at work each day at 7 a.m., precisely when the security guard comes on duty, to avoid being alone in the office. If this routine proceeds as planned, Sandra would never be alone and her anxiety would be minimal. But if, for example, her boyfriend unexpectedly needs to leave the house earlier than usual (perhaps to go to the airport for a business trip), Sandra would become panic-stricken and unable to shower. If forced to sleep alone in the house, Sandra would usually remain awake all night listening carefully and with apprehension for possible signs of an intruder. She depends on her parents' and her boyfriend's presence to provide a sense of safety and quell her distress. Even as an adult, she occasionally sleeps on the floor in her parents' or sisters' bedrooms when she is afraid during the night. Once, she even borrowed her neighbor's dog overnight to protect her. This dependency extends to other areas in her life. During a business trip to California a few years ago, Sandra insisted that a coworker share her room so she would not have to be alone.

Interestingly, despite her excessive dependence, she remains emotionally aloof from important people in her life, particularly her parents. She has pleasant but superficial relationships with her colleagues that do not extend beyond the work environment. Her relationship with her boyfriend, the second man she has ever dated, is characterized by a sense of uncertainty and a lack of strong feelings. She frequently sleeps at his house, is physically intimate with him, and socializes primarily with him alone. Yet she expresses concerns about her feelings towards him and wonders whether he "really loves" her. A lack of trust seems to permeate all her relationships. In fact, she freely acknowledged, "I don't trust anybody."

In terms of her daily life, Sandra spends a good part of each day worrying about a host of issues. Described by family and friends as a worry-wart for as far back as she can recall, Sandra usually expects the worst to happen. She typically finds herself "jumping from one worry to another" during the course of each day. The objects of her worry include her job, her car, her boyfriend, his job, their relationship, and her biological mother as well as a host of periodic stressors. Her greatest fear remains being hurt or killed by a male assailant. Sandra stated that this fear was reinforced when a drug-addicted neighbor, who was later arrested, broke into her house when she was a teenager. The family was home sleeping during the break-in and fortunately no one was hurt. However, Sandra was extremely disturbed that an intruder was in the home while she was sleeping. Currently, she finds that she "even worries about worrying," fearing that some day she will "have a nervous break-down" as her mother did.

Because Sandra has such a difficult time controlling her worry, it is not surprising that she finds herself in an almost constant state of anxious arousal. She complains of feeling on edge much of the time and suffers from muscle tension in her back, neck, forehead, and jaw. She recently considered seeing her dentist about some TMJ-like symptoms. When she finds herself in situations such as being alone in her house or walking to her car in the dark, she immediately experiences palpitations, pounding heart, and accelerated heart rate. These symptoms are accompanied by sweating, trembling and shakiness, and a fear of dying. Sandra rates all of these symptoms as "very severe" but is not fearful of the symptoms themselves according to her report.

Lately, she finds that she is quick to snap at subordinates at work and her boyfriend has complained that she is overly irritable with him. She wonders if her irritability is due in part to her lack of sleep. She has nightly difficulty falling asleep, and even after falling asleep, her sleep is restless and disturbed. She has frequent nightmares, which often include people threatening and chasing her with weapons and having trouble getting away from them. For example, following a stressful day at work when her boss appeared angry with her, Sandra dreamed about a man stabbing her and killing her parents.

Sandra's childhood was marked by a number of unfortunate events. Born in Illinois, Sandra was the product of a dysfunctional relationship, and her parents became estranged soon after her birth. Her father showed little interest in her during her childhood and Sandra "disowned him." Sandra suspects that he may have had some type of drug problem. Her biological mother cared for Sandra until she was 4. Her real mother, with whom she has infrequent contact, has a chronic, recalcitrant delusional psychotic disorder and has had more than 30 psychiatric hospitalizations. During her childhood and adolescence, Sandra saw her mother during arranged visitations and vividly recalls her mother expressing strong fears for her daughter's safety during these visits. Frequently delusional, Sandra's mother often entreated her to be careful, to avoid the horrible fate she imagined would befall her daughter. Sandra remembers leaving these visits feeling anxious and disturbed. To this day, her mother will express great surprise and relief when she sees Sandra, exclaiming, "I thought you were dead!"

When Sandra was 4 years old, she was placed in foster care with family acquaintances who adopted her several years later. This couple had already adopted twin boys from Columbia and had two daughters of their own, one of whom was legally blind. Sandra's adoptive father, a welder at the local Navy shipyard, is described as "quiet, reserved, and well liked." He suffers from crippling arthritis. Both he and Sandra's adoptive mother were raised in and closely followed the charismatic Catholic doctrine. Sandra's adoptive mother attended Mass daily and worked part-time at a Catholic bookstore. The adoptive mother had seriously considered entering the religious life during late adolescence. Sandra states that her parents appeared to have a satisfactory relationship with common religious and cultural values. Sandra had infrequent contact with her maternal grandmother and grandfather who passed away during her childhood. In contrast, her paternal grandmother, a widow, lived nearby and often visited Sandra's family.

As the youngest child, Sandra states that she was a "daddy's girl" who never felt comfortable with her "very religious and controlling" adoptive mother. Prone to episodes of rage, her adoptive mother frequently used physical discipline, such as hair-pulling and hitting, as well as verbal threats such as "If you don't behave, I'll send you back to the agency." To avoid her adoptive mother's wrath, Sandra recalls slipping out of the house early on summer mornings with her siblings and spending the day playing outside the home.

Sandra's familial difficulties were compounded from ages 8 to 12. During this time, she was repeatedly fondled by her two brothers and forced to look at their genitals. Sandra's unhappiness with her home was evident when at the age of 10, she ran away from home with two of her neighborhood friends. When she was brought back home, Sandra reluctantly told her parents about her brothers' sexual overtures. She remembers that her parents did not believe her "stories." Sandra was very fearful at this time that the agency might take her away from her parents if people outside the family found out about the sexual abuse. Her school counselor arranged a psychological evaluation for Sandra, but after the family had several sessions with a therapist, the matter was dropped.

Subsequently, Sandra was very cautious in the presence of her brothers. However, she recollects getting along fairly well with them and her sisters despite some occasional teasing for her excessive anxiety. Also, like many adopted children, she described often feeling "apart" from the family or like an "outsider." When she was 12, Sandra again became fearful of one of her brothers who reestablished his pattern of sexually fondling her. On one occasion, she remembers that he threw her down on the ground while in the garage and tried to have intercourse with her but she was able to fight him off. Sandra told her mother and a parish priest, who taught religion at her school, about these experiences but reports that the situation remained unchanged.

On another occasion while on a family vacation in New Mexico, Sandra's adoptive father made a sexual advance toward her while inebriated. She remembers that he fondled her breasts but stopped when she became upset. He never repeated this type of behavior. However, as Sandra says, "the damage was done." Her idealized image of her father "was shattered." Given that her father was the only member of the household with whom Sandra felt close, she experienced this incident as "devastating" and felt that it "ruined" her life. Sandra did not discuss this incident with anyone at that time. Instead, she told her mother about her brother's sexual overtures in a letter, pleading with her mother to intervene. Her mother responded by accusing Sandra of lying.

Furious with her mother's response, Sandra felt "completely abandoned" in time of need. The tension and anger between Sandra and her mother fueled daily arguments between them throughout Sandra's teenage years. Sandra found that her anger spread to other relationships in her life. She relates feeling competitive with other children and upset when they were more successful than she was. She described herself during her adolescence as "an angry, vicious person" who argued and fought with her peers, leading her to be rejected and ostracized. An above-average student in high school, Sandra graduated in the upper 25% of her class. She describes having a number of acquaintances but no close friends throughout her youth.

When Sandra was 19, her parents announced that they were planning to adopt a young Chinese child. Sandra recalls figuratively "exploding in anger" at that very moment. She recollects fearing that this child would suffer as she had in the family and feeling helpless to stop it. Sandra fled to a friend's house. During this time, she shared the secret about her brothers with her friend's older cousin. The local division of human services became involved. The mother of her friend's cousin, a psychiatric nurse practitioner, also confronted the parish priest and reported him to his superior for failing to report the sexual abuse. He was subsequently removed from the parish and the local congregation "found out" about Sandra's story. Sandra reports feeling that the reputation of the family "was smeared" and that her family blamed her for this. Eventually, Sandra's brother and father did admit their wrongdoing and were forced to seek counseling. As an adult, Sandra had the option of prosecuting but decided against it. Her father secretly told her that if she decided to prosecute, he would kill himself.

When asked about her brothers' and father's sexual contact with her, Sandra matter-of-factly discusses what happened to her as she remembers it. However, she feels she has "resolved" the issue. She remembers feeling guilty and fearful about the issue in the past but no longer feels the experience's impact on her life.

After graduating from high school, Sandra took several courses at a local business college and later took a position as a bank teller. Over the past several years, she has distinguished herself as a committed employee and earned several promotions to her current position as a manager of a large bank. She supervises 12 employees in her department. Working an average of 60 hours per week, she often has to work under time pressure and on weekends. Sandra devotes almost all her energy to her job, a job she finds fulfilling yet highly stressful. Her supervisor relies heavily on Sandra who tends to do his work as well as her own. Completely focused on her work and perfectionistic, Sandra is constantly fearful that she may make a mistake or do a poor job. She feels she has to be "number one" in her boss's eyes and stated, "If I'm not, I'm nothing."

Generally cautious in her interpersonal relationships, Sandra tends to remain aloof and wary of others. Beneath her pleasant demeanor, she harbors a deep sense of mistrust. Fearing the negative and expecting the worst contributes to a chronic sense of apprehension and a pervasive anxiety-ridden state. Steeped in a history of what she perceives as negative life events and disillusionment with her family, she has worked hard to achieve a sense of satisfaction in her life. She struggles with anger toward her adoptive mother by whom she has never felt accepted or loved. Her anger is bound with a sense of guilt for failing to meet her mother's expectations and win her approval. At 26 years of age, she still lives at home with her parents who frequently badger her about her lifestyle and boyfriend. Although frustrated with this living situation, she feels "trapped" by her phobia. The thought of going home alone to an empty apartment each night "forces" her to tolerate living with her parents.

Sandra was administered the Multimodal Life History Inventory, the Anxiety Disorders Interview Schedule-Revised, the Michigan Alcohol Screening Test, the Beck Depression Inventory, the Beck Anxiety Inventory, the Fear Survey Schedule, the Millon Clinical Multiaxial Inventory-II, and a mental status exam. A synopsis of the findings reveals that Sandra is an intact young woman suffering from a moderately severe level of phobic anxiety and avoidance, generalized anxiety, and chronic worry in her daily life. Though exhibiting dependent features, there is no evidence of a personality disorder or depression at this time. She currently meets *DSM-IV* diagnostic criteria for specific phobia and generalized anxiety disorder. She does not meet criteria for post-traumatic stress disorder or panic disorder. In terms of her physical health, Sandra does not take medication or suffer from any serious ailments. She reports that she has never used drugs or alcohol. A recent physical by her family physician revealed no significant medical problems although she occasionally suffers from upper respiratory problems related to her allergies.

The following are short excerpts from initial sessions in which Sandra describes some of her presenting symptoms.

EVALUATION SESSION EXCERPT

Sandra:	My whole life is just one big fear.
Therapist:	Tell me what you mean by that.
Sandra:	Well, you see, almost everything I do in my life and everything I don't do is because of fear. I'm so afraid something bad will happen to me—fear rules my life, fear runs my life.
Therapist:	Give me an example of how fear rules and runs your life.
Sandra:	Well, I could never stay alone in the house. I'm so afraid somebody will break in and hurt me, maybe even kill me.
Therapist:	So, you fear that something horrific will happen to you when you are alone in the house, especially at night in the dark.
Sandra:	That's right. I can't get it out of my mind.
Therapist:	No matter how hard you try.
Sandra:	Right.
Therapist:	In what other ways do your fears impact on your life?
Sandra:	I can't fall asleep at night. I have to fall asleep before my family does.
Therapist:	What happens if you don't?
Sandra:	I'm anxious and fearful that somebody will break in. It takes a few hours for me to get to sleep.
Therapist:	What kinds of situations pull for you to be afraid?

Sandra:	Like I said, when I'm alone in the house, especially at night. If I have to stay late at work and no one else is there—that's bad. If I have to walk to my car at night—I can't even take a walk alone at night. I don't even watch the news. It scares me too much.
Therapist:	Okay, what else?
Sandra:	When I shower—I can't do it if no one is home.
Therapist:	So, it sounds as if your fear impacts tremendously on your life.
Sandra:	It does.
Therapist:	What things do you do to comfort yourself or make the fear go away?
Sandra:	It depends on the situation.
Therapist:	Let's go through each situation. How about when your parents go away on a trip?
Sandra:	I stay at my boyfriend's house until they get back.
Therapist:	Suppose they go out in the evening.
Sandra:	I won't go home 'til I'm sure they're home. But if I have no choice, like if my boyfriend is out with his friends, I'll go in and check the entire house and then call my grandmother. I'll stay on the phone until my parents come home.
Therapist:	What about showering?
Sandra:	Well, I always shower when somebody is home with me. I'll even wake up two hours earlier than I need to in the morning to be sure somebody is there when I shower.
Therapist:	You also mentioned that you have to fall asleep before your parents do.
Sandra:	That's right. If I don't, it takes me hours to fall asleep.
Therapist:	What do you do to get to sleep?
Sandra:	Usually, I'll just go into their bedroom and sleep on the floor, that helps.
Therapist:	How about leaving work in the evening?
Sandra:	First of all, I get to work early so I can park my car as close as possible to my building.
Therapist:	Anything else?
Sandra:	Oh, I always park under a light. I run as fast as I can to my car. I open the door and check the back seat to make sure no one is there. Then I jump into the car and drive away as fast as I can.

4TH SESSION EXCERPT

Sandra: I had some words with my parents last night. I'm just so tired of it. All I hear from my family is criticism. It's like they gang up on me.

Therapist: Sounds really uncomfortable. What do they criticize you about?

Sandra: They're unhappy with the fact that I'm dating Ted. Always have been, you know.

Therapist: What is it about Ted that they don't like?

Sandra: He's not a religious person. They see this as terrible. I guess they think he's influenced me. I haven't been going to church lately. That drives my mom nuts. Maybe that's why I do it.

Therapist: So, you're saying that they are threatened by Ted and his presumed effect on you.

Sandra: Oh, I'd say so. Are they ever!

Therapist: You said something a moment ago that I think is important. You said that your choosing to avoid church drives your mom crazy—"Maybe that's why I do it." Presuming that's the case, are you saying that avoiding church is a way of retaliating against your mom?

Sandra: In some ways I believe so. You see I've never really felt loved by her or accepted by her for that matter. That upsets me. No matter how hard I've tried, no matter how much I've done, it's never good enough. In a strange way I'd like her approval, her acceptance.

Therapist: I think I understand. You would like to have unconditional love and acceptance and you just can't seem to get it, can you?

Sandra: Right, no matter what. Well then, you see, I also ruined her perfect world when I admitted the abuse in the past.

Therapist: So she's never recovered from the past. Is that it?

Sandra: That's true and I've been paying for it ever since.

Therapist: How about *your* recovery from the past?

Sandra: Oh, it was a long time ago. I realize now that it is a part of my past, it happened. I didn't like that it happened. I've accepted it and moved forward. It's something bad that happened to me and is not my fault. I used to think so in the past, but not anymore.

QUESTIONS FOR CONTRIBUTORS

The case of Sandra is actually a composite of several individuals who have presented with anxiety problems. This case was constructed to represent a patient commonly seen in clinical practice. Any likeness to an actual person is purely coincidental. The contributors in this volume were asked to consider the case of Sandra and respond to the following questions based on their theoretical orientation.

I. **Treatment Model.** Please describe your treatment model succinctly.

II. **The Therapist's Skills and Attributes.** Describe the clinical skills or personal attributes most essential to successful therapy in your approach.

III. **The Case of Sandra.** It is important to the goals and mission of this volume that you answer *each* of the following questions regarding the enclosed case material.

A. *Assessment, Conceptualization, and Treatment Planning*

1. **Assessment.** What further information would you want to have to assist in structuring this patient's treatment? Are these specific assessment tools you would use? What would be the rationale for those tools?

2. **Therapeutic Goals.** What would be your therapeutic goals for this patient? What are the primary and secondary goals of therapy? What level of coping, adaptation, or function would you see this patient reaching as an immediate result of therapy? Please be as specific as possible.

3. **Timeline for Therapy.** What would be your timeline for therapy? What would be the frequency and duration of the sessions?

4. **Case Conceptualization.** What is your conceptualization of this patient's personality, behavior, affective state, cognitions, and functioning? Include the strengths of the patient that can be used in the therapy.

B. *The Therapeutic Relationship*

1. **The Therapeutic Bond.** What are the important considerations in the bond or affective relationship between therapist and client? Examples would include the development of trust, boundaries and limit-setting, self-disclosure, transference, and countertransference.

2.   **Roles in the Therapeutic Relationship.** What are the appropriate roles of the therapist and the patient in your model of treatment, and what might you do to facilitate these roles? For example, what is the therapist's degree of directiveness and activity level, and what is the therapist's role as an expert providing specific instruction? To what extent is the therapeutic relationship collaborative, and what are your expectations of the patient in her role?

C.   *Treatment Implementation and Outcome*

1.   **Techniques and Methods of Working.** Are there specific or special techniques that you would implement in the therapy? If so, what would they be? What other professionals would you want to collaborate with on this case, and how would you work together? Would you want to involve significant others in the treatment? Would you use out-of-session work (homework) with this patient, and if so, what kind?

2.   **Medical and Nutritional Issues.** How would you handle the medical and nutritional issues involved in the work with this client?

3.   **Potential Pitfalls.** What potential pitfalls would you envision in this therapy? What would the difficulties be, and what would you envision to be the source(s) of the difficulties? Are there special cautions to be observed in working with this patient? Are there any particular resistances you would expect, and how would you deal with them?

4.   **Termination and Relapse Prevention.** What are the issues to be addressed in the termination process? How would termination and relapse prevention be structured?

5.   **Mechanisms of Change.** What do you see as the hoped-for mechanisms of change for this patient, in order of relative importance?

3

Cognitive-Behavioral Treatment

Elizabeth A. Meadows and Kelly A. Phipps

TREATMENT MODEL

Cognitive-behavioral therapy (CBT) has a rich tradition grounded in experimental animal learning research and empiricism. Two specific learning theories, classical conditioning and operant or instrumental conditioning, greatly influenced the development of behavior therapy. In classical conditioning, associations are made between two stimuli: an unconditioned stimulus (UCS) that automatically elicits a reflexive response; and a conditioned stimulus (CS), a previously neutral stimulus that comes to elicit the same response via repeated pairing with the UCS. This form of learning was discovered by Pavlov (1927), and is thus sometimes referred to as Pavlovian conditioning. In operant conditioning, associations are made between a behavior and the consequence of that behavior, so that behaviors that are rewarded or reinforced increase. These associations were first reported by Thorndike (1898) in his law of effect and then capitalized upon by Skinner (1938), who demonstrated that Thorndike's law of effect could be used not only to explain the frequency of behaviors emitted naturally, but also to manipulate the frequency of those behaviors via deliberate reinforcement. This reinforcement can be both positive, in which an appetitive or pleasant stimulus is contingently presented, or negative, in which an aversive stimulus is contingently removed; both positive and negative reinforcement would have the effect of increasing the behaviors reinforced. Punishment—the contingent presentation of an aversive stimulus or contingent removal of a positive one—would have the converse effect of decreasing the punished behaviors. The effects of punishment appear to be more variable than reinforcement, due to aspects such as the reinforcement that can be provided by the attention (even if negative) that punishment provides.

The phenomena of classical and operant conditioning form the basis of much of behavior therapy. In its early forms, the learning theories were translated directly into models of etiology and intervention, models that continue to be used to this day. For example, one etiological pathway to development of a phobia is through traumatic conditioning. If a person is bitten by a dog, for example, dogs may then become associated with a fear response. In this example, the dog is initially a neutral stimulus; it does not elicit any response from the person. The dog bite, however, is frightening, and automatically elicits a fear response (automatically in that the person does not need to "learn" to be afraid of the dog bite). As the presentation of the dog and the presentation of the dog bite occur contiguously, the two stimuli become associated in the person's mind, and thus the automatic response of fear to the dog bite becomes a conditioned response of fear to the dog as well, making the dog a conditioned stimulus.

The intervention for such an acquired fear logically follows from the learning literature. After demonstrating that responses can be conditioned via pairing with an unconditioned stimulus, Pavlov (1928) further demonstrated that these responses do not persist indefinitely. He noted that the newly conditioned stimulus will eventually cease eliciting the conditioned response if it is not reinforced by pairing with the UCS, a process known as extinction. Using this paradigm, presentation of the CS (in this example, the dog) without the pairing of the UCS (the dog bite) should lead to extinction of the fear response to the dog. This led to the intervention known as exposure, one of the primary treatment methods used for anxiety-based disorders.

Operant conditioning can similarly be shown to explain the development of psychopathology and to lead to logical interventions. For example, a child who wants a candy bar might be told no initially. If the child then starts screaming, the parent may ignore the screams and continue to deny the child the candy bar, or may instead give in and allow the candy. If the parent gives in, the child's screaming has been reinforced; the child learns that the behavior of screaming will lead to the presentation of something positive, in this case, the candy bar. Operant conditioning theory states that behavior that is reinforced will increase, and so the parent in this case has inadvertently taught the child to have a temper tantrum as an effective means of getting what he or she wants.

As in the case of classical conditioning, operant conditioning also leads to appropriate interventions for its outcomes. In the example above, if the parent stops reinforcing the behavior (i.e., lets the child scream without providing the candy or other desires of the child), and does so consistently, the child will eventually learn that the screaming no longer brings about the desired consequence and will stop that behavior. On the other hand, if the parent begins reinforcing more appropriate behaviors, such as politely asking for candy, those behaviors would then increase. Such patterns of deliberate reinforcement and lack of reinforcement form the basis for many behavior modification programs.

Mowrer's (1939) two-factor theory, which combines classical and operant conditioning, has been especially influential in theories of anxiety disorders. This theory states that fears can be acquired via classical conditioning, as described above, and then maintained via operant conditioning in the form of avoidance learning. Avoidance learning is a form of negative reinforcement, in which by escaping or avoiding an anxiety-provoking situation, one learns that the anxiety quickly decreases. As the anxiety is considered aversive, its termination serves as a negative reinforcer of the avoidance that led to its decrease, thus leading to more avoidance in the future. It is this theory that forms the basis for many cognitive-behavioral models of anxiety disorders and their treatments.

Initially, behavior therapists did not focus on thoughts or cognitions as they are not observable behaviors. However, largely due to the work of Albert Ellis and Aaron T. Beck in the 60s, the impact of thoughts on emotions and behaviors began to be emphasized. Beck's cognitive theory (1967) stated that we do not respond to events in our environment directly, but rather to our interpretation of these events. Thus, the same event, say, a noise in the middle of the night, could lead to many different emotional and behavioral responses. If one were to attribute the noise to an intruder breaking into one's home, the emotional response would likely be one of fear, and the behavioral response one of calling 911 or getting a baseball bat to try to scare the intruder away. If instead the noise were attributed to one's cat knocking over a bottle, the emotional response might be anger or frustration at having been awakened, and the behavioral response might be to mutter "stupid cat," and fall back to sleep. In this example, the event itself, a noise in the night, is exactly the same; the responses differ greatly, depending upon the interpretation of the event. As was the case for the learning theories reviewed above, the cognitive explanation for psychopathology—that erroneous beliefs or interpretations lead to pathological emotions and behavioral patterns—leads to a logical intervention: By challenging the erroneous beliefs and replacing them with more rational or adaptive ones, the adaptive emotions and behaviors would follow.

Today, many theorists have combined the cognitive theories and learning-based behavioral theories into cognitive-behavioral theory, noting that cognitions are in fact a form of behavior, albeit a covert form, and that if treated as behaviors they respond as such. In addition, more modern views of learning theories incorporate cognitive components rather than relying solely on automatic unthinking processes. For example, Rescorla (1988) stated that classical conditioning is not simply a function of contiguous pairing of stimuli, but rather results from the change in meaning to which the pairing leads. Specifically, he noted that the CS comes to signal the UCS, and that it is this contingent pairing, rather than contiguous pairing, that leads to the learned associations. For example, suppose one student was presented with a bell followed by a cupcake for 10 trials, and another student was presented with the same 10 trials, but also received 10 trials of the bell with no cupcake interspersed throughout the first 10 trials. Traditional views of classical conditioning would suggest the development of similar responses between the two students, as each had 10 reinforced trials of bell-cupcake. However, the more cognitive view would suggest that the second student did not experience the same contingent association, in that the bell did not necessarily signal the arrival of a cupcake. For the first student, a bell always meant a cupcake would follow. In this example, we might expect that the first student would develop a stronger conditioned response to the bell, having learned a cupcake would surely follow.

Cognitive explanations have also been used to explain the mechanisms underlying interventions such as exposure. Foa and Kozak (1986) theorized that exposure does not work simply due to the breaking of associations between a situation and the fear with which it had become associated, but rather is due to the emotional processing that occurs as a result of the exposure. Specifically, they noted that it is the introduction of corrective information during the exposure that accounts for the decrease in fear. If this information is not incorporated into the exposure (that is, if the person is so dissociated during imaginal exposure that they feel as if they are literally reliving the frightening event rather than simply remembering it), fear reduction would not be expected to occur.

Much of current CBT attempts to understand the relationships among a host of different variables including thoughts, behaviors, sensations, and emotions. This process is often referred to as a functional analysis, as it is the function, rather than the form, of each variable that is seen as important (Cone, 1997; Kanfer & Saslow, 1969). This approach acknowledges that not every behavior, for example, holds the same meaning for everyone, and that it is important to understand how the different variables interact and impact each other to develop an effective plan of intervention.

Although a true functional analysis would be tailored to each individual, general functional models of anxiety disorders have been developed that have led to theoretical-based interventions. These often include a three-component, or three-system, model of anxiety in which the anxiety construct is broken into behavioral, cognitive, and physiological components (Rapee et al., 1991). Each component plays a role in the disorder, as does the interaction among the components. To use generalized anxiety disorder as an example (Craske, Barlow, & O'Leary, 1992), the physiological component might consist of muscle tension, increased heart rate, queasiness, and trembling, symptoms often related to sympathetic nervous system arousal. The cognitive component might include thoughts that something bad will happen: A job might be lost, one might not have enough money, or others might disapprove. This cognitive component, worry, forms the key feature of GAD. Finally, the behavioral component might include various safety behaviors in which one engages to forestall the content of the worries, such as checking one's work meticulously, calling home to ensure everyone is safe, or asking others for their opinions. These components can interact to create a cycle of increasing and continuing anxiety. For example, one might worry about performing badly at work, which could then lead to physiological arousal symptoms, which could then lead to a decreased ability to focus on one's work, thus in fact leading to small errors. The safety behavior of checking one's work might then be reinforced when the errors are found (increasing the likelihood of such checking behavior), thus also leading to the worry that if the work had not been checked, perhaps the boss would find out and the person would be fired. By intervening in the specific components (e.g., using physical control methods to target the physiological responses, cognitive challenging to target the cognitive responses, and exposure to target the behavioral responses), this cycle could be broken and more adaptive patterns developed.

THE THERAPIST'S SKILLS AND ATTRIBUTES

A good CBT therapist must possess a number of skills both generally applicable to clinical work and specific to CBT, as well as several relevant personal characteristics. Obviously, one of the most important qualities is that the therapist be well grounded in cognitive-behavioral conceptualization. Second, the therapist must be competent in the implementation of the various techniques used within CBT, such as exposure or cognitive restructuring. Neither of these skills alone is sufficient, but together they provide the therapist with a powerful way of understanding a client's problems and intervening appropriately.

Another important skill a CBT therapist must possess is the ability to work collaboratively with his or her clients. CBT is fairly directive and also fairly structured. In that sense, it is the therapist's job to keep sessions on track. However, the therapist must be able to do so by working with the client toward common goals, rather than by forcing the client to follow a specific agenda. At times, the therapist may need to interrupt a client to keep a session's focus. However, the therapist must do so in a way that is clear to the client why refocusing is important for their own goals, rather than simply the therapist's goals. This requires both general interpersonal skills and also the self-confidence to know when to redirect.

One of the most important attributes a CBT therapist must possess is the ability to engender trust in one's clients. Although trust is obviously important within most therapy relationships, there are some aspects of CBT in which a lack of trust in the therapist would absolutely inhibit the therapy. Specifically, many of the methods used within CBT require clients to directly face the sources of their distress. CBT for anxiety disorders, for example, requires clients to confront the very fears for which they are seeking help; an oft-heard response to this request is "If I could do that, I wouldn't need therapy!" It is the role of the therapist in this situation to convey the therapist's firm belief that the client can in fact face these fears, and that by doing so, the fears eventually can be overcome. There are several ways in which this trust can be developed. One of the most important is by virtue of the therapist's competence and experience. Clients are far more likely to trust a therapist enough to confront difficult situations if they believe the therapist knows what he or she is doing and have seen this method work in the past. This trust is also engendered by the therapist's ability to communicate that he or she understands why the client may not yet believe, on a gut level, that these methods will work, and also that the client is likely to be terrified of doing what is being asked in exposure. Many CBT therapists combine this empathy for the client's distress with the confidence that the client can in fact face his or her problems and overcome them. They support this confidence with their experience of many past clients who, though initially as reluctant as the current client, were able to confront and overcome their problems.

Because of CBT's emphasis on empiricism, another important therapist attribute is the willingness to question what one is doing, to test the results of each hypothesis and intervention, and to teach one's clients how to do the same. The ability to think logically and to apply this logic to the therapeutic situation is invaluable in doing good CBT. This issue arises in the area of assessment and case formulation. For example, the therapist must sort through many potentially relevant variables to construct a formulation of the client's problems that explains the problems and suggests places to intervene. Logical thought also becomes important in using many CBT techniques. Cognitive restructuring is based on the ability to apply rational thinking, to identify when one's thoughts may be irrational, erroneous, or simply unhelpful, and to challenge such thoughts with cold logic, so that more adaptive ways of thinking may be put in their place. A therapist who is weak on logical ability would likely have difficulty in this task.

THE CASE OF SANDRA

Assessment, Conceptualization, and Treatment Planning

Assessment

The assessment conducted with Sandra included a number of clinician-administered and self-report measures. In addition to the outcomes of these measures, it would also be important to examine the entire proto-col. This is especially true of the ADIS-R, a semistructured interview that provides a diagnostic profile as an outcome but includes considerable additional information in the body of the interview. For example, in examining the ADIS-R, we could see why Sandra did not meet criteria for post-traumatic stress disorder (PTSD). This question is important, given Sandra's history of traumatic events and the similarity of her symptoms, especially the primary symptom of fear of physical assault, to symptoms commonly seen in PTSD. In fact, Sandra's diagnosis of specific phobia (presumably, of being alone for fear of assault) might better be conceptualized, depending on her responses to the PTSD module of the ADIS-R, as part of a PTSD-related syndrome. Closer examination of other symptoms reported by Sandra, such as nightmares, estrangement from others, irritability, difficulty sleeping, and avoidance, might indicate whether treating these symptoms as part of a PTSD-like syndrome is warranted.

Given Sandra's diagnosis of GAD, it might also be important to include a measure specifically targeting GAD symptoms, such as the Penn State Worry Questionnaire (Meyer et al., 1990). This measure would provide useful information in determining the severity and nature of the disorder, and would also be an excellent method by which to measure Sandra's progress in treatment.

Finally, one of the most important assessment tools for treatment planning and treatment evaluation is self-monitoring. Initial self-moni-toring of content, frequency, severity, and context of various symptoms (that is, worry, physical symptoms, fears) can provide a baseline against which later monitoring can be compared. Self-monitoring can also provide important information regarding Sandra's symptoms that may impact significantly upon the treatment. Such monitoring is commonly used in treatment programs for most anxiety disorders, including spe-cific phobias (Antony, Craske, & Barlow, 1995) and generalized anxiety disorder (Craske et al., 1992).

In addition to the aforementioned anxiety assessment information, it is important to note that Sandra's biological mother has a history of hospitalization for paranoid schizophrenia. Information regarding her mother's problems should be obtained as her mother's illness is likely to have influenced the development of Sandra's current problems in several ways. For example, Sandra has been told throughout her life that the world is a dangerous place from which she must always take care to protect herself. This pattern continues into the present when

Sandra's mother greets her with statements such as "I thought you were dead!" Such statements can fit into a formulation of Sandra's fears as learned via modeling (of her mother) and experience (of her abuse and of the intruder). It is also important to consider the possibility of schizophrenia or a related process in Sandra herself. No psychotic symptoms were reported in the case study, and these would have been screened in several of the instruments used during the assessment. Additionally, Sandra's fears of danger have been in existence for quite some time and are accompanied by many other symptoms of anxiety unrelated to such danger. However, a more detailed assessment of prodromal schizophrenia may be warranted given that children of individuals with schizophrenia are at higher risk for developing the disorder (Goldstein, 1987; Gottesman, McGuffin, & Farmer, 1987; Heston, 1966) and that Sandra's age falls within the median age of schizophrenia onset in women (*DSM-IV*, 1994).

Therapeutic Goals

The primary therapeutic goal would be to reduce Sandra's fear of being alone. Sandra stated that this is her biggest problem, and it appears to be creating the most difficulties in her daily functioning. Reducing this fear would likely have a number of beneficial effects. In addition to decreasing Sandra's anxiety level, it would allow her to become more independent. She would be able to sleep alone, move out of her parents' house, travel for work without relying on colleagues, and free her from the need to plan her movements (such as when to arrive at work or to shower) based on the schedules of those around her. Finally, it is probable that many of the panic-like sensations Sandra currently experiences will disappear once the fear of being alone is reduced, as these sensations appear to develop in response to phobic stimuli, rather than to be coming from "out of the blue" as would be the case in panic disorder.

An advantage to targeting the fear of being alone first is that the skills used to reduce this fear are the same or similar to those that might be used to target some of Sandra's other symptoms. Thus, a secondary goal would be for Sandra to apply skills, such as confronting her fears and challenging her maladaptive thoughts, to other areas (e.g., her pervasive worries about her job and her family). Reducing Sandra's tendency to worry in general would also likely relieve some of her physical symptoms, such as muscle tension, and would also target her perfectionism, as many of her worries appear to stem from the perfectionist tendencies.

An early goal of treatment would be to help Sandra sleep with less difficulty. It does not appear that her sleep difficulties are primary, but rather are in response to both her fears of being alone and the generally high arousal levels she experiences. However, lack of sleep can clearly exacerbate many problems, making otherwise manageable ones seem insurmountable. An early intervention such as sleep hygiene or breathing retraining might allow Sandra to reduce her sleep problems, providing her with much-needed rest and allowing her to develop a sense of mastery over at least one problem quickly. This experience of control could then increase her willingness to tackle more difficult problems in therapy.

Finally, Sandra appears to have interpersonal problems that may be an appropriate target for treatment. She reports a pervasive lack of trust, which may be part of a PTSD-like constellation and might be reduced by targeting trauma-related difficulties. She also reports a lack of close relationships, which obviously may be related to the lack of trust, but which may also stem from other problems as well. Increasing Sandra's social sphere and her sense of connection to those in her life may be an appropriate secondary goal, as would be increasing her ability to accept and in some way resolve the anger and guilt she experiences with her family.

As an immediate result of therapy, Sandra should be able to meet the primary goal—reducing her fear of being alone—as demonstrated by a reduced fear level and an ability to remain alone in a variety of situations. She should also be able to control her worry levels and have considerably reduced levels of physical arousal and muscle tension. Together, these results would also allow Sandra to function far more independently than she is currently able to. It is very likely that she can achieve these goals via a relatively brief course of CBT.

The other secondary goals—increasing Sandra's emotional engagement with those around her and managing the complex relationships with her family—may require more time to change and thus might not be resolved upon termination of therapy for the primary problems. In concluding therapy with her major fears under control, with more independence, with more of a sense of control over her life, and with the skills she learned in therapy to obtain this control, Sandra would be well positioned to continue making progress in this area on her own. Alternatively, it may be advisable at some point, depending on her desire for better family relationships and family members' willingness to return for family therapy in the future.

Timeline for Therapy

As is the case with most CBT, therapy should be time-limited. This has several advantages, one of the most important being the decreased likelihood of wasting session time. Knowing that therapy will end within a few months allows the client to focus on the work of therapy for those months without the concern that he or she must continue doing so indefinitely and without the luxury of knowing that taking a week or more off from working will not affect the outcome. The time-limited nature of CBT would also address one of Sandra's primary problems, that of dependency. Built into CBT is the knowledge that the client must learn these skills and be able to apply them on her own, not just in response to the therapist's request. In this case, Sandra would be working toward independence not just as a treatment goal, but also as part of the process of CBT.

Most empirically supported treatment programs for anxiety disorders are designed to last for approximately 10 to 15 weeks. Although circumscribed, specific phobias have often been treated in just a few sessions, or even in a single extended session (Muris, Merckelbach, van Haaften, & Mayer, 1997; Öst, 1996; Öst, Brandberg, & Alm, 1997); Sandra's fear of being alone does not seem a likely target for such a brief treatment. Treatment sessions generally occur once a week, although some programs (Borkovec & Costello, 1993) have held twice-weekly sessions, sometimes decreasing frequency toward the end of therapy. Session duration is often longer than the typical 50-minute hour, especially when exposure is used. Research has consistently shown that prolonged exposure is more effective in reducing fear than are shorter exposure sessions (Antony & Swinson, 2000). A general guideline for exposure sessions is that the exposure continue until fear ratings drop by at least 50% (Meadows & Foa, 1998) or until they reach only mild levels (Antony & Swinson, 2000). In addition to the exposure itself, time must be allotted for review of homework, discussion of the exposure session, and assignment of new homework. Thus, therapy sessions are often conducted in 90 to 120 minute periods.

Case Conceptualization

Sandra's pervasive fears of being alone lest she be physically harmed by an assailant appear to be shaped by a number of life experiences.

From early childhood, she was exposed to her mother's pathological fears of danger. These fears continue to this day, so that each visit with her mother reinforces Sandra's own fears when she is greeted with statements like "I thought you were dead." In addition, Sandra has experienced multiple incidents demonstrating that she is at risk: She was sexually abused by her brothers and her father; was told in no uncertain terms that others, such as her mother and parish priest, would not protect her from such abuse; and had her home broken into by an intruder while she slept. Each of these experiences likely contributed to what Janoff-Bulman (1992) refers to as a shattering of assumptions. Janoff-Bulman describes three core assumptions we hold about ourselves and the world: The world is benevolent, the world is meaningful, and the self is worthy. Sandra's experiences, however, may have taught her that the world is dangerous, and that she is not worthy of protection from such dangers. According to Janoff-Bulman, these beliefs are likely to lead to many of the symptoms we consider part of PTSD, such as hypervigilance, as well as basic feelings of insecurity, lack of trust, and powerlessness.

In addition, that Sandra continues to live with her parents, who are described as fairly demanding and rigid, may also contribute to her worrying and perfectionism. Although she reports that she has "resolved" the issue of the abuse, living with people who abused her and failed to protect her may be further contributing to Sandra's feelings of danger in a general sense, even if she is not currently in danger of being abused by family members. Finally, some of her arousal level may stem from a biological predisposition. This information must also be taken into account especially when explaining to Sandra the possible etiology of her symptoms, such as in a *psychoeducational* component of therapy on the physiology of anxiety and worry (Craske et al., 1992). Such psychoeducational activities will help to make her symptoms seem more understandable.

As discussed earlier, in CBT conceptualizations, etiological and maintaining variables are not necessarily the same. In Sandra's case, it is likely that her early life experiences and biological predisposition played a critical role in the development of her anxiety. However, the anxiety is likely maintained through other factors, primarily her severe avoidance of frightening situations. Each time Sandra refuses to sleep alone, to shower when no one else is home, or to arrive at work before the security guard, her fears of danger are reinforced by the thoughts that if she *were* to do any of those things, she would clearly be at high risk of assault, and that it is only because of her vigilance that she has protected herself from these assaults. Thus, a crucial role of therapy would be to demonstrate to Sandra how these behaviors and thoughts and experiences interconnect, and how she can now break these long-standing patterns of avoidance to teach herself that she is quite safe being alone in most places.

Sandra also exhibits a number of strengths that should be of use in therapy. Despite overwhelming fears and pervasive anxiety, Sandra has been able to perform very well in life. She graduated in the top quarter of her high school class and currently holds a demanding job in which she performs at a high level, having earned several promotions. As a teenager, she was able to mobilize available resources when her family announced plans to take in another foster child and she believed the child might be at risk for the same abuse she herself suffered. When it fell on her to protect another, she persisted in telling her story until she reached people who took action. Each of these examples points to Sandra's ability to accomplish her goals regardless of whatever anxiety she experiences. This ability will help her enormously as she confronts her fears directly in CBT. She has already demonstrated the ability to function well while feeling very anxious and can be reminded of this if, as is often the case, she is doubtful about her ability to conduct the exposure practices that will be such an important part of her treatment.

Overall, Sandra's current difficulties can be seen as a combination of her early traumatic experiences and her interactions with her biological mother leading to schemas of danger and threat, a possible biological predisposition toward physiological arousal, and a behavioral pattern of avoidance. These factors may also reinforce each other, leading to a cycle of fear and anxiety.

The Therapeutic Relationship

The Therapeutic Bond

As described earlier, one of the most important considerations in the therapeutic relationship is a high degree of trust between therapist and client. In most CBT programs, therapists ask their clients to confront directly their most challenging problems, and to do so repeatedly. For clients to agree to these challenges, they must trust that their therapists have the knowledge and experience to guide them through these experiences. Moreover, they must believe that their therapists have an understanding of why it may be quite difficult for them to engage in this direct confrontation of their problems.

Although the concepts of transference and countertransference are not generally emphasized in CBT, there are many times when a therapist will use his or her own reactions to a client to help conceptualize the client's problems. In behavioral terms, the client's presentation in session is simply another sample of his or her behavior in general, but one that is being directly observed by the therapist and thus can be used as an example when it is happening.

Depending on the problem for which CBT is being used, the therapeutic relationship may take on more or less importance. In some cases, especially those in which concrete problems are addressed with specific techniques, such as in vivo exposure for a spider phobia, there may not be a need for much of an affective relationship at all. In our experience, many clients in CBT for anxiety disorders have referred to their sessions as their "anxiety classes," viewing the therapist as more of a teacher or guide. In other cases, of course, the affective elements take on more importance, either because of the nature of the problem or because of the interpersonal needs of a client.

In Sandra's case, it seems likely that her therapist would need to use a certain amount of interpersonal skills to ensure that Sandra feels understood and safe enough to confront her many fears and worries. Modeling or limited self-disclosure can be very helpful in establishing such a safe and trusting relationship. For example, clients who are hesitant to perform exposure initially are often more willing to do so if the therapist first models the procedure for them. It has been suggested that therapists should not ask a client to do anything they would not be willing to first do themselves (Antony & Swinson, 2000). Similarly, disclosing to one's clients ways in which CBT methods have helped to manage one's own fears, or even the fact that the therapist has had his or her own excessive fears, can be quite helpful. Such disclosure serves to demonstrate the effectiveness of the techniques and the therapist's willingness to use them him- or herself as well as to normalize the experience of anxiety.

One potentially important role of self-disclosure in Sandra's case might be in acknowledging that although the world is not as dangerous as Sandra acts, it is not perfectly safe either. Thus, there are some realistic precautions one might take to avoid unnecessary risk. This issue comes up often in trauma-related problems, as the client has already experienced danger in the world. In such cases, it is important to assess with the client which of their fears seem appropriate, thus warranting precautions, and which fears or precautions appear to be based more upon erroneous beliefs or associations than on actual danger. For example, if Sandra's workplace were in a crime-ridden neighborhood where her officemates were regularly attacked when alone or at night, then her behavior of ensuring the presence of a security guard before arriving at work would not be considered an unreasonable anxiety behavior but rather a realistic precaution. In making such distinctions, especially if the therapist is female, it can be useful for the therapist to disclose some of her own safety behaviors, noting how these behaviors acknowledge the possibility of danger yet do not interfere with daily functioning. A common example of this would be carrying one's car keys in hand, rather than in a purse or pocket, so that the key is readily available and the car can be entered quickly. Many women probably engage in this behavior on a regular basis, as a simple precaution that does not take extra time or interfere with one's life. It is possible that if Sandra's therapist shared such behaviors, Sandra might feel a bit more understood than if she encountered a therapist who appeared to live his or her life as if the world were completely safe.

Roles in the Therapeutic Relationship

The active, directive nature of CBT is reflected in the behavior of the therapist and the role of the therapeutic relationship. In most CBT, clients and therapists act as a collaborative team. The clients are the experts on their own experiences and feelings and are the ones who do the important work of practicing skills learned in therapy and keeping track of these practices in sufficient detail so that they can be reviewed in session. The therapists are the experts in CBT conceptualizations, analyzing the roles of the various factors that may play a part in the etiology and maintenance of clients' problems, in the development of appropriate treatment plans based upon these conceptualizations, and in the implementation of CBT techniques. Both the clients' and therapist's areas of expertise must be recognized within the collaborative nature of CBT. Both client and therapist must work as a team, each playing an active role in therapy.

   A CBT therapist is generally very directive in structuring sessions and ensuring that each session remains on task. Given the expertise of the therapist in knowing what methods are likely to reduce the client's anxiety, the therapist must be directive in suggesting particular activities for session time and between-session practices. The therapist is also aware of which client behaviors are likely to reduce the effectiveness of treatment and must take action if these behaviors arise. For example, clients often prefer talking about their problems or reviewing their week to conducting the often difficult work of exposure or cognitive restructuring. The therapist must be careful to avoid this trap (Persons, 1994) and to point out how the client's preferences might be viewed as avoidance behavior, so that the client can increase his or her own awareness of subtle avoidance that arises in daily life.

In Sandra's case, both client and therapist will play critical roles in therapy. Sandra will need to carefully monitor her fears, worries, and physical sensations on a daily basis throughout therapy and to conduct daily practices of skills learned in session. As CBT cannot work without the active participation of the client, the expectation that she will complete all these assignments will need to be conveyed to her at the onset of treatment, along with the rationale for doing so. It is important to note, however, that as each new assignment or skill arises, its specific rationale is again reviewed in treatment, and the importance of regular practice emphasized. If Sandra fails to conduct these practices, the therapist would need to address this issue immediately. Together, the therapist and Sandra would attempt to determine the reasons for noncompliance and formulate ways in which she could better practice her CBT skills. In the end, Sandra must be willing to do these tasks or therapy will fail. There is nothing magical about CBT or a CBT therapist that will allow a client to improve without considerable effort and regular practices.

Treatment Implementation and Outcome

Techniques and Methods of Working

A CBT treatment plan should follow logically from the case conceptualization, so that the relationships among variables thought to be responsible for the client's problems are addressed in a way that changes the client's patterns. There are several ways this might be done. In the initial stages of treatment plan development, it can often be helpful to develop a problem list, itemizing the problems a client wishes to address (Persons, 1989). In Sandra's case, her problem list might read as follows:

1. Fear of being alone (includes avoidance of such situations), fear of being harmed by an assailant
2. Trouble sleeping—difficulty falling asleep and nightmares
3. Being a "worrywart"—worrying about job, family, car, etc.
4. Constant anxious arousal and frequent muscle tension
5. Irritability
6. Perfectionism
7. Interpersonal problems, including lack of trust in relationships and not feeling close to others

From this list, several items are likely related, as would follow from the case conceptualization and also from the *DSM-IV* diagnostic criteria. For example, worrying, muscle tension, and perfectionism can all be seen as part of generalized anxiety disorder, as can potentially the trouble sleeping. The fear of being alone, if less severe, might simply be conceptualized as another sphere of worry, although in Sandra's case it is separated out into the diagnosis of specific phobia. This fear also seems to encompass the nightmares, given their content of physical harm by an assailant.

There are several strategies that might be used in developing Sandra's treatment plan. Nelson (1988) outlines several ways in which assessment and treatment are linked within CBT. The first is functional analysis, as described earlier, in which the relationships among the variables in Sandra's life are viewed as leading to her current problems, with the treatment plan then consisting of intervening in these relationships. The second strategy outlined is the keystone target-behavior strategy, in which one problem is targeted for treatment with the assumption that improvement in that area will lead to improvements in other areas as well. Finally, there is the diagnostic strategy, in which a treatment package that has been shown to be effective for a specific disorder is selected on the basis of the client's diagnosis with that disorder. Each of these approaches has its advantages and disadvantages, yet there is also considerable overlap in how they would actually be implemented. For example, the treatment programs that have been developed for specific disorders have generally been based on theoretical conceptualizations of how the disorder developed initially, thus combining, in part, the first and third strategies.

The diagnostic strategy is the least idiographic of the three, assuming that the pathway to a disorder is similar among all clients. It is also the strategy most emphasized in today's health care field. For example, the lists of empirically supported treatments compiled by the American Psychiatric Association's Division 12 Task Force on Psychological Interventions (available on-line at www.sscp.psych.ndsu.nodak.edu/est_docs/tf_docs.htm), along with the proliferation of treatment guidelines published by numerous organizations, focus largely on manualized treatments targeting specific *DSM-IV* diagnoses. One approach, the one we favor personally, uses the diagnostic strategy first; this assumes that Sandra's disorders will respond to the same treatments that have been most effective with others with the same disorders. In this case, treatment programs that have been shown to be efficacious for GAD and specific phobia would be used. Given that actuarial judgement tends to be more accurate than clinical judgement (Meehl, 1954, 1986) this strategy allows the best odds for treatment to work, by capitalizing on the large numbers of clients who participate in the treatment outcome studies used to support these programs. This strategy also capitalizes on a finding by Schulte et al. (1992) that standardized exposure treatment outperformed individualized treatment for phobic patients. Acknowledging that no treatment is effective for everyone, should the treatment package based on diagnostic strategy not work as planned the therapist would then employ a functional analytic method to determine why that might be and make accommodations accordingly.

To use this two-pronged approach with Sandra, the available treatments for GAD and specific phobia would be reviewed and one selected. Of the available treatments, exposure is considered the treatment of choice for anxiety disorders in general (Antony & Swinson, 2000; Barlow, 1988) and is the only treatment with considerable support for the treatment of specific phobia (Antony & Swinson, 2000). An exposure-based treatment appears to be appropriate for both of Sandra's primary diagnoses as well as for the alternate conceptualization of a PTSD-like syndrome described earlier.

Many exposure treatment programs include components such as psychoeducation in addition to the exposure itself. Psychoeducation can serve a number of purposes: reassuring clients that there are reasons for their problems or that they are not "crazy"; beginning the process of cognitive restructuring by providing alternative explanations for symptoms; and providing a framework for the remaining components of treatment, so that clients fully understand how the treatment will be conducted and why each component is thought to be relevant for their problems. In this case, providing information-conditioning processes and the ways in which avoidance serves to maintain fear will allow

Sandra to understand how her avoidance of being alone, while reducing her anxiety in the short term, serves to strengthen it in the long term. This knowledge may make it more likely that confronting her feared situations, such as showering while alone in the house, will be acceptable to her.

A number of exposure treatments include teaching some form of coping strategy prior to beginning the exposure. As just noted, psychoeducation can serve as a form of basic cognitive restructuring and could thus fall into this category; in some treatment packages, more in-depth cognitive challenging skills are taught prior to exposure onset. Two relatively easy coping skills include breathing retraining and progressive muscle relaxation. In Sandra's case, either or both of these skills might be quite appropriate. Given her frequent muscle tension, a progressive muscle relaxation component, in which one systematically tenses and releases various muscles in the body (Bernstein & Borkovec, 1973), may allow Sandra not only to reduce such tension when it arises, but also to recognize muscle tension at milder levels and implement relaxation skills before the tension becomes a problem.

As noted earlier, breathing retraining may be quite helpful as an initial treatment component due to Sandra's sleep difficulties. In our experience treating women with PTSD or PTSD-like symptoms, particularly following sexual assault, we find breathing retraining (slow rhythmic breaths that the client focuses on) very useful in falling asleep initially and in falling back to sleep after waking from nightmares. In addition, it is relatively quick and easy to learn for most clients, so that in just one session Sandra might leave therapy with a useful skill to give her some relief in the following week.

The bulk of Sandra's treatment, however, would focus on confronting her fears via prolonged exposure. The first step in doing so is to develop a hierarchy of feared situations, so that Sandra can begin by confronting relatively easy situations and then gradually move on to confronting more difficult ones. The rankings of situations are determined by Sandra's assigning each a SUDS rating (subjective units of distress/discomfort; Wolpe & Lazarus, 1966), where 0 = not at all anxiety-provoking and 100 = as anxiety-provoking as imaginable. SUDS ratings will also be used while carrying out the exposure practices, to quantify Sandra's responses during exposure and to indicate when habituation has occurred. In developing the hierarchy, it is useful to have items that range widely on the SUDS scale; this can often be accomplished by varying the aspects of a few items. For example, by using just a few situations that are currently being avoided according to the case presentation, one possible list of items to be ranked into a hierarchy for Sandra might look like this:

1. Showering with parent or boyfriend outside house (i.e., in garage or backyard), but no one inside house
2. Showering with no one at home
3. Arriving at work shortly before security guard is scheduled to come on duty, with guard to call Sandra upon his or her arrival
4. Same as #3, but with no phone call
5. Arriving at work at least an hour before security guard is on duty (or staying at least one hour after guard goes off duty)
6. Staying at home alone, during the daytime, knowing where parents or boyfriend are
7. Staying at home alone, during the daytime, not knowing where parents and boyfriend are
8. Staying home alone at night before bedtime, knowing where parents or boyfriend are
9. Staying home alone at night before bedtime, not knowing where parents and boyfriend are
10. Sleeping alone in bedroom, with others elsewhere in house
11. Sleeping alone in bedroom with others elsewhere in house initially, but with their leaving while Sandra is asleep
12. Sleeping alone in house
13. Sleeping in hotel room alone, with coworker or other in room next door
14. Sleeping in hotel room alone, with coworker or other not next door, but with Sandra knowing where they are in same hotel
15. Same as #10, but with Sandra not knowing which room coworker or other is in
16. Sleeping in hotel room with no one Sandra knows staying at same hotel

In examining this list of situations, we might expect that the easiest (or lowest ranked) situations and thus the ones slated first for exposure would be numbers 6, 7, and 8, perhaps followed by 10, 13, 1, or 3. The hardest situations, and thus the ones that would be assigned only after the easier ones had been mastered, might be numbers 2, 5, 12, and 16.

The types of situations of which Sandra is afraid do not lend themselves readily to in-session exposure practice, and thus the actual exposure would take place between sessions, with session time devoted to reviewing assignments, troubleshooting, and developing new assignments. Sandra would be instructed to place herself in the assigned situation each day, to monitor her SUDS level before starting and at regular intervals during the practice, and then to remain in the situation until her SUDS rating had dropped by at least 50% or to only mild levels. For situations in which it is difficult to remain for long periods of time (such as showering), Sandra might need to repeat the practice several times throughout the day.

In some cases, it can be helpful to use imaginal exposure as well. Unlike the in vivo exposure described above, imaginal exposure is easily done in session and can be particularly useful in cases of frightening memories. Sandra denies being bothered by specific memories of the childhood abuse or the intruder incident so exposure to such memories may be unnecessary. However, imaginal exposure can also be useful as a precursor to more difficult in vivo exposure practices, and if Sandra finds it difficult to confront some of her listed situations initially, the therapist might lead her through the confrontation imaginally first, with the in vivo practice coming after initial decreases in anxiety. Imaginal exposure is conducted similarly to in vivo exposure in the sense of using SUDS ratings throughout the practice and remaining with the exposure until the ratings drop. Sandra would be instructed to narrate her feared scenario (such as showering while alone in the house) while picturing it vividly, and doing so in as much detail as possible.

Given the nature of the situations listed in Sandra's hierarchy, it is obvious that other people would need to be involved in her treatment. Sandra's boyfriend and parents would need to agree to remain in the house when called for by that week's exposure, and also to stay out of the house as the exposure practices progressed. These significant others might also be called upon as coaches, to remind Sandra of her assignments and encourage her to perform them regularly and correctly, but while still following her lead (i.e., it is not the role of a coach to "force" clients to do their homework). Other people, such as the security guard or coworker, would need to be incorporated into the treatment plan as well, although it is likely that Sandra could readily involve them in her exposures without their knowing that it was part of her treatment plan. For example, she could inform the security guard as she leaves work one day that she may arrive early the next morning and ask the guard to give her a call upon arriving. In this way, hierarchy item 3 could be accomplished without explicitly telling the security guard that Sandra is conducting an exposure practice.

Given the need for prolonged, repeated exposure practices and the types of situations to be confronted in Sandra's case, it is clear that between-session homework would be an integral part of treatment. It is often the case in CBT that the bulk of the work of treatment is conducted by the client between sessions, with sessions serving largely to review the past week's practices and assign new homework for the coming week, and that would appear to be likely in Sandra's treatment as well.

It should be noted that although it addresses Sandra's primary fear of being alone, the described treatment plan does not directly address many of her other concerns such as general worrying, anxious arousal, and perfectionism, which comprise the GAD diagnosis she also met. It seems likely that if she masters her fear of being alone, much of her other worrying will decrease. Such anxiety has been shown to decrease via generalization from other treatment programs (Brown, Antony, & Barlow, 1995). Additionally, many of the techniques that Sandra learns in this treatment program can be applied to treating her other fears. For example, the imaginal exposure that targets her fear of being alone could also be used to target her other worries; such methods are referred to as "worry exposure" in Craske et al. (1992) treatment program for GAD. Similarly, the physical relaxation skills Sandra learns initially in the treatment would also be applicable to feelings of anxious arousal even when the arousal does not occur in response to fears of being alone. Finally, if significant general anxiety remains following the described treatment, it may be worthwhile to add a component of cognitive restructuring (CR). CR is included in many treatment programs for anxiety disorders, as well as forming a treatment program in its own right. It was not included in the initial treatment program for several reasons. First, there are more studies attesting to the consistent efficacy of exposure than there are studies of other therapies for most of the anxiety disorders. Second, exposure is especially indicated for specific phobia, one of Sandra's two primary diagnoses. However, if Sandra's general anxiety remains clinically significant even after her phobic fear decreases, treatment might then explicitly target this anxiety via worry exposure and CR. Similarly, it is possible that Sandra's general lack of trust and her difficulties in interpersonal relationships might decrease during this treatment, as she develops a greater sense of safety in her world. However, these feelings may also require additional therapy sessions that target schemas related to these problems. For example, she may believe she is not worth the love and attention of others, perhaps as a result of the abuse in her family and the abuse remaining unaddressed when she reported it. In this case, an additional course of CR might be very appropriate.

Medical and Nutritional Issues

According to her initial evaluation, Sandra does not take medication, has no medical problems other than allergies, and does not use drugs or alcohol. Thus, it is unlikely that there are any medical factors either contributing to her current problems or that need to be taken into account in treatment. Had Sandra not had a recent physical, it would be wise to refer her for one prior to beginning treatment, to ensure that medical problems that can mimic anxiety (such as hyperthyroid) were not present. The records of Sandra's recent physical should be reviewed. If tests for these types of medical problems were not conducted, it might be useful to refer her back to her physician for a fuller medical examination. Similarly, if Sandra had had any medical problems that might need to be considered in treatment (such as a heart problem that would contraindicate increasing her heart rate above a given level), it would be important for the therapist to consult with Sandra's physician to determine, for example, what the maximum allowable heart rate would be so that exposure practices could be tailored accordingly.

Another area that can be helpful to examine is caffeine intake. Although Sandra stated she does not use drugs, many people exclude caffeine from this category, and thus it is important to inquire directly about caffeine use. Sandra clearly has anxiety problems beyond those that can be explained even by high levels of caffeine, but if she consumes excessive amounts, it might contribute to her constant anxious arousal and sleep difficulties, and also to her worries that she is potentially headed for a "nervous breakdown."

Potential Pitfalls

One of the most common problems in CBT is client adherence to treatment tasks. Because CBT is such an active form of therapy, requiring both in- and between-session work of clients, client adherence is a critical problem that must be dealt with immediately. It can arise for many reasons, including fear, lack of confidence in the therapy or therapist, lack of time, and lack of support of others. If Sandra has difficulty completing any therapy assignments, a discussion of the reasons for this difficulty would become the first priority in therapy so that these reasons can be addressed and the assignments completed. Adherence is such an important issue that potential clients are often warned in advance about the heavy demands of time and effort required by the treatment. If they are not in a position to meet those demands currently, it is recommended that they postpone therapy (or select a less demanding form of therapy) until such a time as compliance becomes possible.

The various techniques used with CBT can also be associated with certain problems. For example, while relaxation is generally a method for reducing anxiety, some people actually find that relaxation increases their anxiety, a phenomenon known as relaxation-induced anxiety (Heide & Borkovec, 1984). If this proves to be the case with Sandra, it can be addressed either by reviewing possible reasons for the anxiety (such as the increased attention to her physical state) or by dropping this component. Alternatively, changing the relaxation procedure or using other forms of relaxation training may be useful in this situation. Sandra may also benefit from using cognitive restructuring to decrease any relaxation-induced anxiety.

Exposure can also be associated with problems, such as dissociation or numbing (failing to experience the fear during the exposure, or becoming overwhelmed with fear), frustration (with lack of progress or continued anxiety), or other emotions arising instead of anxiety, such as anger or shame. Often, these can be addressed as they arise by reviewing the rationale and method of exposure and addressing any misconceptions the client has (such as that the level of anxiety should come down immediately). In some cases, modifications to the exposure might be made, such as helping the client titrate his or her emotions by introducing additional safety cues (such as breaking into the exposure practice with brief reassurance). Finally, if the exposure brings on emotions primarily of shame or anger and these emotions cannot be put aside during practices despite review of exposure rationale, switching to another form of treatment might be warranted, as exposure has not been shown to be effective in reducing these emotions (Meadows & Foa, 1998).

In some cases, even successful treatment can be associated with problems. For example, if a client's family or social network has become accustomed to working around his or her anxiety and avoidance, the elimination of these problems could prove disruptive and new relationship patterns might need to be negotiated. In Sandra's case, it is possible that her parents or boyfriend might feel less needed or important if Sandra were to become able to stay alone in the house. This can be true even if her current need for their presence is seen as an imposition. Thus, the impact of therapy on Sandra's relationships might be assessed throughout treatment, with any negative responses addressed early on so that progress could continue.

Similarly, Sandra's personal life appears to be somewhat limited in part because of her many restrictions. It is possible that once these restrictions are lifted (such as Sandra's becoming able to travel alone), she might become more aware and less tolerant of this limited social life. Her awareness could lead to depression or other negative responses. It is possible that Sandra could simply decide to increase her social network, but it is likely that she would need some assistance with this task. She has already complained of her inability to trust others, and her lack of trust would likely interfere with the development of new relationships. Also, Sandra may not have developed the various social skills needed to maneuver her way through a wider social world due to her reliance on a few significant others. Such problems, should they arise, could be addressed by cognitive restructuring or social skills training, as appropriate. If such problems are anticipated and Sandra prepares for them, they may have a less negative impact than if she expected the rest of her life to fall into place upon overcoming her fears.

Termination and Relapse Prevention

There are several issues that arise at the termination of CBT. One matter is attributing progress only to the therapy sessions, rather than to the effort and new skills learned by the client. As part of the termination process, then, it would be important to assess Sandra's view of her progress and what she sees as the reasons for that progress. Should she refer to the therapist's efforts rather than her own, this would be addressed directly, with the emphasis on the work she herself has done and on the times she has used her skills on her own throughout treatment. Similarly, clients may report concern that once they stop therapy they will not be able to continue their practices as they will not be reporting back to the therapist. This concern can be addressed in several ways. First, as an interim measure, the client can suggest other people to whom he or she can discuss practices. However, it would not be advisable for this practice to continue long term. The second way of addressing this (either alone or with the first measure) would be to point out the problems in working only when reporting to others. If Sandra only conducts her exposure exercises because she fears the disapproval of others for *not* doing them, she continues to be as dependent on others as if she needed their physical presence. The importance of self-motivation must be emphasized, and if needed, ways to develop this motivation can be discussed (such as recognizing the progress made by virtue of her own efforts). Finally, a common way of addressing this fear is by stretching out the final sessions, perhaps by holding the last two sessions on a biweekly rather than weekly basis. This provides additional time for the client to practice independently while still having the buffer of knowing that a therapy session is upcoming.

Relapse prevention is also an important part of termination. Toward the end of treatment, Sandra and her therapist could discuss possible obstacles that might arise, such as situations that are more difficult than the ones practiced in therapy. One such situation might be an extended business trip abroad; another might be an actual attack by an assailant. Sandra and her therapist could discuss ways she might deal with such situations, so that Sandra could feel more prepared for future eventualities. Further, the likelihood that such situations would lead to a temporary setback should be addressed explicitly with plans for how to deal with such a setback. For example, if Sandra finds herself responding with increased anxiety to future situations, she might deliberately return to conducting formal practices of the skills she learned in therapy. These skills often become rusty once the client feels and is functioning better. To encourage the practice and use of skills in future situations, Sandra might be given extra copies of her monitoring forms to use periodically after therapy ends. Another possibility would be to return for booster sessions as needed. One of the most important issues to address is the difference between a setback or lapse and a relapse. Sandra should be prepared for the possibility of increased anxiety at times, but also should be reminded she now has skills to deal with anxiety that she did not have previously, and that even if the skills are rusty, they will return upon being used and practiced again. Reminding herself of this fact can prevent one incident of increased anxiety from developing into a full-blown relapse, in which Sandra feels she has lost all the ground gained in treatment.

Mechanisms of Change

The primary mechanism of change by which Sandra would be expected to overcome her fears is the breaking of erroneous or maladaptive associations. Her current fears have likely been maintained via avoidance learning. Specifically, each time Sandra escapes or avoids an anxiety-provoking situation such as being alone, the subsequent immediate reduction in anxiety serves as a negative reinforcer, increasing the likelihood that the avoidance will continue. This avoidance also prevents Sandra from learning that even if she remained in the situation, eventually her anxiety level would come down on its own. Thus, by confronting her feared situations and remaining in them despite her anxiety, via controlled exposure practices, the associations Sandra has learned between avoidance and the reduction in anxiety would be broken. In addition, Sandra will have the opportunity to learn new information, namely, that being alone is not necessarily dangerous, and that even if she sleeps or showers alone, she will in all likelihood remain quite safe and unharmed.

Another mechanism of change is the increased sense of control Sandra would be expected to develop. As reviewed earlier, a sense that one does not have control over one's environment, especially over potentially threatening events, has been proposed as a major etiological factor in generalized anxiety disorder (Barlow, 1988). By learning that she does not need to avoid being alone to feel safe or decrease her anxiety, Sandra is likely to feel more in control of both her behaviors (such as choosing to confront her fears and approach frightening situations) and her emotions (by observing how her own actions of remaining in frightening situations over time leads to a decrease in anxiety).

Finally, whether addressed explicitly via formal cognitive restructuring or indirectly by the introduction of new or corrective information via psychoeducation and exposure, Sandra's erroneous beliefs would be challenged in treatment and replaced with more realistic or adaptive thoughts as an additional mechanism of change. Sandra now approaches the world as if there is danger around every corner and as if there is considerable probability that if she were to, say, shower while alone in the house, she would be attacked by an assailant. It seems apparent in this example that Sandra is greatly overestimating the chances of being attacked while in the shower. She relies on the emotional reasoning that feeling something is dangerous makes it so. Examining the *realistic* probabilities of such an assault—based on objective evidence such as assault rates in her neighborhood or on comparing the number of times Sandra and others she knows have been assaulted in the shower versus the number of times they have showered in their lives—directly addresses whether Sandra's avoidance behavior makes sense given the actual situation. Similar challenging methods can be used for Sandra's other fears and worries. For example, she is likely overestimating the probability of something bad happening if she makes any mistakes at work, viewing such a possibility as a recipe for disaster rather than as a common occurrence experienced by everyone.

CONCLUSION

The cognitive-behavioral treatment plan described in this chapter would be expected to address Sandra's problems in several ways. Imaginal and in vivo exposure would break the erroneous associations she has made between being in the presence of others and being safe and would demonstrate that her anxiety will eventually decrease even if she does not avoid frightening situations. Realizing that she does not have to live in constant fear and rearrange her life to avoid this fear would provide Sandra with an increased sense of control, which would then be expected to generalize to ameliorate many of Sandra's other anxieties. Finally, challenging Sandra's emotion-driven rather than logic-driven beliefs would decrease her excessive fear. This challenge must be accompanied by the acknowledgement that nothing is completely safe and that in situations where the realistic probabilities of harm are quite high, greater precautions might be expected. This comparison of probable versus improbable harm would allow Sandra to again gain greater control over her life and to make conscious decisions about her reactions and behaviors in a variety of potentially anxiety-provoking situations.

REFERENCES

American Psychiatric Association (1994). *Diagnostic and statistical manual of mental disorders* (4th ed.). Washington, DC: Author.

Antony, M. M., Craske, M. G., & Barlow, D. H. (1995). *Mastery of your specific phobia*. San Antonio, TX: The Psychological Corporation.

Antony, M. M., & Swinson, R. P. (2000). *Phobic disorders and panic in adults: A guide to assessment and treatment*. Washington, DC: American Psychological Association.

Barlow, D. H. (1988). *Anxiety and its disorders: The nature and treatment of anxiety and panic*. New York: Guilford Press.

Barlow, D. H., Rapee, R. M., & Brown, T. A. (1992). Behavioral treatment of generalized anxiety disorder. *Behavior Therapy, 23,* 551–570.

Beck, A. T. (1967). *Depression: Causes and treatment.* Philadelphia: University of Pennsylvania Press.

Bernstein, D. A., & Borkovec, T. D. (1973). *Progressive relaxation training.* Champaign, IL: Research Press.

Borkovec, T. D., & Costello, E. (1993). Efficacy of applied relaxation and cognitive-behavioral therapy in the treatment of generalized anxiety disorder. *Journal of Consulting and Clinical Psychology, 61,* 611–619.

Brown, T. A., Antony, M. M., & Barlow, D. H. (1995). Diagnostic comorbidity in panic disorder: Effect on treatment outcome and course of comorbid diagnoses following treatment. *Journal of Consulting and Clinical Psychology, 63,* 408–418.

Cone, J. D. (1997). Issues in functional analysis in behavioral assessment. *Behaviour Research and Therapy, 35,* 259–275.

Craske, M. G., Barlow, D. H., & O'Leary, T. (1992). *Mastery of your anxiety and worry.* San Antonio, TX: The Psychological Corporation.

Foa, E. B., & Kozak, M. J. (1986). Emotional processing of fear: Exposure to corrective information. *Psychological Bulletin, 99,* 20–35.

Goldstein, M. J. (1987). Psychosocial issues. *Schizophrenia Bulletin, 13,* 157–171.

Gottesman, I. I., McGuffin, P., & Farmer, A. E. (1987). Clinical genetics as clues to the "real" genetics of schizophrenia. *Schizophrenia Bulletin, 13,* 23–47.

Heide, F. J., & Borkovec, T. D. (1984). Relaxation-induced anxiety: Mechanisms and theoretical implications. *Behaviour Research and Therapy, 22,* 1–12.

Heston, L. L. (1966). Psychiatric disorders in foster home reared children of schizophrenic mothers. *British Journal of Psychiatry, 112,* 819–825.

Janoff-Bulman, R. (1992). *Shattered assumptions: Toward a new psychology of trauma.* New York: The Free Press.

Kanfer, F. H., & Saslow, G. (1969). Behavioral diagnosis. In C. M. Franks (Ed.), *Behavior therapy: Appraisal and status* (pp. 417–444). New York: McGraw-Hill.

Meadows, E. A., & Foa, E. B. (1998). Intrusion, arousal and avoidance: Sexual trauma survivors. In V. M. Follette, J. I. Ruzek, & F. R. Abueg (Eds.), *Cognitive-behavioral therapies for trauma* (pp. 100–123). New York: Guilford Press.

Meehl, P. E. (1954). *Clinical versus statistical prediction: A theoretical analysis and a review of the evidence.* Minneapolis: University of Minnesota Press.

Meehl, P. E. (1986). Causes and effects of my disturbing little book. *Journal of Personality Assessment, 50,* 370–375.

Meyer, T. J., Miller, M. L., Metzger, R. L., & Borkovec, T. D. (1990). Development and validation of the Penn State Worry Questionnaire. *Behaviour Research and Therapy, 28,* 487–495.

Mowrer, O. H. (1939). Stimulus response theory of anxiety. *Psychological Review, 46,* 553–565.

Muris, P., Merckelbach, H., van Haaften, H., & Mayer, B. (1997). Eye movement desensitisation and reprocessing versus exposure in vivo. A single-session crossover study of spider-phobic children. *British Journal of Psychiatry, 171,* 82–86.

Nelson, R. O. (1988). Relationships between assessment and treatment within a behavioral perspective. *Journal of Psychopathology and Behavioral Assessment, 10,* 155–170.

Öst, L.-G. (1996). One-session group treatment of spider phobia. *Behaviour Research and Therapy, 34,* 707–715.

Öst, L.-G., Brandberg, M., & Alm, T. (1997). One versus five sessions of exposure in the treatment of flying phobia. *Behaviour Research and Therapy, 35,* 987–996.

Pavlov, I. (1927). *Conditioned reflexes.* Oxford, England: Oxford University Press.

Persons, J. B. (1989). *Cognitive therapy in practice: A case formulation approach.* New York: W. W. Norton.

Persons, J. B. (1994). Is behavior therapy boring? *The Behavior Therapist, 17,* 190.

Rapee, R. M., Craske, M. G., Meadows, E. A., Moras, K., & Barlow, D. H. (1991). *The Physiology of Panic and Anxiety.* Center for Stress and Anxiety Disorders, Albany, New York. Unpublished manuscript.

Rescorla, R. A. (1988). Pavlovian conditioning: It's not what you think it is. *American Psychologist, 43,* 151–160.

Schulte, D., Kunzel, T., Pepping, G., & Schulte-Bahrenberg, T. (1992). Tailor-made versus standardized therapy of phobic patients. *Advances in Behaviour Research and Therapy, 14,* 67–92.

Skinner, B. F. (1938). *The behavior of organisms.* New York: Appleton-Century-Crofts.

Thorndike, E. L. (1898). Animal intelligence: An experimental study of associative processes in animals. *Psychological Review Monograph Supplement, 2* (Whole Number 8).

Wolpe, J., & Lazarus, A. A. (1966). *Behavior therapy techniques.* New York: Pergamon Press.

4

Problem-Solving Therapy

Stephanie H. Felgoise, Christine Maguth Nezu, and Arthur M. Nezu

TREATMENT MODEL

Background and Introduction

Problem-solving therapy (PST) is an empirically supported, cognitive-behavioral treatment paradigm. Several different fields of psychology and areas of research influenced the development of PST, which accounts for its widespread applicability today. The historical routes of PST are embedded in early research on human problem-solving conducted in the fields of experimental cognitive psychology, educational psychology, and industrial psychology (D'Zurilla & Goldfried, 1971). In the late 1960s and early 1970s, the field of cognitive-behavioral therapy expanded, and research supported the use of problem-solving-skills training as a therapeutic intervention to facilitate social competence in persons exhibiting psychopathology or in need of therapy (see D'Zurilla & Nezu, 1999, for a historical review).

Since the early 1980s, expansive theory development on problem solving and coping (D'Zurilla & Nezu, 1982; Lazarus & Folkman, 1984) and high-quality research, including treatment-outcome studies, have demonstrated the multiple applications and efficacy of problem-solving-skills training (C. M. Nezu, Nezu, & Houts, 1993). This approach has been applied in various modalities (for example, individual, group, couples) and has been used in prevention programs, community interventions, child development and school programs, in the treatment of substance abuse and family- and health-related problems, and as therapy for various psychological disorders (for a review see D'Zurilla & Nezu, 1999). Specific to the treatment of anxiety disorders, PST has been used successfully for the treatment of social phobia (DiGiuseppe et al., 1990), and generalized anxiety disorder (GAD) (D'Zurilla & Belzer, 1998; D'Zurilla & Maschka, 1988). Other studies differentiated persons with anxiety disorders or symptoms from the general population ("normals") based on social-problem-solving deficits, including post-traumatic stress disorder (A. M. Nezu & Carnevale, 1987), persons with agoraphobia (Brodbeck & Michelson, 1987), chronic worriers, and GAD patients (Dugas, Gagnon, Ladouceur, & Freeston, 1998; Ladouceur et al., 1998).

Overview

Problem-solving therapy (PST) is an empirically supported, cognitive-behavioral intervention that focuses on the emotional, cognitive, and behavioral processes that direct or interfere with individuals' efforts to cope with problems in daily living. This model is often referred to as "social problem-solving" due to its emphasis on the social and interpersonal context in which problems and problem solving often occur (A. M. Nezu, Nezu, Houts, Friedman, & Faddis, 1999). The problem-solving model offers a rational and systematic way for individuals to think about their personal, interpersonal, and objective or impersonal problems and initiate self-directed and purposeful action to change the nature of their problems, their reactions to problems, or both (A. M. Nezu, 1987).

The importance of identifying and focusing on individuals' problem-solving processes as a point of intervention is grounded in our problem-solving model of stress (D'Zurilla & Nezu, 1982; A. M. Nezu, Nezu, Friedman, Faddis, & Houts, 1998). This model was developed concurrently, and is largely consistent with Lazarus's transactional/relational model of stress (D'Zurilla & Nezu, 1999; Lazarus, 1981, 1999; Lazarus & Folkman, 1984). Our problem-solving model proposes that stress and distress result from the reciprocal and interacting relationships among stressful life events (major life events and daily problems), negative emotional mood states, and problem-solving coping (D'Zurilla & Nezu, 1999; A. M. Nezu & D'Zurilla, 1989). Ineffective coping with stressful life events and negative mood states is proposed to lead to distress and maladaptive psychological and physical responses (Neal & Heppner, 1982; A. M. Nezu, 1985, 1986a; Sherry, Keitel, & Tracey, 1984; see A. M. Nezu et al., 1998 for a review). Conversely, effective problem-solving has been shown to mediate or moderate the effects of the stress-distress relationship, specifically with regard to depression and anxiety (Belzer, D'Zurilla, & Maydeau-Olivares, 1998; Kant, D'Zurilla, & Maydeau-Olivares, 1997; A. M. Nezu & Ronan, 1985, 1988; Nezu et al., 1986).

Operational Definitions

Simply defined, a *problem* is a discrepancy between the reality of a current or anticipated situation and the individual's desired goal, or between the current state of a specific task and the aspired goal for completion of that task (A. M. Nezu, 1987). The discrepancy arises due to an obstacle that interferes with the person's ability to produce an adaptive response to the demand presented by the situation or task. Obstacles may include novelty, uncertainty, unpredictability, competing demands, actual or perceived skill deficits, inadequate psychosocial or tangible resources, or maladaptive thinking that prevents initiation of effective action. Problems may become stressful when the requirements to overcome the obstacles involved are perceived as difficult or affect the individual's well-being (D'Zurilla & Nezu, 1982; Lazarus & Folkman, 1984).

Problems may be isolated events (e.g., theft of personal belongings), a series of similar or related events (e.g., panic attacks in crowded locations, sexual abuse), or a pervasive difficulty that occurs for a short or long duration (e.g., chronic worry, lack of trust). Problems may generate from demands originating within the individual (the need to please others, say, or perfectionism) or from the environment (objective work-related tasks or scheduling conflicts). One of the key tenets to PST is the ideographic nature of problems, in that what constitutes a problem is defined individually by the person who is experiencing it. (The process of determining the nature of one's problem will be explained further later.)

Solutions are defined as *any* coping response (cognitive or behavioral) designed to change the nature of a problem situation, one's negative emotional reaction to it, or both (A. M. Nezu, 1987; A. M. Nezu, Nezu, & Perri, 1989). Solutions are also individualistic and are therefore not determined to be right or wrong or inherently positive or negative. *Effective solutions,* however, meet three specific criteria: (a) they solve the problem (meet the desired goal state), (b) maximize the resultant positive consequences, and (c) minimize the negative consequences. In general, the quality, effectiveness, and results for a given solution will depend on the person, environment, and person-environment relationship, and the judgment of the problem-solver (D'Zurilla & Nezu, 1999).

According to the problem-solving model, the cognitive-behavioral process by which individuals understand the nature of problems in living and direct their efforts at finding solutions to them is called *social problem-solving* (D'Zurilla & Nezu, 1999; A. M. Nezu, 1987). This problem-solving process occurs on three different levels: the meta-cognitive level, the performance level, and basic cognition and information-processing level (D'Zurilla & Nezu, 1999, p. 13). However, little is known about the exact cognitive abilities necessary for effective social problem-solving (for a review and hypotheses, see D'Zurilla & Nezu, 1999). Thus, therapeutic intervention occurs at the meta-cognitive level and performance levels. The remainder of the discussion of this treatment model will focus on these two core components.

The Problem-Solving Process

Problem solving is conceptualized as a set of five semi-independent yet interacting processes: problem orientation, problem definition, generation of alternatives, decision-making, and solution implementation and verification (D'Zurilla & Goldfried, 1971; D'Zurilla & Nezu, 1982). Each of these components is significant to the overall process of understanding and effectively dealing with major and minor problems in living. Problem orientation appeals to the way one thinks about one's problems (meta-cognitive level), and the four rational problem-solving skills address the measures taken to solve problems (performance level) (D'Zurilla & Nezu, 1999).

The problem-orientation component of problem solving is a motivational process (D'Zurilla & Nezu, 1999; A. M. Nezu et al., 1999) that addresses the individual and immediate cognitive-affective reactions that arise in response to the initial presentation of a problem. Problem orientation is often referred to as one's "world view," or the habitual way of perceiving, thinking about, and reacting to problems, in general. One's world view consists of a set of orienting responses such as the tendency to approach versus avoid problems and the propensity to interpret information automatically based on past learning experiences, or schemas. Problem orientation variables include assumptions, various beliefs, appraisals, and expectations concerning problems in daily living and one's ability to solve them. Approach tendencies and production of positive emotions characterize a *positive problem orientation* and facilitate effective problem solving. Conversely, avoidant or impulsive reactions to problems and resultant negative emotions typify a *negative problem orientation* and inhibit effective problem-solving. Problem-orientation variables have significant implications for anxiety disorders and will be discussed below.

Problem definition, generation of alternatives, decision making, and solution implementation and verification comprise what is referred to as problem-solving proper or rational problem-solving skills (D'Zurilla & Nezu, 1999). In brief, use of rational problem-solving skills provides a systematic way for persons to identify problems and set goals, find and implement the most effective solutions, evaluate the outcome of solutions implemented, and, finally, troubleshoot or reward oneself upon completion of the process. There are specific goal-directed tasks, strategies, and steps to consider within each of these rational problem-solving-skills components that enable effective problem resolution. Despite presentation in a stepwise fashion, real-life problem-solving sometimes requires that the five components in the social problem-solving process are accessed nonsequentially, concurrently, or recursively, as needed. The specifics of each problem-solving component will be detailed later in this chapter.

Problem-Solving Therapy

PST assumes a skills-building approach to helping individuals cope more effectively with major or minor problems in daily living. This approach to therapy is provided in the immediate context of clients' presenting problems. Oftentimes in PST, however, the presenting problems are viewed as *responses* to current antecedent problems (D'Zurilla & Nezu, 1999). Thus, the therapist helps the client to identify and resolve the cause of the chief complaint, change the reaction to this problem, or both. Problems in the client's history are addressed to the extent that they continue to be problematic or contribute to the client's current concerns.

PST serves to enhance individuals' adaptive skills and attributes and minimize maladaptive functioning. As previously mentioned, intervention occurs at various levels of psychological processes, including affect/emotion, cognition, and behavior. The emphasis in therapy is dictated by the identified needs of each client. However, all clients are assumed to benefit from instruction, discussion, and practice of each of the five core components: problem orientation and the four rational-problem-solving skills.

Overall, the goals of PST are to improve individuals' problem-solving skills, increase their sense of control and self-efficacy, decrease their emotional distress, improve their overall quality-of-life (A. M. Nezu et al., 1998), and increase social competence (D'Zurilla & Nezu, 1999). Guidelines, sample explanations, session excerpts, exercises, and worksheets for problem-solving therapy and each of its five core components are available in several problem-solving manuals (D'Zurilla & Nezu, 1982, 1999; A. M. Nezu et al., 1998) and are beyond the scope of this chapter. However, the fundamental aspects of each process and the general therapeutic techniques used will be described in discussing the case example that is the focus of this book.

THE THERAPIST'S SKILLS AND ATTRIBUTES

Knowledge-Base and Skills

Warmth, genuineness, empathy, and positive regard are considered core elements for establishing a good rapport with clients in most therapeutic alliances, including PST. Social-learning and cognitive-behavioral theories of human behavior provide the rationale for why change is expected based on this therapeutic approach to treatment. In general, problem-solving therapists must possess skills and competency with techniques necessary for effective intervention with most cognitive-behavioral treatment models, as well as additional skills specific to this paradigm.

Problem-solving therapy requires the use of psychoeducational techniques such as didactic instruction and homework throughout therapy. These techniques are aimed to teach problem-solving skills and to encourage practice and infusion of new learning into everyday life. Therapists should have experience applying specific cognitive strategies such as imagery, Socratic questioning (to guide clients through the process of identifying self-statements and challenging their own thoughts and beliefs), and broader levels of cognitive restructuring (see Nezu et al., 1998, for a detailed description of the various techniques involved in cognitive restructuring). Fluid use of behavioral techniques such as role-playing, shaping, modeling, coaching, positive reinforcement, rehearsal (i.e., practice exercises), exposure, relaxation training, communications-skills training, and social-skills training, is also essential.

Although cognitive and behavioral theory and skills are necessary to effectively conduct problem-solving therapy, therapists also need to be flexible in their thinking to identify each client's individual needs. Therapists must be able to tailor the problem-solving protocol accordingly, for example, by extending the time spent on problem orientation variables or by recognizing when adjuvant interventions (e.g., medication, family sessions) are warranted. Thus, we firmly believe that flexibility is best guided by a rational and systematic approach to clinical decision-making. In our opinion, sound clinical decision-making skills are perhaps the most critical assets for effective conduct of PST or any other treatment. To that end, we advocate a problem-solving approach to clinical decision-making regarding assessment, case conceptualization, and treatment (A. M. Nezu & Nezu, 1989; A. M. Nezu et al., 1997).

Clinical Decision-Making

The adoption of a problem-solving approach to clinical decision-making positions clinicians in the role of problem solver (A. M. Nezu & Nezu, 1989, 1993; C. M. Nezu & Nezu, 1995). To achieve the goals of therapy, therapists must navigate their way through many clinical tasks or subproblems. A. M. Nezu and C. M. Nezu (1989) describe these tasks according to four main stages of therapy that each presents with unique "problems" to be solved and goals to be achieved: screening and problem identification (assessment), problem analysis and selection of focal target problems (case formulation), treatment design, and treatment implementation and evaluation. The problem-solving process is employed at each of these stages, thereby guiding clinicians to decrease judgmental biases and heuristics (A. M. Nezu & Nezu, 1989), seek out all necessary available facts about the client and possible means of intervention, make more effective decisions throughout the therapeutic process, conduct time-series assessments to monitor the progress in therapy, and adjust the therapy plan as necessary.

In general, clinicians' problem-orientation variables consist of thoughts, beliefs, and assumptions that influence therapy (e.g., theoretical orientation, biases, and heuristics). The main problems to be solved are the clients' reasons for seeking therapy (e.g., reduction of symptoms, desire to increase the likelihood of meeting a life partner) or the discrepancy between their current state of being and desired state. The obstacles that have prevented independent achievement of clients' goals (e.g., skill deficits, physical limitations, or emotional reactions) are considered throughout the stages of therapy. Ultimately, the therapists' goal is to empower clients to achieve their desired outcome of betterment, as operationally defined in collaboration by clients and therapists alike (e.g., reduction of panic symptoms, increase in social competence, improvement in quality of life). The goal of therapy, therefore, is to identify and implement the most effective treatment plan available to help each client overcome identified obstacles, achieve designated goals, and prepare for the future. Whenever possible, the clinician's problem-solving process will be highlighted throughout the clinical decisions made with regard to assessment and treatment of Sandra, the identified client in chapter 2.

THE CASE OF SANDRA

Assessment, Conceptualization, and Treatment Planning

Assessment

Overview. The therapist as a problem-solver attempts to gather all available facts and to test hypotheses and assumptions during the assessment phase of treatment. The information that is obtained through various methods helps (a) to define the client's problems and factors that are etiologically or functionally related to these problems and (b) to establish the therapeutic goals and identify and precisely specify the obstacles to achieving these goals (A. M. Nezu & Nezu, 1989). Obstacles may be characterized as behavioral or affective excesses or deficits, maladaptive thought processes, problems in the social or physical environment, or a combination of all of these.

We would approach Sandra's assessment from a biopsychosocial systems framework, consistent with the multimodal method that is encouraged in cognitive-behavioral assessment. This framework promotes collection of data on intrapersonal variables (such as biological, cognitive, affective, or behavioral excesses or deficits), interpersonal variables (as relationships) and environment variables (e.g., lack of physical or social resources) (Hayes & Follette, 1993). Furthermore, emphasis on cognitive-behavior therapy prescribes an empirically based, multimethod (observation, interview, physiological assessment) and multiinformant (self- and other-report) measurement of lower-level (frequency of panic attacks versus experiences of anxiety), precisely specified behavior (overt or covert) and contemporaneous causal variables (Haynes, 1998; Nelson & Hayes, 1981; O'Leary & Wilson, 1975). Sandra's case history and intake information is comprehensive and provides much of this necessary information. However, there are several areas that would require additional inquiry from our viewpoint.

Mood-monitoring.   Three aspects of an empirically based assessment are the use of empirically validated measures, time-series assessment, and clinical hypothesis-testing. Psychosocial functioning is dynamic and therefore should be continually monitored to track changes (progress, decline, or stability) over time. Therefore, in addition to the historical and current baseline data already provided by Sandra, more specific details regarding the antecedents, consequences, and frequency of her panic attacks, somatic arousal, and depressive symptoms (lower-level variables) would be acquired through self-monitoring and record keeping. A mood monitoring measure would be selected from a vast array of available instruments to serve as an aid in gathering this information. Collection of data serves to define Sandra's problems further and confirm or disconfirm hypotheses about symptom severity, stimuli, maintaining variables, and coping attempts. Data will also be used for psychoeducational purposes to facilitate the client's understanding of her problems and as a monitoring tool throughout therapy.

Specific Coping History.   There are several specific topics that need to be addressed with regard to Sandra's coping abilities. For example, how did Sandra process or "resolve" her history of sexual abuse with her brothers and father (as stated in the case description)? Although she does not meet criteria for post-traumatic stress disorder, does she have symptoms of this diagnosis? Has she ever experienced dissociative reactions? How did she cope with the apparent lack of support provided to her by her church when she requested help? How does she cope with daily interactions with her parents, visits with her biological mother, and the stressors at work? Has she tried other means to reduce her fears about being alone in the house? How does she believe her family could protect her if there were an intruder? Conversely, in what situations or with whom does Sandra feel safe? Are there situations in which she feels a stronger sense of control or more capable of dealing with external stressors? What aspects of her life make her feel proud? Additionally, information about daily activities and habits, such as Sandra's exercise routine and caffeine intake, would also be acquired.

Answers to some of these questions and others that may arise would be sought from independent reports from Sandra and her significant others (boyfriend, family). Data collection from multiinformants allows for a comparison of their subjective reports or observations and Sandra's perception of the same events or situations. Such comparisons may aid in the clearer identification of objective problems, problem-orientation variables, or both.

Current Records of Coping. Self-report information about Sandra's specific thoughts, feelings, emotions, and behaviors would be obtained through completion of daily "records of coping" (D'Zurilla & Nezu, 1999; A. M. Nezu et al., 1998; A. M. Nezu et al., 1989). Self-collected records of reactions to contemporaneous problem situations would be used to help Sandra recognize the connections among thoughts, feelings, and actions and provide her with the responsibility of self-directed participation in the assessment process. Because Sandra's self-reported history seems to emphasize or highlight maladaptive situations, she also may be advised to complete records of thoughts, feelings, and actions pertaining to pleasant events. Data collected from these records of coping will help the clinician gain a better assessment of Sandra's strengths and weaknesses in coping and will be used in problem-orientation sessions. Identification of strengths and adaptive skills will be important to increase her self-efficacy and hope for the future and to motivate her to learn new ways of thinking and coping.

Sandra's history reveals several incidences of avoidant coping strategies, escape, heightened physiological responses, overcompensation, and excessive cognitive worry in response to stressful situations. In some cases, perhaps, these responses may have been adaptive (e.g., avoidance of sexual abuse or mother's threats) when alternative coping strategies (e.g., confiding in her mother and parish priest) proved ineffective. However, obtaining a fuller history of coping efforts will inform the case formulation and would allow the clinician to test this and other hypotheses regarding Sandra's coping style.

Objective Measure of Coping. The administration of the Social Problem Solving Inventory-Revised (SPSI-R; D'Zurilla, Nezu, & Maydeau-Olivares, in press) provides a valuable objective assessment of coping skills. This 52-item Likert-type self-report measure consists of five major scales: Positive Problem Orientation scale, Negative Problem Orientation scale, Rational Problem-Solving Skills scale, Impulsivity/Carelessness Coping Style, and Avoidance Coping Style (D'Zurilla & Nezu, 1999). This objective assessment permits comparison of client data to normative scores for various psychological, medical, and normal populations (D'Zurilla, Nezu, & Maydeau-Olivares, in press). The benefits of this comparison are twofold. First, empirically based nomothetic information may positively influence the direction of PST and the clinician's approach to treating clients with similar symptomatology. Second, the client's data gleaned from the SPSI-R will highlight particular areas that should be emphasized during the course of the problem-solving therapy.

Sandra's clinical history, for example, seems to suggest that negative problem-orientation variables and avoidance dominate her coping style and may contribute to or maintain her anxiety disorder. In general, persons with a negative problem orientation tend to maintain maladaptive belief systems and attributions concerning problems, are likely to overestimate the magnitude or impact of problematic situations (Lazarus & Folkman, 1984), and underestimate their ability to solve problems (poor self-efficacy, Bandura, 1997; Hamberger & Lohr, 1984). These individuals generally tend to devote less effort and persistence to overcoming problems. As a result, a negative problem orientation tends to produce more destructive worrying and anxiety, less tolerance for frustration and uncertainty, and less productive problem solving (see D'Zurilla & Nezu, 1999 for a review of this literature). Thus, evaluation of Sandra's problem orientation is considered critical to treatment planning.

Further rationale for assessing Sandra's problem-solving process is drawn from research specifically on problem solving in persons with generalized anxiety disorder (GAD). Research has shown that negative problem orientation correlates with GAD symptoms and differentiates persons with GAD symptoms from moderate worriers (Ladouceur et al., 1998). Another recent study of social problem solving and anxiety conducted by D'Zurilla and colleagues (D'Zurilla, personal communication, March 28, 2000) found that problem orientation is a predictor of both worry and trait anxiety. Specifically, problem-solving efficacy and negative problem orientation had "direct effects on trait anxiety and indirect effects via worry." According to D'Zurilla's report, these findings suggest that worriers are unsuccessful problem solvers due to their poor problem orientation. Worriers in this sample did not have deficient rational problem-solving skills.

Sandra clearly classifies as a "worrier," and completion of the SPSI-R will likely confirm her negative problem orientation. The SPSI-R will also reveal important information about her coping style and whether or not she is deficient in rational problem-solving skills. Objective measurement also serves to minimize the clinician's biases and assumptions by providing empirically based results. Hence, the SPSI-R would be administered to Sandra before treatment began, and again toward the end of therapy to measure changes. If follow-up sessions are indicated, the SPSI-R may be subsequently readministered to assess maintenance of treatment gains.

Therapeutic Goals

Goals can be defined on two levels: ultimate outcomes and instrumental outcomes (Mash & Hunsley, 1993; Rosen & Proctor, 1981). The client's specified reasons or goals for seeking therapy, in part, constitute the ultimate outcomes desired (e.g., decrease in anxiety). Instrumental outcomes are comprised of the cognitive, behavioral, emotional, social, or environmental changes deemed necessary to achieve the ultimate outcomes (e.g., increase problem-solving skills, improve communication between client and partner) and are delineated by the therapist's case formulation (A. M. Nezu et al., 1997).

Ultimate Outcomes/Long-term Goals.   There are several hypothesized, functionally related long-term goals for Sandra. Although not specifically stated and obviously in need of verification, Sandra seems to hope for the ultimate outcomes of decreased fear of harm (by an assailant), decreased cognitive, behavioral and somatic symptoms of anxiety, improvement in her relationships, and an improved sense of trust in others. Sandra's anxieties dictate her daily rituals and obsessive behaviors; as such, an obvious goal for therapy is to significantly reduce these activities. Additional ultimate goals related to improvement of her general coping skills would include the following: (a) increase Sandra's sense of control over problems in her daily life, and her subsequent emotional, cognitive, and physical responses to these actual or perceived problems; (b) decrease Sandra's avoidant behaviors; (c) decrease Sandra's feelings of helplessness and powerlessness; (d) increase Sandra's self-sufficiency and decrease her dependence on others; (e) decrease Sandra's guilt and anger, and facilitate adjustment related to her past experiences with her family; (f) facilitate the improvement in the quality of Sandra's relationships; and (g) facilitate Sandra's future functioning and improvement in the quality of her life.

Instrumental Outcomes/Short-term Goals. Short-term therapeutic goals for Sandra include facilitating change from a negative problem orientation (assuming the data supported this) to a positive problem orientation and consistent use of rational problem-solving skills to help her cope with her problems. Adopting a positive problem orientation, as mentioned previously, will likely lead to positive affective changes and will facilitate an adaptive approach to solving problems. More specifically, adopting a positive problem orientation will likely lead Sandra to better understand her anxiety reactions as problems to be solved, rather than as symptoms to avoid. As needed, Sandra will also learn specific skills (i.e., communication skills, relaxation techniques, assertiveness skills) to facilitate use of rational problem-solving skills and to provide her with the means to overcome deficiencies that are identified as obstacles to achieving her personal goals. Because the emphasis in her treatment would likely be on problem-orientation variables, discussion of rational problem-solving-skills training is deferred to the section on techniques and methods of working.

For Sandra, an adaptive change in problem orientation is seen as the instrumental mechanism for change in her overall clinical presentation and achievement of the ultimate outcomes delineated above. Persons with a positive problem orientation believe that problems are (a) "normal" and to be expected, (b) present challenges in living rather than hopeless circumstances (obstacles versus barriers), (c) are "solvable" in general, and (d) are solvable by oneself in particular (self-efficacy) (D'Zurilla & Nezu, 1999). Accurately identifying problems when they occur and changing the interference of emotional reactions to useful personal experiences that can help later define the problem are essential components to a positive problem orientation. In contrast, Sandra seems currently to maintain a negative problem orientation. A negative problem orientation is characterized by (a) the tendency to avoid dealing with problems and to react impulsively to problems, (b) the expectation that problems are unsolvable, and (c) the belief that one lacks the ability to solve problems.

Problem-orientation training is the process by which Sandra would learn to use and view emotions in a more productive and adaptive framework. Goals for Sandra include becoming more able to recognize the connection between her thoughts, feelings, and behaviors and restructuring her maladaptive thinking patterns (assumed from the case history) by use of self-directed cognitive techniques. Acquiring the ability to self-monitor emotions and her thinking processes would enable Sandra to engage in more productive thinking (e.g., focus on the achievement of personal goals), more rational thinking (i.e., likelihood of being harmed by an assailant; evaluation of fears about showering in the house alone), and setting more realistic expectations for herself and others (expectation for perfection, high need to please others). Consistent with these goals, problem-orientation training ideally would facilitate Sandra's establishment of a more adaptive core belief system (i.e., not all persons are untrustworthy; self-worth is not measured by others' appraisal). Her therapist may begin to reprocess the abusive events in her life to help her understand her current problems. Revisiting these significant negative life events will be likely initially to increase Sandra's negative emotions. By virtue of PST, however, Sandra will learn new ways of thinking about her past situations (history of abandonment and sexual abuse), new ways of coping with the initial increase in negative emotions, and new ways of controlling the effect her past will have on her future. Despite its presentation in a unilateral fashion, problem orientation permeates the problem-solving process, and therefore some of the therapy directed at these variables would occur in concert with rational problem-solving training.

Rational problem-solving-skills training (or honing existing skills) would be prescriptive to maximize Sandra's self-directed use of newly learned skills and techniques (cognitive and behavioral) to manage her anxiety and daily problems and to increase daily positive experiences. Sandra's increased self-reliance on rational problem-solving skills will optimally lead to problem-solving successes, which will, in turn, further improve her positive orientation, problem-solving self-efficacy, and willingness to engage in prosocial activities. Thus, the cyclical nature of problem-orientation variables and rational problem-solving skills becomes apparent.

Predicted Long-term Outcome Subsequent to Ending Therapy. PST, in general, is geared toward improving social competence and facilitating effective coping with daily stressors and problems. Throughout the course of therapy, clients are encouraged and assigned to practice implementation of new skills. Compliant individuals, therefore, should ideally experience at least minimal problem-solving success weekly. The built-in process of skills building and practice facilitate increased levels of coping, sense of control, and functioning almost immediately. In fact, numerous outcome studies show that PST clients show significant improvement in mood, coping skills, distress level, and quality of life in 8 to 12 PST sessions (see D'Zurilla & Nezu, 1999 for a review). Thus, expectations for Sandra's coping ability are positive; however, the amount of effort required in therapy and independently for her should not be underestimated. Her lack of trust for others and the longevity of her symptomatology present obvious challenges to the therapy process.

Based on findings from several treatment-outcome studies with other populations (i.e., depression, agoraphobia), it is predicted that Sandra would be able to maintain gains from treatment over time. These studies have demonstrated maintenance of gains from problem-solving therapy at 3 to 6 months following completion of treatment for depression (Arean et al., 1993; Mynors-Wallis et al., 1995; Nezu, 1986b; Nezu & Perri, 1989), agoraphobia (Jannoun, Munby, Catalan, & Gelder, 1980), and stress-management workshop participants (D'Zurilla & Maschka, 1988). To date, no long-term follow-up data from PST treatment-outcome studies on GAD or specific phobia can be found in the literature.

The long-term outcome of PST for Sandra will depend on her commitment to practicing and adopting the problem-solving model and becoming more independent in her thinking and functioning. Furthermore, her willingness to enlist the support of her family and friends will be a partial determinant. Specifically, their current behaviors seem to contribute to or maintain Sandra's current level of functioning; and therefore, effective change for Sandra will require some change in her significant others' responses to her when she manifests anxiety symptoms.

Timeline for Therapy

Sandra's complex developmental and learning history, constellation of anxiety disorders and symptoms, and high level of family and significant-other involvement may dictate more than the average number of therapy sessions (8 to 12) described in most PST treatment-outcome studies. Perhaps this also may be true for others with predominant symptoms of anxiety, because D'Zurilla and Belzer (1998) propose a PST program for GAD that consists of 10 to 16 sessions. Additional sessions for Sandra will allow for more in-depth problem-orientation training, gradual exposure to avoided situations, and inclusion of her family and boyfriend in some of the therapy sessions. Sessions would mostly occur once weekly for 1 to 1 1/2 hours, unless an increase in frequency becomes indicated. The weekly spacing of sessions is usually preferable to allow clients to do homework between sessions and practice applying the new skills or strategies learned in session.

Therapy might follow the following timeline as specified. The initial therapy session following assessment would focus on (a) reviewing the therapist's case formulation and educating Sandra about her clinical symptoms, (b) socializing Sandra to PST, (c) establishing the goals of her therapy, and (d) continuing to build a positive therapeutic alliance. It is estimated that at least six sessions would focus exclusively on problem-orientation variables. Subsequently, discussion of problem-orientation variables would be integrated with rational problem-solving-skills training. An estimated one to three therapy sessions would focus predominantly on each of these four problem-solving skills, for an average of eight additional problem-solving therapy sessions. During these sessions, however, previously learned skills are always reviewed and incorporated into discussion of newly discussed problems, homework, and training in new problem-solving skills. Finally, six sessions of Sandra's problem-solving therapy would be devoted exclusively to the practice and application of the entire problem-solving process and termination issues.

Case Conceptualization

Case formulation in cognitive-behavior therapy results from a synthesis of previously collected biopsychosocial client information collected by self-report, therapist interviews and impressions, and reports by others. The therapist creates a functional analysis of the causal or contributing factors that have led to the identified problems and their consequences. Specifically, a functional analysis represents the therapist's hypotheses about the relationships among the client's developmental history, current or recent stressors, relevant stimuli that trigger or exacerbate the target problems, and maintaining variables or the "current dysfunctional system" (A. M. Nezu et al., 1997). The Clinical Decision-Making Model suggests that the hypothesized relationships among these client variables may be depicted by the creation of a clinical pathogenesis map (CPM; A. M. Nezu & Nezu, 1989). A CPM is a visual representation of the case formulation with suggested causal paths between different phenomena that are maintaining the patients' problem. A CPM may be shared with the client, if deemed appropriate. Case formulations and CPMs are likely to change due to client improvement, disconfirmation of hypotheses, or discovery of new information.

According to the available information, Sandra evidences difficulties across several domains: cognition, affect, behavior, biology/physiology, and social-interpersonal areas. Several factors in Sandra's developmental history are hypothesized to have had a significant impact on her current functioning. The numerous serious negative life events described in the case presentation are likely to have shaped Sandra's beliefs about relationships, trust (or mistrust), danger of harm, and her inability to please key figures in her life. Sandra seems to have developed maladaptive schemas about herself, her own self-worth, and others. She manifests these beliefs in her irrational cognitions, worries and fears, perception of excessive vulnerability, and maladaptive behaviors that interfere with her daily functioning. Sandra's anxiety is routinely reinforced, and therefore maintained, by her boyfriend, her family, others in her immediate social environment, and by the moderate relief she experiences from performing compulsive, ritualistic behaviors.

Sandra was raised in an unstable environment where she could not depend on consistent support, love, or encouragement from her biological or adoptive parents. During Sandra's formative years, her biological mother was continuously hospitalized for paranoid schizophrenia and Sandra was apparently rejected by her father. She was separated from her biological parents at age 4 and placed in the care of a foster family, therefore again being removed from key figures in her life. Little is known about the transition to her new family; however, it seems that Sandra feared her adoptive mother and relied on her adoptive father for comfort. Yet this once trusted relationship with her adoptive father was betrayed when she was 13. Sandra similarly reported that each of her family members (biological and adoptive) has independently betrayed her trust, abandoned or threatened to abandon her, physically or sexually abused her, or threatened her safety. Sandra apparently did not have positive role-models in her childhood and adolescence, and she seems to have learned and generalized beliefs that the world and people are to be feared and that people are not trustworthy. Sandra's biological mother clearly stated these messages to her when she was younger, and her experiences with her adopted family, social worker, and priest reinforced the veracity of these claims.

Sandra has maintained maladaptive beliefs about herself and others for many years, and it is hypothesized that she tends to focus only on experiences that validate these beliefs and disregards experiences that may contradict her world view. Beck et al. (1979) describe this maladaptive pattern of thinking as comprised of filtering and biased search strategies that serve to maintain anxiety and depression. Sandra reported several other situations that exemplify reinforcement of her fears of harm and mistrust of others. The entrance of an intruder into her home during her teenage years, for example, is lasting evidence for Sandra that her fears are justified. Furthermore, her biological mother routinely emplored her to "be careful" and expressed great surprise that she has continuously avoided "the horrible fate she imagined would befall her." According to the information gathered, Sandra did not report any situations that disconfirmed her fears or provided evidence against her beliefs. In fact, being alone or the thought of being alone are stimuli for her fears of harm and lack of safety.

Sandra's current pattern of avoiding or escaping problems also appears to have been learned at an early age and reinforced continuously throughout her life. Sandra's avoidant coping style seems to have developed in response to experiences that proved alternative coping strategies ineffective. For instance, Sandra's effort to gain protection from abusive situations by reporting them to persons with authority resulted in significant negative consequences. Sandra was not believed, was accused of lying, was threatened to keep silent and was "abandoned" by her mother, father, priest, and social worker in her times of need. Thus, Sandra reports frequent escapes or running away to avoid her "mother's wrath," her brothers' abuse, and her feelings of helplessness and upset in response to her parents' decision to sponsor another foster child.

Experiences such as these seem to have taught Sandra that escape, avoidance, and remaining on the offense were the only ways she could protect herself from harm or cope with unpleasant and feared situations.

She could not rely on others and could not let her guard down. Based on the provided information, in fact, these coping responses may have been the most adaptive choices available to her at those young ages. Or, perhaps Sandra gave up on problem solving in these situations due to feelings of hopelessness and fear of consequences. Regardless, these experiences of helplessness and inability to initiate effective action seem to have strongly influenced her current poor problem-solving self-efficacy and failure to implement more effective problem-solving skills in other situations throughout her life.

Constant worrying seems consistent with Sandra's pattern of coping, so much so that worry seemed to serve a protective function for Sandra. Focusing her attention on feared situations seems to provide the unrealistic expectation that she can ward off the feared outcomes. Likewise, Sandra's current ritualistic behaviors—for example, parking her car in a specific place—seem to serve the same function of seeking a sense of control. Finally, her aloof presentation and lack of expressed emotion may also represent Sandra's effort to maintain her guard and not reveal her vulnerabilities to others. Her poor sleep accompanied by frequent nightmares seem to be an outlet for her feelings and emotions. Likewise, the physical symptoms that co-occur with her persistent worry and fear represent other manifestations of her difficulties and are by-products of her inability to cope with the multiple stressors in her life. Thus, coping strategies (i.e., avoidance, inhibition of emotions and feelings) that may have been adaptive for Sandra in specific instances in the past appear to have been become generalized beliefs and behaviors.

Sandra's irrational thoughts, emotional responses, and maladaptive beliefs and behaviors are hypothesized to lead to misperception of events and to excesses of anxiety, avoidance, lack of trust, and need for control. These negative feelings and emotions reinforce her need to engage in extreme behaviors and worry, and they inhibit her ability to engage in effective action. The description of recent events and level of functioning also suggests that she has little endurance for uncertainty and a low frustration tolerance as evidenced by her recent anger outbursts. These maladaptive ways of coping continue to be reinforced or maintained in new ways. Sandra's routines to avoid being alone in her home and to maintain a sense of safety, as examples, are maintained by her parents', boyfriend's, and others' availability to her in support of her excessive needs (i.e., sleeping on her parents' floor, showering only when others are home). Thus, the cyclical nature of her difficulties becomes evident.

Sandra's past experiences of "failing to meet her mother's expectations," failing to gain approval from her family, and fearing the consequences of misbehavior seem connected to current beliefs and behaviors described in her work place. For example, Sandra reportedly works extra hours, strives for extreme perfection, and fears making mistakes at work. Sandra seems to fear that the consequences of evaluation will be rejection or abandonment. Perhaps she has learned that she must "behave" and "please others" to retain her position at the bank just as she had to behave to prevent her return to the adoption agency and has had to submit to others' demands throughout her adolescence and young adulthood. Thus, it seems possible that Sandra sets unrealistic goals for herself to achieve more than is expected in order to avoid the negative consequences she anticipates in accordance with her maladaptive beliefs established from her past learning experiences. Sandra did not report any evidence that the consequences she fears are realistic. However, she did acknowledge that her boss relies on her to do his job as well as her own and that she has earned several promotions during her tenure as at the bank. Alternatively, Sandra may be seeking to maintain approval and positive reinforcement for her efforts at work. If so, her attempts to gain approval and positive feedback are extreme.

Despite Sandra's anxiety related to work and her performance, her position as a loan manager reveals several of her strengths that will be useful in therapy. Sandra has "worked hard" to achieve a sense of satisfaction in her life and finds her job fulfilling. She manages to function well at work with regard to supervising 12 employees. Although details were not provided, it is likely that until her recent increase in irritability Sandra had been effectively coping with the pressures at work, conflicts that arise among employees, and frequent decisions that require her attention. If she had not been functioning adequately, it is unlikely that she would have earned several promotions and retained employment in the same place for so many years. Identifying the positive thoughts, feelings, and behaviors that had allowed Sandra to function more efficiently in her work environment could be generalized or called upon to improve her functioning in other situations.

Sandra has remained in a committed relationship with her boyfriend for 5 years. This long-standing relationship seems to be troubled by poor communication and lack of certainty about her feelings and trust in him, yet he has remained loyal to her. Learning what positive attributes he perceives in Sandra may provide insights into other strengths of hers. It is clear that among her strengths, Sandra has a strong will to survive.

In summary, Sandra's troubled developmental, relationship, and coping history are viewed as antecedents to current problems in functioning and daily living. As such, Sandra needs to learn new ways of coping in contrast to what has been learned in the past. Emotion-focused coping, therefore, will be employed to restructure maladaptive thoughts and feelings that have remained connected to these past experiences. These factors that are core components of Sandra's negative problem orientation are coupled with either deficient or dormant problem-solving skills to overcome current stressors. Thus, establishing new beliefs, experiencing more positive experiences, and implementing effective problem-solving skills are prescriptive goals for Sandra's treatment.

The Therapeutic Relationship

The Therapeutic Bond

Problem-solving therapy requires a collaborative, teamwork approach to treatment. The therapeutic relationship, therefore, is an important element of the therapeutic process and must provide support, instruction, trust, and safety. Therapists gain their clients' trust by exhibiting general therapeutic skills such as warmth, empathy, genuineness, and positive regard (Rogers, 1957). In addition, problem-solving therapists are advised to establish the credibility of the therapeutic approach by conveying their knowledge of the relevant empirical research that supports their work. Providing a simple yet solid rationale, PST serves to normalize the clients' problems in the context of others who seek treatment and fosters clients' confidence in PST.

The development of a strong therapeutic alliance is critical in early sessions, as is the establishment of therapeutic limits and boundaries. The therapeutic alliance is emphasized because problem-solving therapists will be guiding clients to leave their habitual ways of thinking or to engage in new behaviors that may initially be anxiety-provoking and stressful. Facilitating this change may involve confrontation, and suggesting that clients change their long-term patterns of reacting to stress and distress may be interpreted as a criticism of one's personality or character. Therapists must, therefore, adeptly express acceptance and respect for clients while recommending that they modify their ways of coping that have thus far been counterproductive for them. This is especially important for Sandra, who experienced profound betrayal by other people in her life from whom she expected help. We would continually assess her predictable interpersonal fears of the therapist's betrayal or lack of approval as a "problem to be solved." Shared with the client in this way, problem-solving skills could be directed toward various incidents that occur in this context and provide a model for how she will problem-solve similar fears with relationships outside the therapy situation.

Trust in the therapist's skills and the therapeutic process will also minimize the likelihood that therapeutic techniques and instructions will be dismissed or resisted. For example, without a proper understanding of the rationale for therapy or the role of the therapist, patients are likely to get frustrated with therapists' unwillingness to "give" them answers, "define" problems for them, or endorse their goals as "good" or "bad," right or wrong. On the contrary, clients who trust their therapists may feel more accountable to therapy with regard to homework and implementation of solutions in anxiety-provoking situations.

Self-disclosure.   Due to the collaborative nature of PST, clients who are beginning therapy may be inclined to ask, "What would you do?" Or to say, "The options are sort of neutral, tell me which you think is better!" Self-disclosure is not recommended, however, due to the potential for the therapists' decisions and behaviors to interfere with clients' individually relevant problem-solving efforts. It is generally recommended that therapists respond in a nonevasive, nonpunitive manner by reviewing the individualistic nature of problem solving and the idiosyncratic determination of goals and effective solutions. The therapist may wish to explain that the best use of session time is to focus on the client's goals and decision-making process. Therapist self-disclosure, therefore, may actually serve as an obstacle to achieving the goals of therapy. It should be noted, however, that therapist self-disclosure should not be confused with the therapist's *modeling* the use of problem-solving skills as problems in the therapy process arise. In fact, therapists are encouraged to model the problem-solving process as often as possible and appropriate and to share their relevant thoughts to the extent that it is clinically indicated. Examples include engaging clients in problem solving for problems such as frequent client cancellations, client's inability to continue to pay for therapy sessions, or stating the "problem" of perceived client anger or frustration.

Transference/Countertransference.   Although these terms are not generally adopted in cognitive-behavior therapy, most cognitive-behavioral therapists identify and acknowledge the tendency for interpersonal patterns that occur in clients' lives to emerge in the therapeutic relationship. Therapists' goals are to help clients identify adaptive and maladaptive ways of thinking and behaving, and therefore the therapeutic relationship and in-session behaviors provide samples of clients' reactions to situations or feelings that should be discussed in session with regard to problem solving and coping. For example, clients who exhibit dependent behavior in their interpersonal relationships may try to solicit more effort from the therapist. Likewise, clients who feel isolated or abandoned by their families may maintain schemas that lead them to perceive therapists' actions as consistent with those who have betrayed them. Identifying these thoughts and feelings provides excellent opportunities for demonstration and implementation of problem-orientation strategies directly to the context of the therapeutic relationship. This may indeed represent some of the most significant work with Sandra.

The challenge of PST for clinicians is to maintain objectivity, support, and acceptance of clients who choose to make decisions or engage in behaviors that are contrary to their own world views. For example, clients provide therapists with their own problem to be solved when they choose to drop out of therapy, continue to stay in dysfunctional relationships, are promiscuous, or select alternative therapy over a proven and effective medical intervention. Therapists have to identify their own limits to which they can provide therapy effectively without compromising their own values or their clients' treatment. Given these considerations, therapists must recognize that while remaining within the legal, ethical, and professional guidelines of protecting clients and themselves, their roles are to maintain objectivity, help individuals evaluate *all* the consequences of their decisions, consider all options available, and reach confident decisions that are best for them. Ultimately, clients have the right to make "bad" decisions, and therapists therefore have the obligation to recognize when their own biases or reactions may interfere with the clients' choices or best interests.

Roles in the Therapeutic Relationship

As previously stated, the PST model prescribes a collaborative therapeutic treatment alliance. The therapist is an expert in problem solving and the client is the expert in his or her own particular life circumstances and personal experiences. Thus, therapists and clients both make valuable contributions to therapy and to the achievement of the clients' goals. The expectations for these roles are established in the first session of therapy. Included in this discussion will be the therapist's and client's adherence to appointment times and commitments to therapy (i.e., completion of homework assignments), routine mutual agenda-setting for each session, mutual respect, confidentiality, and the agreement that the client will vocalize concerns or questions about therapy as they arise. Clients have a high level of responsibility for their progress and achievement in therapy, which requires their willingness to be an active participant in therapy, both in and out of sessions. However, therapists should consider motivational problems as a challenge to understand in the context of the client's clinical mapping, and not as a "resistance" on the patient's part.

The therapist's role requires continuous adjustment and modification of directiveness and activity level in therapy, in accordance with the goals of each individual session. During problem-orientation training, for example, the therapist may engage in more Socratic questioning or direct confrontation to help the client recognize and modify maladaptive thought patterns. In portions of problem-orientation training or rational problem-solving skills training, the therapist initially takes a more didactic approach to the therapy session and incorporates more teaching metaphors, relevant examples, and learning tools such as handouts and work sheets. Yet in some aspects of problem-solving therapy, the therapist functions as a team member or coinvestigator of the nature of the client's problems. During practice sessions or homework review, the therapist's role may emphasize provision of corrective feedback or prompting of alternative considerations, more similar to a coach. There likely will be times when the therapist may find interactive role-plays to be the most effective means of assisting a particular client, while in other situations subtle prompting and reflective listening may be the operative techniques to facilitate the client's adoption of problem-solving principles and improvement of coping skills. Thus, problem-solving therapists' level of involvement will vary throughout the course of therapy, but is generally typified by a moderate to high level of activity. The challenge for the therapist, in sum, is to strike the optimal balance between being an active and directive practitioner, and functioning as a team member collaboratively seeking to investigate the client's problems and overcome the challenge of the client's clinical dysfunction.

Treatment Implementation and Outcome

Techniques and Methods of Working

The question of what specific or special techniques are implemented in PST can be answered in several ways. From a general cognitive-behavioral perspective, a variety of anxiety-management skills would be used to target Sandra's cognitive, affective, behavioral, physiological, and interpersonal responses to anxiety-provoking stimuli, in accordance with the assessment data and case formulation. Such techniques might include cognitive restructuring strategies already discussed as part of problem-orientation training, exposure treatment, covert desensitization, behavioral exercises and role-plays, relaxation training, and diaphragmatic breathing. However, the vast repertoire of anxiety reduction and cognitive restructuring techniques would likely differ depending on the nature of a particular client's presentation. These general therapeutic techniques are considered within the framework of PST. The therapist as problem-solver considers the alternative cognitive-behavioral techniques and skills that could be introduced into therapy in response to obstacles that are preventing the client from achieving particular goals. For example, exposure therapy may be the technique chosen as one solution to implement in an effort to help the client overcome the clinical problem identified (i.e., anxiety) and achieve the therapeutic goals outlined. Furthermore, the therapist and client also may consider adjuvant interventions such as medical treatment or spiritual consultation when problem-solving treatment strategies result in these options.

An alternative answer to the question of what methods and techniques are used in PST addresses the specific components of problem-solving-skills training. The remainder of the discussion will focus on the techniques used to teach each of the problem-solving skills, because this will somewhat differentiate this chapter from the other cognitive-behavioral-therapy chapter in this book. Problem-orientation training was elucidated in the treatment goals discussion, so the reader is referred back to that section for a review of the techniques and approaches used to facilitate a positive problem orientation. Training in problem-solving skills proper typically includes individual sessions for each of the four components: problem definition and formulation, generation of alternatives, decision making, and solution implementation and formulation. As mentioned, each of these skills involves attention to problem-orientation variables to some degree, and review of other problem-solving skills proper also occurs throughout the course of treatment. Although more comprehensive rationales for each of these steps are typically given in therapy (see D'Zurilla & Nezu, 1999; A. M. Nezu et al., 1998), provision of this detail is beyond the scope of this chapter. As such, only a brief reference to the significance of each component is now made.

Problem Definition and Formulation. There are several tasks involved in problem definition and formulation: (a) defining the nature of the problem for oneself, (b) gathering factual information about a problem situation and separating facts from assumptions, (c) identifying *why* a situation is a problem (evaluating personal or impersonal obstacles), (d) determining realistic problem-solving goals for the successful resolution of the problem, and (e) assessing the cost-benefit ratio of solving and not solving the problem. A well-defined problem will increase appropriate and directed efforts to generating relevant alternative solutions, making accurate decisions about solution options, and objectively evaluating the results of one's efforts. Thus, in order to solve a problem, individuals must first understand clearly what the problem is, why the situation or task presents a problem for them, and what their goals are for solving the problem. The therapist employs the client to adopt an "investigative-reporter" approach to identifying the facts of a problem and separating them from assumptions that may be clouding an objective appraisal of a problem situation. Problems are defined in concrete and objective terms. Likewise, goals are clearly specified with consideration of how realistic the goals are for the individual.

Generation of Alternatives. The problem solver is positioned to begin the process of finding a solution to a problem once the goals, and obstacles to achieving those goals, have been identified in problem definition and formulation. The "generation of alternatives" stage of problem solving promotes the use of brainstorming to maximize the potential solution options available to the individual. While brainstorming, clients are taught to defer judgement of ideas in order to enable development of more options. The underlying rationale is that generating a larger quantity of solution options than would naturally occur through habit or routine increases the likelihood that a good or better alternative will be discovered.

Use of brainstorming methods engages individuals in productive thinking, decreases impulsive problem solving, and empowers individuals by developing new or existing skills that enable them to move beyond their previous level of ability to discover problem solutions. Brainstorming will be helpful throughout the problem-solving process. Such methods may be used to explore all obstacles involved in understanding the nature of problems, or in predicting all possible consequences from implementing specific solution options. In therapy, creativity and brainstorming are fostered by instruction and use of in-session practice with benign or hypothetical problems, perspective-taking, and imagery.

Decision Making.   After constructing an exhaustive list of solution alternatives, clients then begin the process of systematically and rationally evaluating each option to find the most effective solution. This process essentially involves conducting a cost-benefit analysis of the predicted consequences that would occur as a result of implementing each of the solution alternatives. Valences of the predicted consequences are recorded according to a simple rating scale (i.e., positive, negative, neutral; −1, 0, 1; ☺, O, ☹) of the client's choice. Individuals are instructed to consider the likelihood that the alternative would accomplish the specified goal, the likelihood that the client could implement the solution effectively, and the likely resultant personal, social, short-term and long-term consequences. Use of brainstorming strategies may facilitate this process. Once these variables are considered and the most effective solution is selected, the client develops the overall solution plan. This plan may include either a combination of solution options or a contingency plan in case the anticipated consequences do not occur as predicted. Finally, upon completion of the decision-making tasks, the client is ready to proceed to solution implementation and verification, unless none of the identified solutions seem to produce sufficient positive consequences worthy of implementation. In such cases, the individual may need to troubleshoot and recycle back through the previous problem-solving steps, including problem orientation. Oftentimes, clients may need to be guided back to consideration of problem-orientation variables if, for example, the consequences predicted seem unrealistic (positive or negative), are biased, or self-defeating. A poorly defined problem or misdirected goal may also have derailed the problem-solving process.

Solution Implementation and Verification.   This is a critical problem-solving skill because up to this point problems have only been dealt with on a hypothetical basis. The goals of solution implementation and verification are to carry out the solution plan optimally, monitor the consequences, evaluate the consequences, and self-reinforce or trouble-shoot, as indicated (D'Zurilla & Nezu, 1999, p. 32). Thus, individuals are encouraged to plan, rehearse, or practice the implementation of their solution, if feasible, to maximize the likelihood of success. Techniques used to facilitate this process may include role-plays, behavioral rehearsal, positive self-statements for self-encouragement, anxiety reduction techniques, imagery, or others. Clients are encouraged to think about variables such as timing, setting, and circumstances that may impact on their success in implementing their solution plans. Monitoring and evaluation systems are devised prior to implementing a solution, and clients record this information throughout their implementation efforts (i.e., maintain a mood diary while enrolled in yoga classes). Comparison of actual consequences and predicted consequences are made at intervals that may be predetermined in therapy. Reinforcement or troubleshooting is encouraged throughout the evaluation of the verification process. Because many problem orientation variables may interfere with solution implementation, solution verification, or both, the therapist should encourage finding as many opportunities as possible for the client to implement solutions during the course of treatment.

Homework.   Homework assignments commensurate with the goals of each step in the problem-solving process are devised to help the client learn and apply their new skills. In-session and between-session practice is considered crucial to the development and adoption of problem-solving coping skills and the development of a positive problem-solving self-efficacy (see Nezu et al., 1998 for examples of homework assignments and corresponding handouts). Thus, as each new set of skills is learned, the client is responsible for systematically practicing and completing work sheets on the entire problem-solving process learned to date. Initially, less complex problems are used for the purpose of learning the sets of skills, and then attention to more complex problems is encouraged. Practice of additional skills or techniques introduced throughout the course of PST (i.e., assertiveness skills, relaxation training) occurs concurrently, sequentially, or independently, depending on the nature of the relationship between the problems addressed.

Participation of Others.   Sandra would be encouraged to invite her parents and boyfriend into therapy once treatment goals and the treatment plan have been established. Their cooperation will be necessary to support Sandra's move toward independence and reduction of her specific phobias. Specifically, because her family's and boyfriend's behaviors are hypothesized to inadvertently maintain Sandra's dependence and ritualistic behaviors, they will need to be informed about what changes she will make and how they can facilitate rather than hinder this process. Likewise, her treatment may require changes in their behaviors. The explanation and rationale for these changes therefore must be discussed and agreed upon. Perhaps a behavioral contract might be devised to create consensual rules and boundaries regarding the involvement of the family and boyfriend and the responses each of them, including Sandra, are expected to provide in various situations. Provisions would be made for extreme behavioral or emotional reactions and the initial exacerbation of Sandra's fear and anxiety that may be expected during certain components of therapy (i.e., exposure). If the family or boyfriend is not cooperative or is resistant to involvement, the therapist would engage in problem solving to generate alternative approaches to Sandra's treatment that would minimize the potential for the family to sabotage or negatively influence treatment.

Medical and Nutritional Issues

Four main concerns with regard to medical and nutritional issues arise in consideration of Sandra's treatment and dictate the need for a psychiatric or additional medical consultation. The first medical issue is the high level of anxiety reportedly experienced by Sandra during the initial phase of assessment and upon beginning therapy. Sandra would be referred to a psychiatrist willing to collaborate in her care for possible psychopharmacological management of anxiety symptoms initially. If deemed appropriate, one advantage of the medication plan would be to treat Sandra's anxiety symptoms with psychiatric medication to allow her to experience more immediate relief from her present high level of constant arousal and possibly glean more benefits from therapy. Among the potential risks of this dual treatment might be Sandra's attribution of improvements to the medication rather than to her own efforts; however, this could effectively be addressed in therapy, as necessary.

Second, it is also worth considering if Sandra is biologically predisposed to anxiety and paranoia, given that her mother has a diagnosis of paranoid schizophrenia. Although this predisposition may not be changeable or validated, it may prove useful for treatment planning and consideration of medication. In addition to feeling "anxious and disturbed" about comments made by her mother, Sandra may also fear that her anxieties will develop into the severity of her mother's condition. Exploring this topic may lead to psychoeducation about her mother's clinical diagnosis. Alternatively, discussion about Sandra's exposure to her mother and its impact on her may be relevant regarding the adoption of her mother's fears and development of learned maladaptive behaviors.

Third, Sandra reports poor sleep, which has obvious implications for her health and general functioning. A less restrictive intervention regarding Sandra's sleep problems would be to introduce a nonpharmacological intervention such as relaxation training. However, if sleep disturbance appeared to significantly impact upon mood and her ability to work with the problem-solving strategies introduced during sessions, referral for a short-term antidepressant may be indicated. The fourth issue of caffeine and nutritional intake needs to be explored with Sandra. Although the family physician reports no "serious ailments," general health behaviors can impact Sandra's overall well-being. Depending on the outcome of further assessment and the medical consultation, sleep hygiene and health behaviors may be incorporated into problem-solving therapy or addressed by adjuvant medical intervention.

Potential Pitfalls

Potential pitfalls in PST, in general, include the following (see A. M. Nezu et al., 1998, D'Zurilla & Nezu, 1999, for a comprehensive explanation of PST "do's and don'ts"):

1. Viewing PST as only skills training and not psychotherapy
2. Presenting PST in a mechanistic manner
3. Delivering a generic treatment that does incorporate relevant life experiences of a given patient
4. Forgetting to review or assign homework
5. Using humor injudiciously
6. Overlooking complex psychological, emotional, existential, and spiritual problems or overemphasizing superficial problems
7. Focusing only on specific skills training or minimizing the importance of patient's feelings
8. Rushing through or minimizing training in solution implementation or losing sight of the overall PST goals
9. Equating problem-focused coping with problem-solving coping

Potential pitfalls to Sandra's treatment are connected more specifically to her personal constellation of problems. First, failing to adequately address the issues of trust and safety would surely sabotage her therapy. Sandra's current method of coping with frightening, anxiety-provoking, or threatening situations is avoidance or escape. Thus, a strong therapeutic relationship and ongoing discussion about safety and trust will be critical to prevent her attrition.

Second, Sandra's feelings have been disregarded in the past. Validating the magnitude of her past experiences and current difficulties, therefore, may elicit significant emotional responses that the therapist must be prepared to address. On the contrary, if Sandra's feelings are seemingly inaccessible to her, or her thoughts and feelings are indistinguishable, failure to dedicate a sufficient amount of time in therapy to this problem will inhibit her potential for a successful outcome in therapy.

Third, Sandra's daily activities involve several family members or significant others. Underestimating the impact Sandra's therapy could have on these other individuals would potentially create numerous problems for her and for them. Including key persons in occasional therapy sessions, as described above, and monitoring and evaluating the impact of therapy on Sandra's relationships with these individuals will allow for implementation of appropriate interventions, as necessary. Finally, if one of Sandra's therapeutic goals is to decrease her dependency on her family and boyfriend, the therapist should be cautious of Sandra's increasing her reliance on therapy and the therapist in their place.

Resistance to change or to engage in anxiety reduction strategies such as exposure treatment, for example, is expected from an individual such as Sandra who has maintained her extremely maladaptive coping style for an extended period of time. Her lack of trust of others, general anxiety, and fears are suspected to be core contributing factors to the anticipated resistance. Likewise, Sandra's poor self-efficacy and her disbelief that problems can be solved or that she can be helped may also represent barriers to engaging her in therapy. The recommended approach to dealing with such anticipated resistance is to address the issues directly with Sandra in the initial sessions of therapy and as the resistance becomes evident. Discussion of her expectations, the therapist's expectations, and other clients' reactions in similar situations may serve to normalize Sandra's fears, enhance her trust in the therapist, and increase her feeling of safety in the therapeutic process.

Termination and Relapse Prevention

Sandra's history reveals a pattern of dependence on others that signifies reason for concern that she may become overly dependent on her therapist. Sandra may be motivated for change and increased self-reliance, but development of her independence will be challenged by her typical pattern of functioning. Thus, termination for Sandra should be an issue that remains in the therapist's mind almost from the beginning of treatment.

Toward the middle to end of therapy, the therapist should open discussion about Sandra's thoughts and feelings regarding termination. It is possible that Sandra may fear her independence and therefore show an increase in symptoms as termination draws near. Another possibility may be that she becomes angry, reverts back to avoidant behaviors, and discontinues treatment prematurely. However, proper discussion and problem solving regarding termination issues should minimize the likelihood of these or other negative outcomes. The therapist must be sure to communicate his or her confidence in Sandra's coping abilities and substantiate these claims with a review of her progress. Sandra and the therapist must also realistically consider anticipated difficulties she may experience in general, and with regard to termination specifically. Thus, termination may be viewed as the "problem" and an operational definition for Sandra's optimal independent functioning is the identified goal. Together, Sandra and the therapist may problem-solve anticipated obstacles, generate options to overcome or cope with them, and decide on a hypothetical plan that may be implemented if such problems arise.

One option that may be advisable to facilitate termination is to taper Sandra's treatment off toward the end of therapy. Spacing out Sandra's last few sessions may provide her with an opportunity to experience daily life without the frequency of weekly sessions and to problem-solve difficulties that occur in the interim. If termination induces substantial anxiety in Sandra, it may also be useful to provide her with the safety of having scheduled follow-up appointments or booster sessions. Caution is advised in offering this option, so that Sandra does not misperceive the therapist's preventative measure as a lack of faith or trust in Sandra's coping ability. Finally, Sandra should be provided with extra handouts, work sheets, and copies of her completed homework assignments for future reference.

Mechanisms of Change

The expected mechanism of change for Sandra centers on the improvement of problem-solving coping, which incorporates changes in problem orientation and rational problem-solving skills. Sandra's improvement in problem-solving skills and anxiety management strategies learned in PST (i.e., relaxation techniques, use of positive self-statements) is expected to lead to an improved sense of control and problem-solving self-efficacy, use of proactive coping methods, decreased use of avoidant coping strategies, increased trust in others, and increased involvement in prosocial and enjoyable activities. Changes in these aspects of Sandra's current thoughts, feelings, behaviors, and ways of coping are predicted to improve her relationships, daily functioning, and overall quality of life.

CONCLUSION

Social problem-solving skills, techniques, and therapy have many clinical applications for therapists and clients alike. Problem solving is recommended as a framework for therapists' clinical decision-making and for clients' enhancement of social competence and reduction of distress related to major and minor life events. Ongoing clinical research continues to build on the existing empirical support for using a problem-solving approach to treatment of various clinical disorders, enhancement of coping skills, and improvement of quality of life.

The prescribed PST intervention for treatment of Sandra's anxiety and clinical symptoms demonstrates the flexibility of this cognitive-behavioral paradigm and its appropriateness for the treatment of persons with complex intra- and interpersonal problems. Discussion of assessment, conceptualization, treatment planning and implementation, and the therapeutic relationship with Sandra highlight the individualistic nature of this therapy modality. Recommendations made to increase the likelihood of effective treatment, avoid pitfalls, and overcome obstacles are intended to be generalizable to therapy with persons with anxiety disorders and other difficulties.

REFERENCES

Arean, P. A., Perri, M. G., Nezu, A. M., Schein, R. L., Christopher, F., & Joseph, T. X. (1993). Comparative effectiveness of social problem-solving therapy and reminiscence therapy as treatments for depression in older adults. *Journal of Consulting and Clinical Psychology, 52,* 687–691.

Bandura, A. (1997). *Self-efficacy: The exercise of control.* New York: W. H. Freeman.

Beck, T. A., Rush, A. J., Shaw, B. F., & Emery, G. (1979). *Cognitive therapy of depression: A treatment manual.* New York: Guilford.

Belzer, K. D., D'Zurilla, T. J., & Maydeau-Olivares, A. (1998). *Correlations between the Social Problem-Solving Inventory-Revised and measures of worry and state and trait anxiety.* Unpublished data, State University of New York at Stony Brook.

Brodbeck, C., & Michelson, I. (1987). Problem-solving skills and attributional styles of agoraphobics. *Cognitive Therapy and Research, 11,* 593–610.

DiGiuseppe, R., Simon, K. S., McGowan, L., & Gardner, F. (1990). A comparative outcome study of four cognitive therapies in the treatment of social anxiety. *Journal of Rational-Emotive and Cognitive-Behavior Therapy, 8,* 129–146.

Dugas, M. J., Gagnon, F., Ladouceur, R., & Freeston, M. H. (1998). Generalized anxiety disorder: A preliminary test of a conceptual model. *Behaviour Research and Therapy, 36,* 215–226.

D'Zurilla, T. J., & Belzer, K. D. (1998). Problem-solving therapy for generalized anxiety disorder. In A. M. Nezu (Chair), *Social problem-solving therapy: State-of-the-art and future directions.* Symposium presented at the 32nd Annual Convention of the Association for Advancement of Behavior Therapy, Washington, DC.

D'Zurilla, T. J., & Goldfried, M. R. (1971). Problem solving and behavior modification. *Journal of Abnormal Psychology, 78,* 107–126.

D'Zurilla, T. J., & Maschka, G. (1988, November). *Outcome of a problem-solving approach to stress management: I. Comparison with social support.* Paper presented at the Association for Advancement of Behavior Therapy Convention, New York.

D'Zurilla, T. J., & Nezu, A. M. (1982). Social problem solving in adults. In P. C. Kendall (Ed.), *Advances in cognitive-behavioral research and therapy (Vol. 1).* New York: Academic Press.

D'Zurilla, T. J., & Nezu, A. M. (1999). *Problem-solving therapy: A social competence approach to clinical intervention.* New York: Springer.

D'Zurilla, T. J., Nezu, A. M., & Maydeu-Olivares, A. (in press). *Manual for the Social Problem-Solving Inventory-Revised.* North Towanda: Multi-Health Systems.

Hamberger, L. K., & Lohr, J. M. (1984). *Stress and stress management.* New York: Springer.

Hayes, S. C., & Follette, W. C. (1993). The challenge faced by behavioral assessment. *European Journal of Psychological Assessment, 9,* 182–188.

Haynes, S. N. (1998). The changing nature of behavioral assessment. In A. S. Bellack & M. Hersen (Eds), *Behavioral assessment: A practical handbook* (pp. 1–21). Boston: Allyn & Bacon.

Jannoun, L., Munby, M., Catalan, J., & Gelder, M. (1980). A home-based treatment program for agoraphobia: Replication and controlled evaluation. *Behavior Therapy, 11*, 294–305.

Kant, G. L., D'Zurilla, T. J., & Maydeau-Olivares, A. (1997). Social problem solving as a mediator of stress-related depression and anxiety in middle-aged and elderly community residents. *Cognitive Therapy and Research, 21*, 73–96.

Ladouceur, R., Blais, F., Freeston, M. H., & Dugas, M. J. (1998). Problem solving and problem orientation in generalized anxiety disorder. *Journal of Anxiety Disorders, 12*, 139–132.

Lazarus, R. S. (1981). The stress and coping paradigm. In C. Eisdorfer, D. Cohen, A. Kleinman, & P. Maxim (Eds.), *Theoretical bases for psychopathology*. New York: Spectrum.

Lazarus, R. S. (1999). *Stress and emotion: A new synthesis.* New York: Springer.

Lazarus, R. S., & Folkman, S. (1984). *Stress, appraisal, and coping.* New York: Springer.

Mash, E. J., & Hunsley, J. (1993). Assessment considerations in the identification of failing psychotherapy: Bringing the negatives out of the darkroom. *Psychological Assessment, 5*, 292–301.

Mynors-Wallis, L. M., Gath, D. H., Lloyd-Thomas, A. R., & Tomlinson, D. (1995). Randomized controlled trial comparing problem solving treatment with amitriptyline and placebo for major depression in primary care. *British Medical Journal, 310*, 441–445.

Neal, G. W., & Heppner, P. P. (1982, March). *Personality correlates of effective problem solving.* Paper presented at the annual meeting of the American Personnel and Guidance Association, Detroit, MI.

Nelson, R. O., & Hayes, S. C. (1981). Nature of behavioral assessment. In M. Hersen & A. S. Bellack (Eds.), *Behavioral assessment: A practical handbook* (2nd ed., pp. 3–37). New York: Pergamon.

Nezu, A. M. (1985). Differences in psychological distress between effective and ineffective problem solvers. *Journal of Counseling Psychology, 32*, 135–138.

Nezu, A. M. (1986a). Effects of stress from current problems: Comparisons to major life events. *Journal of Clinical Psychology, 42*, 847–852.

Nezu, A. M. (1986b). Efficacy of a social problem solving therapy approach for unipolar depression. *Journal of Consulting and Clinical Psychology, 54*, 196–202.

Nezu, A. M. (1987). A problem-solving formulation of depression: A literature review and proposal of a pluralistic model. *Clinical Psychology Review, 7*, 121–144.

Nezu, A. M., & Carnevale, G. J. (1987). Interpersonal problem solving and coping reactions of Vietnam veterans with posttraumatic stress disorder. *Journal of Abnormal Psychology, 96,* 155–157.

Nezu, A. M., & D'Zurilla, T. J. (1989). Social problem solving and negative affective conditions. In P. C. Kendall & D. Watson (Eds.), *Anxiety and depression: Distinctive and overlapping features* (pp. 285–315). New York: Academic Press.

Nezu, A. M., & Nezu, C. M. (Eds.). (1989). *Clinical decision making in behavior therapy: A problem-solving perspective.* Champaign, IL: Research Press.

Nezu, A. M., & Nezu, C. M. (1993). Identifying and selecting target problems for clinical interventions: A problem-solving model. *Psychological Assessment, 5,* 254–263.

Nezu, A. M., Nezu, C. M., Friedman, S. H., & Haynes, S. N. (1997). Case formulation in behavior therapy: Problem-solving strategies and functional analytic strategies. In T. D. Eells (Ed.), *Handbook of psychotherapy case formulation* (pp. 368–401). New York: Guilford.

Nezu, A. M., Nezu, C. M., Friedman, S. H., Houts, P. S., & Faddis, S. (1998). *Helping cancer patients cope: A problem-solving approach.* Washington, DC: American Psychological Association.

Nezu, A. M., Nezu, C. M., Houts, P. S., Friedman, S. H., & Faddis, S. (1999). Relevance of problem-solving therapy to psychosocial oncology. *Journal of Psychosocial Oncology, 16*(3/4), 5–26.

Nezu, A. M., Nezu, C. M., & Perri, M. G. (1989). *Problem-solving therapy for depression: Theory, research, and clinical guidelines.* New York: Wiley.

Nezu, A. M., & Perri, M. G. (1989). Problem-solving therapy for unipolar depression: An initial dismantling investigation. *Journal of Consulting and Clinical Psychology, 57,* 408–413.

Nezu, A. M., & Ronan, G. F. (1985). Life stress, current problems, problem solving, and depressive symptoms: An integrative model. *Journal of Consulting and Clinical Psychology, 53,* 693–697.

Nezu, A. M., Nezu, C. M., Saraydarian, L., Kalman, K., & Ronan, G. F. (1986). Social problem solving as a moderator variable between negative life stress and depressive symptoms. *Cognitive Therapy and Research, 10,* 489–498.

Nezu, A. M., & Ronan, G. F. (1988). Problem solving as a moderator of stress-related depressive symptoms: A prospective analysis. *Journal of Counseling Psychology, 35,* 134–138.

Nezu, C. M., & Nezu, A. M. (1995). Clinical decision making in everyday practice: The science in the art. *Cognitive and Behavioral Practice, 2,* 5–25.

Nezu, C. M., Nezu, A. M., & Houts, P. S. (1993). The multiple applications of problem-solving principles in clinical practice. In K. T. Keuhlwein &

H. Rosen (Eds.), *Cognitive therapy in action: Evolving innovative practice.* San Francisco: Josey-Bass.

O'Leary, K. D., & Wilson, G. T. (1975). *Behavior therapy: Application and outcome.* Englewood Cliffs, NJ: Prentice-Hall.

Rogers, C. R. (1957). The necessary and sufficient conditions of therapeutic personality change. *Journal of Consulting and Clinical Psychology, 21,* 95–103.

Rosen, A., & Proctor, E. K. (1981). Distinctions between treatment outcomes and their implications for treatment evaluations. *Journal of Consulting and Clinical Psychology, 49,* 418–425.

Sherry, P., Keitel, M., & Tracey, T. J. (1984, August). *The relationship between person-environment fit, coping and strain.* Paper presented at the 92nd Annual Convention of the American Psychological Association, Toronto, Ontario, Canada.

5

Acceptance and Commitment Therapy

Steven C. Hayes, Julieann Pankey, and Jennifer Gregg

TREATMENT MODEL

Acceptance and commitment therapy (pronounced *act*, not a-c-t) is a contextual behavioral psychotherapy approach (Hayes, Strosahl, & Wilson, 1999) that views psychopathology as a relatively frequent and statistically normal side effect of human language processes. According to the theory of language underlying ACT (relational frame theory; see Hayes, Barnes-Holmes, & Roche, in press; Hayes & Hayes, 1992), human verbal behavior is based on the learned ability to relate events arbitrarily, mutually and in combination, and to transform the stimulus functions of one event based on its relation to another. This simple verbal process gives rise both to the human ability to think, reason, and verbally problem solve and to the equally characteristic ability to amplify suffering.

The acronym FEAR expresses four of the key concepts in an ACT approach—fusion, evaluation, avoidance, and reason-giving (Hayes et al., 1999). Cognitive *fusion* refers to the tendency for verbal knowledge to dominate over other sources of behavioral regulation. In certain contexts, verbal symbols begin to assume many of the functions of the events to which they are related. When this is excessive, people become heavily rule-governed—colloquially they live their lives "in their heads"—and show notable insensitivity to the contingencies they experience directly.

Evaluation involves the application of a comparative relation to two or more verbal events. When combined with temporal verbal relations, this verbal process allows the comparison of conceptualized consequences, or the comparison of experienced events to feared or wished for events. Unlike the comparisons made by nonverbal organisms, which must all be based on experience, evaluation for human beings can be entirely based on verbalized events that have never been contacted. This greatly amplifies the capacity for human suffering. For example, a relatively successful life can be considered a failure compared to an imagined ideal. Similarly, it is a very small step from "That's bad" to "I'm bad," requiring only sufficient perspective-taking to talk about oneself as an object. If "I'm bad," then I cannot be good until I change. Unfortunately, often the grounds for the evaluation are difficult or impossible to change, and the very effort to change may contradict the desired outcome, as will be explained in this chapter.

Experiential *avoidance* occurs when a person is unwilling to remain in contact with a particular private experience (e.g., bodily sensations, emotions, thought, memories, behavioral predisposition) and takes steps to alter the form, frequency, or situational sensitivity of these events even when doing so causes psychological harm (Hayes et al., 1996). The combination of cognitive fusion and evaluation leads naturally to experiential avoidance. Consider a person who experiences a frightening event and becomes anxious. For a verbal organism, it is not just the original situation that now may be avoided, but also the memory of it, talk about it, anxiety itself, or other situations that give rise to anxiety because all of these can be conceptualized and evaluated verbally.

Unfortunately, experiential avoidance has negative consequences. Avoidant coping strategies such as denial, repression, and suppression are consistently associated with negative health outcomes (see Suls & Fletcher, 1985 for a meta-analysis). Suppression of unwanted thoughts increases their frequency, and if they are linked to negative mood it increases the degree to which this mood evokes and is evoked by the troublesome thought (Wegner, Erber, & Zanakos, 1993; Wegner & Zanakos, 1994).

Reason-giving is the attempt to create literal explanations for problematic behavior that make sense of its occurrence without leading directly to its alleviation. Clients who can offer good reasons for their pathological behavior are more severe and more difficult to treat than others (Addis & Jacobson, 1996). Reason-givers ruminate more, particularly in response to negative moods (Addis & Carpenter, 1999), in an effort to find and formulate better reasons. Ruminative worry reduces uncertainty (Dugas et al., 1998), avoids more distressing topics (Borkovec & Roemer, 1995), and reduces arousal (Wells & Papageorgio, 1995). Unfortunately, although the worrier believes that rumination will help deal with the situation, it has, in fact, no such instrumental benefit (Borkovec, Hazlett-Stevens, & Diaz, 1999) in part because reason-giving tends to focus on internal events (Bloor, 1983). Worry and reason-giving tend to be another form of experiential avoidance.

ACT interventions are designed

- to undermine the experiential avoidance agenda
- to break up the fusion of event and symbol and to deliteralize language representations (Hayes et al., 1999)
- to teach acceptance and willingness as responses to unwanted private events and to other domains in which direct change is not helpful or possible (e.g., the past)
- to help the client maintain contact with a transcendent sense of self
- to clarify life values and directions
- to help the clients behave in accord with chosen values through behavioral commitment strategies

These goals are approached through a wide variety of specific techniques. In general terms, ACT relies heavily on nonanalytic forms of verbal interaction: metaphor, paradox, and experiential exercises. The experiential avoidance agenda is challenged by a detailed examination of the workability of the client's past practices in that area. Defusion is fostered by meditation and mindfulness exercises, by the use of paradoxical and process-oriented language in therapy, by creating contexts in which literal meaning is diminished, and by the use of language conventions that decrease the degree to which private verbal behavior is taken literally. Acceptance is fostered by deliberate exposure through the use of experiential and Gestalt procedures and by exercises that allow the client to go through exposure while in contact with a transcendent sense of self. Behavioral commitment linked to chosen values occurs in a very behaviorally sensible way (have clear goals, break down behavior change into steps, take one step at a time, etc.), but all the while with an attempt to delink behavior change from an unnecessary and counterproductive attempt to change private events.

From an ACT perspective, psychological health refers to an increasing ability to live life in accord with chosen values, while simultaneously maintaining a nondefensive contact with historically produced private reactions (thoughts, feelings, memories, bodily sensations). The acronym "ACT" refers to the key steps involved: Accept, choose, and take action. In this view, health is not a state, but a process of change in specific domains (acceptance and valued action). Psychological health of this kind is available to anyone. No one's history is so horrific that it is impossible to do a better job of noticing the reactions produced by it, while taking at least some positive behavioral steps.

A small but growing body of literature supports the empirical value of ACT (see Hayes et al., 1999, for a review). In the area directly relevant to this chapter, ACT has been shown in recent randomized controlled study to be useful in the treatment of workplace anxiety and stress (e.g., Bond & Bunce, 2000), and a protocol largely based on the ACT manual has been shown to be useful in the treatment of generalized anxiety disorder (Orsillo & Roemer, in press). ACT was developed originally with anxiety disorders as its focus, and a series of case studies in that area presented the first empirical support for its use (Hayes, 1987). Furthermore, training therapists in ACT has been shown to produce generally better clinical outcomes across the range of client problems normally encountered in outpatient settings, including anxiety problems (Strosahl et al., 1998). Thus, there is some evidence in support of the efficacy and effectiveness of ACT in the area covered by this chapter.

THE THERAPIST'S SKILLS AND ATTRIBUTES

ACT therapists adopt a posture of *radical acceptance*, in which any private experience can be observed, felt, and explored without evaluations about these experiences being taken literally. Central to an ACT therapist's skills is the ability to accept compassionately no reason-giving on the client's part, but rather to encourage the client to come into contact with the workability of their behaviors, the valued life they wish to live, and the behavioral steps needed to move in that direction.

The therapeutic relationship in ACT is one between equals. Clients are not "broken" and therapists "together." Rather, therapist and client are like two persons climbing separate mountains that are within shouting distance across a deep canyon. From the point of view of the client— the climber—the barriers ahead seemingly may prevent progress. From the point of view of the therapist—the person across the canyon—it may be clear that there is a path ahead. But this difference in view comes from an advantaged perspective, not from psychological superiority. On his or her mountain, the therapist's own barriers present the same challenge as that facing the client. The therapist may or may not have had a history as difficult as the client's, but still must learn how to dissolve his or her own barriers and move ahead. The therapist and the client share the experience of being human, and that means that both are tempted by human language itself to do what does not work.

Being able to contact and accept their own difficulties, especially in therapy, is a powerful asset for ACT therapists. For example, suppose an ACT therapist is working with a client who is anxiety-disordered, and an impasse is reached. The therapist feels confused, on the spot, awkward, and somewhat incompetent at the moment. In the normal scheme of things, therapists would be tempted to hide their lack of confidence, to ignore their own confusion, and to cover up their fears. This is very likely exactly what the client is doing, and it is a major reason the client is losing control over his or her life. Instead of hiding, able ACT therapists would instead notice their own thoughts, as thoughts (not as what they say they are), and notice their own feelings, as feelings, and then do what needs to be done clinically. This might include sharing their feelings with the client—which models exactly what the therapist is asking the client to do. Instead of trying to *feel* confidence, they would *do* confidence, by feeling what they are already feeling anyway. (This is very much in accord with the etymology of "confidence," which comes from two Latin words that mean with fidelity or with faith.) For example, the therapist might say to the client, "I'm feeling confused and a bit anxious right now—I'm not sure what to say and I guess I think I'm supposed to. I notice that my mind is telling me that I'm a dope for not knowing exactly what to do. So let me just take a moment to thank my mind for that thought and to feel uncomfortable . . . so here I am, wondering what to do." Moments such as these, if genuine, can be powerful moments for clients, because they reduce any sense of one-upmanship and provide a concrete model of what acceptance and defusion might mean.

Understanding ACT treatment strategies at a deep, functional level is very helpful, and it is aided by personal work by therapists using ACT techniques on their own problems. The goal of ACT is to change the function of a client's private events rather than the form. Focusing on this functional level requires being able to consider how a behavior may function for the person rather than becoming too involved with the literal content or topography of the thought, emotion, or behavior.

Detecting the functional level is fostered by the ability to track any event at multiple levels simultaneously. When a client says something it may have meaning at all of the following levels:

- The statement has literal meaning based on its content.
- The statement is part of a therapeutic relationship and has meaning as an event in that relationship. It may have been evoked or shaped by the therapist or may be designed to change the behavior of the therapist.
- The statement is a sample of the client's social behavior and may have meaning as an example of the kinds of things the client does in relationships more generally.
- The statement is situated in the history and the current context of the client and as such reflects the client's past.
- The statement is situated in the history and the current context of the client and as such may serve a dynamic psychological function for the client (e.g., such areas as experiential avoidance or avoidance of the domination of authority).
- The statement is part of an ongoing life story as verbally constructed by the client and may serve the function of perpetuating that story and showing its correctness.
- The statement may be an example of the kind of problematic behavior with which the client is struggling.
- The statement may be an instance of new, more healthy behaviors.

Experienced ACT therapists learn multiple tracking skills, so that all of these levels may be detected and updated continuously. Interventions may thus be directed at the function of behavior, not just its form. For example, a client who is anxiety-disordered may dominate a session with talk about a recent bout with anxiety. The therapist may have noticed that the client talks a lot following any kind of emotional connection in therapy and may formulate the hypothesis that the client avoids a sense of intimacy in therapy by excessive literal talk. Tracking the client's talk at multiple levels may thus allow interventions to occur at these levels rather than that readily reached by the form of the client's verbalizations. Based on the idea that the client is avoiding anxiety in session related in part to the therapeutic relationship, when our talkative anxiety disordered client takes a breath, the therapist may say, "I notice that it is getting a little heady in here. I'm listening to what you are saying about last week, but I'm also noticing what is going on right now. Can we just take a moment to sit silently, noticing that we are both here together in this room? Would you be willing to do that just for a few moments? [sits silently for perhaps 30 seconds]. And as we do that, I'd like you to watch what your body does. If you notice that it does anything, tell me what comes up, being careful not to go off into an interpretation of what that might mean. Just note what shows up and try to stay with it without making it come or go." If the therapist is correct about the function of the talk, such an intervention might elicit some of the emotional reactions that are being avoided and may also do so in a way that increases the client's ability to contact those reactions without having to engage in avoidance behavior. By under-cutting the avoidance, nonproductive and excessively literal talk may begin to drop away.

An ACT therapist maintains a warm, nonjudgmental, direct, honest, and caring therapeutic relationship. The therapist does not offer the "golden fix-it," but rather fosters opportunities for clients to become present to the difficult private events they are experiencing, to accept these without buying into them literally, and to move forward in the valued life direction of their choice.

THE CASE OF SANDRA

Assessment

Broadly speaking, assessment in ACT centers on the function of the client's current and historical symptoms, which requires an examination of the current and historical influences that contribute to the current set of difficulties. The specific form and focus of this assessment is guided by the underlying theory. For that reason, a particular focus will be given to cognitive fusion and experiential avoidance. There will be a detailed examination of the control strategies the client has used, either historically or currently, and whether the client is utilizing any of them in the session. The link between the need for emotional control and specific historical factors will be examined. Because experiential avoidance is assumed to occur readily in normal humans, the purpose of this focus on historical content is more to determine the specific triggers that are likely and to detect the verbal story the client is constructing that supports avoidance behaviors.

In the case of Sandra, much of the general symptom information has been gathered, but further assessment would address the specific function of her avoiding being alone, what the consequences of this avoidance have been, and what the feared or experienced consequences of being alone or vulnerable have been. The functions of worry and worry about worrying would be explored, by examining in detail what happens (e.g., what her body does, what else she thinks of, how her behavior changes) when worry is entered into. The verbal and experiential linkage among events would be explored (e.g., what memories show up when she connects with her fear of abandonment) but not in a way that would suggest this linkage is itself a problem.

Commonly in ACT, this initial assessment is actually done as part of the intervention itself. For example, considerable focus would be given to what she has done to "try to deal with her problem," knowing full well that the client will initially believe that her problem is fear rather than the attempt to control fear as a method of behavioral regulation. In this initial assessment phase, the ACT therapist will gradually formulate what has been said to reveal the experiential avoidance strategy that underlies the symptoms. For example, the therapist in this case asks, "What do you do to get to sleep?" and is told, "I'll go into their [the parents'] bedroom and sleep on the floor." An ACT therapist might later say, "So it sounds as though you are worrying about sleeping and you are feeling somewhat anxious. Then you go to sleep on the floor in your parents' bedroom and your worries and fears subside and you sleep better. Is that right?" If the patient agrees, the therapist might continue, "OK. So how about areas other than worries and fears about sleeping? What else do you do to deal with fears and worries?" This subtle reframing begins to focus the client on the broader functional class, of which sleeping strategies are but a part. This client is engaged in a life-and-death struggle with the private results of her own history. She believes that she must feel *better* in order to live better. ACT assumes that she must *feel* better in order to live better. This is not because feeling feelings is an end in itself, but because the avoidance of feeling feelings prevents behaviors that the client values.

As this history and current behavioral pattern is explored, no attempt is made initially to point to the problematic nature of avoidance and suppression strategies. The therapist will present no evaluation or analysis, staying instead with simple questions and with answers that seemingly are embraced literally. The goal is gradually to widen the focus of assessment to detect the underlying common function and to do so in a way that that function is gradually put on the table. In the case of Sandra, this might include

- the function of always being around people (is it in order to avoid feeling the fear she feels when she is alone?)
- the role and effects of worry
- what does she do with the emotions associated with traumatic life events (her matter-of-fact style of reporting suggesting that she intellectualizes these events)
- the role of anger with coworkers and her boyfriend—are there other feelings that occurred immediately before the anger (e.g., hurt, vulnerability, anxiety) and what happened to them when she acted angrily?
- whether she has difficulties being close to others and if so whether this in order not to feel what she might have to feel if she were close to another person

These and other areas of Sandra's life where she was working to not feel what was there for her to feel would be examined in detail. No emphasis would be placed on whether this avoidance was positive or negative, but gradually the questioning would be done in a manner that itself produces some healthy distance between the avoided emotions and Sandra. For example, the therapist might say, "So it sounds as though you notice yourself feeling afraid and then you start talking to yourself about what you can do to get rid of that feeling. Your mind tells you the problem is that you are alone and you start to strategize how you can get someone here so that the fear will go away. Is that sort of how it goes? OK, good, very nice. So what else do you do to keep fear at bay?" In this little dialogue several subtle methods are used to create psychological distance between Sandra and her problematic psychological content. The use of "mind" as if it is a third person encourages a listening posture, instead of a statement of ontological reality posture; the use of "you notice yourself feeling afraid" (instead of the more common construction of "you are afraid") does the same thing. The phrase "OK, good, very nice" begins to establish a social/verbal context in therapy in which any content is welcome, and it subtly suggests that the problem as the client views it (namely, the presence of fear) is not necessarily the problem as the therapist views it and that the client is doing exactly what might be expected.

A formal assessment measure we have developed to assess experiential avoidance is the Acceptance and Action Questionnaire. The following nine items are rated on a scale of 1 (never true) to 7 (always true):

1. I am able to take action on a problem even if I am uncertain of what the right thing to do is.
2. I often catch myself daydreaming about things I've done and what I would do differently next time.
3. When I feel depressed or anxious, I am unable to take care of my responsibilities.
4. I rarely worry about getting my anxieties, worries, and feelings under control.
5. I'm not afraid of my feelings.
6. When I evaluate something negatively, I usually recognize that this is just a reaction, not an objective fact.
7. When I compare myself to other people, it seems that most of them are handling their lives better than I do.
8. Anxiety is bad.
9. If I could magically remove all the painful experiences I've had in my life, I would do so.

Ratings on items 1, 4, 5, and 6 are reversed for scoring purposes. This simple scale has been validated with more than 3,000 patients in several different validation studies summarized in Hayes, Bissett, et al. (under submission) and has good reliability and validity. The AAQ is regularly used about every month to track progress in ACT.

Some of Sandra's particular experiences should be explored to learn more about what she avoids more specifically. One place to start with is what happened to Sandra as a teenager when an intruder broke into her house. Even though the intruder did not attack Sandra or her family, the trauma of the experience appears to have developed from Sandra's fear about what *could* have happened to her: In many ways, Sandra could be verbally creating a fate worse than any experience she might have endured. Given this trauma, Sandra fears the attack of an intruder, but fearing the attack of an intruder is a relatively adaptive response in and of itself. For Sandra, however, it is not just the healthy fear of an intruder that keeps her from going to dangerous places alone at night, but rather it is the position Sandra has taken that her fear is real, important, and must be eliminated for her to be safe.

After the methods of control are reasonably well explored (which might take half a session or more), the therapist begins to examine whether these strategies are truly working for the client in her life, as judged by the client's experience. Sandra is very aware of the toll that fear is taking on her life, but she may not yet see that the toll comes from her attempt to control the fear, not from the fear itself. Workability would thus be examined in strategy after strategy. The purpose of this part of the assessment is to help the client come into contact with the fact that the current strategies are not working and to open up a bit to the pain they are in. The therapist's opinion is never the arbiter—the client's experience is. After some exploration of workability a dialogue like the following might ensue:

Therapist:	So tell me. When you get someone to come over so you are not alone, how well does that work? Does it in some absolute or final sense remove your fear?
Sandra:	Well, it helps. The fear goes away.
Therapist:	Really? I can see that your mind tells you that it goes away, but let's look at your experience. You have been afraid to be alone for a long time. As you have worked to get the fear to go away, has that fear occurred less and less often? Is it less and less intense? It is less and less central in your life?
Sandra:	. . . Well, it is more central over time—it is taking over my whole life. But I feel better.
Therapist:	Right. So short term you feel less fear, and long-term fear becomes the central theme of your entire life. Is that fair to say? So, you tell me: *Is this strategy working?* In any final, full, or absolute sense, *does this work?*
Sandra:	Ultimately, no, it doesn't work.
Therapist:	But of course when you are afraid and alone your mind tells you that you have to do something, and it tells you that getting someone there would help. So you may have a choice here. Who are you going to be guided by, your mind or your experience? I don't know about you, but I want to do something in here that works.

	And it sounds as though with all of these strategies, bottom line, none of them work. Heck, here you are in therapy . . . because they don't work. In every other area of life if you worked this hard you'd get some benefit. Yet you've somehow worked your way into a situation in which a struggle with fear is the central theme of your life. So what that tells me is that maybe its not just that these things *haven't* worked . . . maybe they *can't.*
Sandra:	Well, then why am I coming to see you?
Therapist:	Oh, I'm not saying your life can't work! Not at all! I'm just asking you to look at the great pain you are in and to acknowledge that your own experience tells you that as you've tried to deal with it, it has gotten bigger, not smaller. It is not your fault. It's more like a big setup. You are doing the logical, reasonable, normal things. But what if all the things your mind has told you are the *solution* to the problem are instead *the problem itself?*
Sandra:	. . . I'm confused, and a bit scared.
Therapist:	Good. Great. We are making progress. See if you can allow yourself just to feel confused and scared for a moment.

The greatest ally clients have in ACT is their own pain. If the logical and reasonable strategy of experiential avoidance worked, no one would ever question it. What makes people ask questions is the painful failure of this coping strategy. Careful assessment of the ultimate workability of avoidant coping strategies is thus both an assessment strategy in ACT and a central ACT intervention.

Often clients are sent home with a daily self-monitoring form that asks the client to rate three things on a Likert-style scale: the intensity of their dominant negative experiential state (in this case, anxiety), how intensely they struggled not to feel that emotion, and the workability of their approach to life during that day if this day was a model for all others. The client will quickly notice that struggle is negatively correlated with workability and positively correlated with suffering or upset. Sometimes clients even notice that the correlation between struggle and workability is more profoundly negative that the correlation between anxiety and workability.

Another major area of assessment in ACT is an assessment of the client's values, including her valued life direction and goals. This assessment involves asking the client to examine his or her values in a number of content areas, such as social, family, and intimate relationships, work, and spirituality, as well as others. A detailed plan for this assessment is presented in Hayes et al. (1999). Values assessment provides the client and therapist with a framework for behavior change goals and allows the client to have clearer access to times when he or she is not living consistently with his or her values.

Relatively little is presented about Sandra's values in the case description. We would anticipate that her avoidance behavior is not consistent with what she would like her life to be about, and that many of the barriers experienced by Sandra are thoughts, feelings, bodily sensations, and other private stimuli that "cause" her to avoid fearful situations. Assessment in these areas might lead naturally to assessment in such areas as her relationship to her boyfriend, her sexual life, relationships at work, career goals, substance use, goals regarding children and family, religious and spiritual views, health practices, citizenship goals, her strengths, and so on. It is these larger issues that form the context of her suffering, and it is the importance of these that makes the attempt to turn and face her own pain something more than masochism.

Some assessment focus would be placed on the verbal glue that holds together her life story: being right. During sessions, clients often lapse into trying to explain the cause of their problems or begin citing personal history as a reason why things can't change. Sandra is no exception. In the context of assessment, the therapist can begin to undermine the degree to which stories are adopted on the grounds of "truth" as opposed to functional utility. It can be helpful to ask things like this:

- And what is that story in the service of?
- Suppose you had a choice: to live a more vital life or to be right about this story. Which would you choose?
- Could you take these same events in your life, and construct a totally different story that integrated them all? Let's see if we could do that right here (this can be repeated several times).
- Have you said these kinds of things to yourself or to others before? Is this story old?
- If God told you that your explanation is 100% correct, how would this help you?

Therapeutic Goals

Sandra presents a fairly classic case from an ACT point of view. She believes that the problem is her fear, saying "fear rules my life, fear runs my life." On closer examination, however, it is not fear that rules and runs her life: It is fear avoidance, hurt avoidance, and vulnerability avoidance that does so. Sandra has a means-end belief that could be stated as follows: "Because my life is constricted by fear, I need to reduce my fear." Unfortunately, the effort to reduce her fears is exactly what is constricting her life (leading to an inability to establish an independent life). There may indeed be deeper dynamics also involved (e.g., driving her parents crazy may be a function of her anger toward them or even her dependency on them), but these dynamics probably have the same avoidance function (e.g., to avoid hurt and vulnerability I will be angry with my parents).

What justifies an ACT therapist's substituting cognitive defusion and experiential acceptance goals for the client's own goals of avoidance of fear is that this change is in the service of the client's ultimate goal. Clients cannot be expected to know the literature on the behavioral impact of various coping strategies. Even some psychologists do not realize, for example, that thought and emotional suppression tend to *increase* the suppressed event. The real problem here is the constriction of a human life. The mainstream culture and human language itself leads the client to target fear as the cause, missing the point that this very process of misdirected cultural influence is the true cause. Often in ACT, we come to this very question of goals in the phase of therapy that puts emotional control on the table as a central problem. The question is asked something like this:

> Suppose it is like this: In the effort to maintain control of your insides you've lost control of your life. And suppose the reverse is also true, that if you let go of the attempt to control the automatic reactions your history serves up, you can gain control over your life direction. If it is like that, and I think it is, which goal is really more important to you: control over your emotions, or control over your life?

Clients virtually never answer "control over my emotions." That target is not an ultimate goal, but a process goal. The goal of ACT is a deep, behavioral *yes* to the ultimate question life itself keeps asking:

> *Given that there is a distinction between the stuff inside you that you are struggling with and the person who is struggling, are you willing to experience that stuff, fully and without defense, as it is and not as what it says it is AND to do what moves you behaviorally in the direction of your chosen values in this situation?*

Thus, the therapeutic goal for Sandra would be for her to abandon the agenda of regulating her private events and choose instead to act effectively (concrete behaviors in alignment with her values) in the presence of difficult private events. Stated another way, the goal for this client is to love herself and her history and to move out into life. As a young child, others rejected and invalidated her and her feelings. Now she does the same to herself in the name of achievement. That is what needs to change.

Timeline for Therapy

There is no specific timeline set for treatment in ACT, and sessions can occur with the frequency that best suits the current situation of the client. Positive effects have been shown for ACT in controlled studies for interventions that average 4 to 5 hours (Strosahl et al., 1998) or even less (Bach, 2000).

That being said, in a normal anxiety case such as that presented by Sandra, the following would be typical:

General assessment	1 hour
Targeted assessment and creative hopelessness	1 hour
Control is the problem	1 hour
Willingness issues	2 hours
Transcendent self	1–2 hours
Defusion and language traps	2 hours
Emotional exposure	2 hours
Behavioral commitment	2 hours
Cycling specific values/goals/barriers/ actions until the process is acquired	4–12 hours

Such a schedule would translate into a 16- to 24-session therapy program, with additional sessions and booster sessions as needed. Usually the initial commitment would be for 10 sessions. If clear progress is not evidenced by then, a change in course is suggested. If a truncated schedule was necessary, these phases could each be touched, but in a more limited way. A bare-bones anxiety package could be delivered in 8 to 12 sessions or even less with support from books, tapes, or client-run groups, but the opportunity to learn acceptance, defusion, and commitment as a habit of living in this area would be more limited.

Case Conceptualization

In order to conceptualize this case from an ACT perspective, it is important to examine what the client is doing now in her life. Sandra is doing what human beings do: She is attempting to make painful thoughts, feelings, memories, and bodily sensations go away by doing all of the things in her life that should work to do this. She is avoiding ever being alone so that she does not have to experience the fear that is present for her when she is alone. She remains aloof in existing relationships in order to avoid feeling what she would have to feel with respect to them if they were real.

These responses of actively attempting to avoid painful private events are incredibly natural responses for human beings, due to their basic resemblance to other responses that take place outside of the skin, such as getting rid of objects that we do not want in our lives. In addition, Sandra comes by her difficulties honestly. She may have an inherited tendency to associate bad outcomes with the current context, and she certainly has a direct history of wounds in relationships and of fearful experiences. Her biological mother directly encouraged and reinforced fearfulness; her abuse history showed her that people who are close to you can wound you or abandon you physically or psychologically; the invalidation of her experiences by her parents leads her to doubt her own feelings and views; her parents presented poor models of consistent caring. The coping strategies she followed—avoidance, suppression, perfectionism, achievement, workaholism, self-attack, ruminative worry, and interpersonal distance—all helped produce an outward appearance of success while exacerbating and expanding the internal trauma. Stated another way, Sandra survived and even succeeded while using these coping strategies. Thus, she will tend to hold onto them as if her life depends upon it, even though they are tremendously costly.

Sandra has an experiential avoidance disorder (Hayes et al., 1996). She does not know that it is safe to feel, to think, and to remember. She does not realize that the vulnerability she needs to feel now in order to have intimate relationship is not the ignorant innocence of her childhood, but the experienced innocence of a person who knows she can be hurt and who chooses to stay open because one must keep the thorn in order to keep the rose. She has not learned to accept and love herself, with her pain, and is trying instead to perform perfectly in the vain hope that this will make her "feel better." A core of her suffering is historical, but the much larger proportion is of her own making, as she allows her life to be crushed in a futile effort to avoid the painful echoes of her own history.

The Therapeutic Relationship

The Therapeutic Bond

From an ACT perspective, the therapeutic bond is strong, open, accepting, mutual, respectful, and loving, with no sense of one-upmanship (Hayes et al., 1999). The relationship between the therapist and the client is particularly important in that it creates an opportunity for in-session modeling and a supportive context for change. Trust enters the relationship as the client comes in contact with the stance of radical acceptance that the therapist introduces. As in any close, disclosing relationship, it may become important for therapists to bring their experiences into the room when therapist self-disclosure is in service of the client's needs.

The boundaries of the therapeutic relationship come out of its functional purpose. The ACT therapist works for the client, not the other way around. The therapeutic relationship is loving but limited. This supports a nondefensive examination of whatever emerges in therapy, because the client is clear that this relationship is totally focused on his or her own goals and purposes. The usual errors on the therapist's part are experiential avoidance, excessive focus on content, advice giving, or excessive reliance on the therapist's own personal experiences. The ACT therapist needs to be aware of the difficult process that clients are being asked to undertake and to do that same process themselves.

Roles in the Therapeutic Relationship

The ACT therapist attempts to change the ground upon which therapeutic work is done. This means that initially the therapist is quite active or even directive until the old, destructive agenda of experiential avoidance is put to one side. What humanizes this initial phase is the therapeutic posture of the ACT therapist. The therapist and the client, from an ACT perspective, are in essentially the same human situation, and thus there is not sense of one-upsmanship. ACT therapists constantly guard against believing their own talk (which would turn ACT into a process of convincing the client) or using ACT techniques to be clever or to show off. The ACT therapist will *challenge with compassion* rigidly held sets of control strategies and reliance on verbal rules, all the while being mindful that these same processes need to be challenged in themselves as well. When practiced in the way it is conceptualized, ACT is a collaborative effort. ACT therapists use the social context of therapy to induce change, but are cautious using the relationship to induce specific forms of rule following (Hayes et al., 1999).

The beginning sessions of ACT are highly verbal on the part of the therapist. As therapy proceeds it becomes more and more experiential. Clients are told of this process and are cautioned not to expect later sessions to be like earlier ones.

Treatment Implementation and Outcome

Techniques and Methods of Working

ACT as a technology is multifaceted and complex. However, at the core of the methodology are specific techniques such as the use of metaphor, paradox, and confusion in order to break up the structural linkages that verbal language creates. Practicing ACT requires flexibility and a nimble sense of specific client needs, for example, paying attention to whether the metaphors are appropriate or are being understood (at least approximately) on the level they are being presented. The ACT therapist seeks multiple examples in the individual's life and to find exemplars across life domains of how various strategies of control or avoidance—not the person—are in fact the problem. Given the broad structure of this method, the treatment is sectioned roughly into six major domains. These are

- Creative hopelessness
- Control as the problem
- Self as context/defusion and deliteralization
- Experiential willingness
- Choice and values
- Commitment to action and change

Each of the domains has specific methodology, exercises, homework, and metaphors. Given space limitations, it is impossible to present a complete examination of the case of Sandra and include all of the techniques available to the ACT therapist. However, Sandra's case will be delineated with an attempt to describe general metaphors, techniques, and homework that would be assigned as she moved through the therapy.

Creative Hopelessness. The point of creative hopelessness is to have Sandra give up current change efforts and focus on worthwhile methods of change. Here we would want to explore the history of her change efforts, her sense of being stuck in her current life, and her current strategies for change. A useful metaphor would be the "person in the hole," which weaves together the importance and yet the irrelevance of history. Additionally, the metaphor brings the client into contact with the possibility that current change strategies are not working and may never work.

Briefly, the person-in-the-hole situation involves the client's imagining being placed blindfolded in a field with a little bag of tools. The goal is to live life, and the person is told to run about the field to do so. Unfortunately, the field is pocked by large holes, into which the person invariably falls. Stuck in the hole, blindfolded and holding the bag of tools, the person eventually reaches into the bag and finds a shovel. The person begins to dig, faster, slower, big scoops and small ones, but no matter what is done it seems that the hole only gets deeper. The suggestion is made that maybe the clients problems are similar, in that no amount of digging will ever get her out of the hole. A variety of similar metaphors are included in the ACT manual (Hayes et al., 1999) that can be used to make the same point.

Useful homework for the creative helplessness module is the self-monitoring of anxiety, struggle, and workability mentioned earlier.

Control as the Problem. The goal with "control as the problem" is to help Sandra delineate how excessive emotional control is a major problem for her. There are a variety of useful metaphors for this section, one being simply to discuss the 95% versus 5% rule, which simply means that in the world outside the skin the usual rule is, "If you don't want something, figure out how to get rid of it and get rid of it." In the world inside the skin and in some external situations as well, the rule is, "If you are not willing to have it, you've got it." A concrete example of this is to tell the client, "I'll give you $10 million to fall in love." This is a powerful way to demonstrate that although we human beings attempt supreme control in our "outside skin" lives, control is not possible in the same way within our own skins.

The point with discussing control as a problem is to begin making the distinction between useful versus useless change efforts. Sandra may know full well that emotional control and avoidance have not worked in her past, but explaining this process more directly opens up the fundamental unworkability of this system.

At this point, it is useful to point out that it is not important for Sandra to run out and begin change efforts that are different from the ones she is trying now. It is more important for her to simply notice the process in which she has been engaged.

Experiential Willingness. At this point in the protocol, willingness is introduced as a possibility and an alternative way of living. The point here is to discuss the nature of emotional acceptance and how abandoning Sandra's literal control agenda can allow her to move ahead in her life. The metaphor of two scales is a core ACT intervention designed to introduce the concept of willingness and its relationship to psychological distress. Here, the client is asked to imagine that there are two scales, like the volume and balance knobs on a stereo. One is called anxiety and the other is called willingness. Here, Sandra would be asked to imagine her hands on both dials. She came into therapy trying to turn down one dial, but in so doing she unknowingly turned up the other. If she turns the willingness dial instead and takes her hand off the anxiety dial, then anxiety is free to move. It may go up or it may go down, but in the posture she was in at first, it could only go up because anxiety was itself the focus of anxiety.

Self as Context/Defusion and Deliteralization. Experiencing the continuity of consciousness decreases the perceived danger of emotional content because it does not change regardless of the content. Experiential exercises, such as the observer exercise, are useful here. In greatly abbreviated form (the full exercise can be found in Hayes et al., 1999, pp. 193–195), Sandra would be asked to close her eyes while the therapist helps her notice how she is feeling and thinking currently. She would then be asked to recall a recent life event, an event in her adolescence, and an event in her childhood; all the while Sandra would be asked to notice what she was doing, as well as her thoughts, feelings, and emotions during the event. The therapist would then help Sandra notice that *she* is noticing these events, and from that "observer perspective" Sandra would be guided through several forms of content (thoughts, roles, emotions, sensations, emotions, behavioral predispositions, and memories). In each case, the therapist notes the distinction between the person who is conscious and the content of which the person is aware.

Discussion and experiential exercises like those mentioned help distinguish the "person from the programming." This distinction helps to establish a sense of self that exists in the present and is not threatened by emotional exposure or by cognitive defusion.

Choice and Values.   In this section of ACT we are asking the client a basic question: "What do you want your life to stand for?" Client values, in turn, stimulate discussion surrounding goals, actions, and barriers in the person's life. Sandra would be asked to describe what she values in her life and to rate these values in importance. The values would be across domains, such as marriage, family, friendships, employment, education, recreation, spirituality, and other areas. An effort is made to minimize compliance (e.g., reporting values in an effort to please the therapist, parents, and so on). Based on these values, concrete goals are developed that instantiate them, and concrete actions that would produce these goals are identified. Finally, the barriers to implementing these goals are specified. In a large percentage of cases, the barriers identified are private events that the client has been attempting to regulate.

The identified collections of values, goals, actions, and barriers define the target of treatment. Defusion, acceptance, and exposure confront the barriers, while commitment and behavior change produce concrete steps to improve one's life situation. These two steps are described next.

Acceptance, Defusion, and Experiential Exposure.   In this phase of ACT, Sandra and the therapist would repeatedly and deliberately enter into previously avoided domains, such as memories, feelings of fear, or situations. This exposure is not designed to reduce arousal or fear, but to increase the capacity and willingness to feel what is there without defense or avoidance and to defuse from thoughts that interfere with that task. For example, Sandra might be asked to spend a night alone and to speak into a tape recorder (to be brought into therapy later and reviewed) about what she feels, thinks, senses, and remembers while practicing acceptant and defusion skills.

Commitment to Action and Change.   Commitment homework and exercises are the central focus of ACT once the dead end of experiential avoidance and excessive cognitive entanglement is resolved. The areas that were addressed during the values work are systematically dealt with in each domain. Sandra would be asked to make some specific behavioral commitments, and concrete behavior-change exercises would be designed. The goal is not merely to produce valued overt behavior, but equally important to develop acceptance and defusion skills. The definition of psychological health described earlier is relevant here. The goal of this phase of ACT is not the static accomplishment of a particular set of overt behaviors. Rather, the key is an ongoing process of accepting, choosing, and taking action.

In this phase, concrete new behaviors would be practiced, while simultaneously keeping the door open to previously suppressed emotions and thought. For example, Sandra might practice new forms of relating to her boyfriend, parents, boss, or the therapist, while letting go of a struggle with the negative thoughts or emotions that may arise as she does so. All the various components of ACT are tied together in this phase.

Medical and Nutritional Issues

ACT is focused on bringing the client in contact with their values. In Sandra's case description, we know that her sleep is disturbed but we know little about her other health-related values and practices (exercise, nutrition, medical care, and so on). If these are issues, it may be useful to bring her into contact with her values regarding her health and to examine what stands between her and healthier behavior.

Sometimes it is assumed that anxiety is itself unhealthy or stressful and thus must be targeted for change. We do not agree. This is like saying that because quicksand is dangerous, one must fight to get out of quicksand if ever one stumbles into it. To the contrary, the thing to do in quicksand is maximize one's surface area that is in contact with it. Similarly, part of what keeps anxiety high is the client's struggling with it. Precisely because anxiety is aversive, the thing to do when feeling anxious is to be more open to one's contact with it. If she is willing to feel anxiety when it appears, the self-amplifying increase of anxiety will in all likelihood be reduced and anxiety will assume a level determined by history. This level is likely (but not certain) to be lower than the level previously experienced. Over time, as new behaviors build a new history, anxiety will go down (paradoxically, that is only likely if such a result is not the direct goal), but long before that process becomes central, a new, more healthful lifestyle will be in place.

Oddly, the actual data show that anxiety does go down when one is more willing to experience it (Hayes, 1987), as does depression (Zettle & Hayes, 1986), stress (Bond & Bunce, 2000), pain (Cioffi & Holloway, 1993), and other supposedly negative private events. Sleep seems to be a similar issue (if it is desperately important to go to sleep, any lack of immediate sleepiness is reason enough to sit bolt upright). If Sandra responds to ACT in the anxiety area, the use of mindfulness, defusion, and acceptance should be included a sleep program to help with any sleep problem that may remain.

Potential Pitfalls

Several potential pitfalls can be identified relative to the case of Sandra. One might be the tendency to be "correct" about the analysis of Sandra's problems rather than focusing on Sandra's experience of her problems. This may show up as a tendency to try to convince Sandra of an analysis of her problems, or as an excessive reliance on the case conceptualization when contradictory evidence arises. It also might be easy to become entangled in the topographical content of Sandra's presenting problems rather than focusing on the workability of her actions and agenda. Additionally, Sandra presents with emotional aloofness and a superficial sense of acceptance surrounding her history. This presentation may be a problem because of the confusion between her current avoidance-based approach and the new approach that ACT would be trying to establish. Sandra's report of acceptance surrounding her history appears to be a form of emotional avoidance, not acceptance in an ACT sense. An ACT therapist would have to tread carefully, being careful not to mistake similar words for similar functions.

This is particularly important because Sandra seems to intellectualize. ACT is not an intellectual exercise, and attempts to persuade acceptance or commitment are antithetical to the treatment. ACT is not about *telling* Sandra she must accept something, but finding ways to help her engage in acceptance directly. If an ACT therapist is in a "reporter" stance, telling ACT stories, then the therapy is being practiced incorrectly. One stumbling block will come if the therapist begins to believe the ACT story about Sandra; the point is to let go of an attachment to *all* the stories, not to find the "correct" one.

Distinguishing the *choices* she makes from the *decisions* she makes may prove to be a challenge for Sandra. Because of her dependence on others around her and her tendency to intellectualize, Sandra may wish to justify and continuously evaluate her choices, which is a sure route into cognitive entanglement. What needs to be evaluated is the workability of actions, not the values themselves. By definition, values allow evaluation; they are not ultimately the result of evaluation. Thus, a significant hurdle may be her ability to pick a direction for change and work towards it without excessive rumination and reconsideration.

Sandra may want to maintain a story in which she is a victim. Although the abuse is not her fault, the continued distortion it has placed in her life is her responsibility. She does not have a choice about whether she has a painful history. Others made that choice for her. She *does* have a choice about whether she will now attempt to avoid that history and produce the life distortion that results. A stumbling block will come when she realizes that living a vital life means coming to terms with her past role in elaborating her own suffering.

Termination and Relapse Prevention

ACT is designed to help clients get unstuck. The goal is a change in process, not a change in a static outcome. Termination is normally a gradual process that involves tapering over time; it is based on a collaborative sense between the therapist and the client that the process of *living* itself is now what is ahead. After the client officially terminates, additional sessions may be necessary. Booster visits are perfectly appropriate.

Relapse is a difficult time, because the client will often verbally formulate these times in ways that are antithetical to the work itself, but the exact same problem emerges from "success" when clients begin to believe that they have it all figured out. Either "success" or "failure" treats one's own life as an object. The entire process of ACT is about defusing from *any* evaluative language as applied internally, and instead living life as a continuous process of carrying one's history forward into a valued, vital life. When clients come back into therapy having "failed" they generally want support in beating themselves up. Better for the therapist to ask, "Gee, exactly when did your values change?" After hearing that the client's values did not change, the therapist helps the client turn again in the direction he or she was heading before the relapse and begin to walk again, one step at a time.

A metaphor is used to explain this posture. Living a life is like riding a bicycle. When we are riding a bike, we are never truly in balance. In one sense of the term, we are constantly falling over. If we can adjust quickly enough to a continuous process of falling out of balance, we will avoid planting our face in the pavement. There is no "success" as a static thing, any more than we can keep a bike in balance without movement. And as long as we are riding, there is no "failure" as a static thing, just a continuous process of catching ourselves as we fall.

In our experience, clients who respond well to ACT will respond well to new issues that emerge later using the same approach. These booster courses of treatment can be quite brief (two to four sessions). ACT is an enormously flexible approach, which is why it has general applicability across a range of problems (Strosahl et al., 1998). Therefore, ACT is very well suited to a "family dentist" style of intervention in which clients comes back periodically over a period of years.

Mechanisms of Change

Several studies have shown that ACT works through its hypothesized processes. For example, Bond and Bunce (2000) found that the clients who showed reductions in anxiety and stress in a worksite-based ACT program were those who learned greater acceptance skills. This process was quite distinct from clients in a more traditional behavioral treatment.

In a similar vein, Zettle and Hayes (1986) and Bach (2000) found that successful ACT clients showed a dramatic drop in the *believability* of problematic private events (depressive thoughts and hallucinations, respectively), but not their frequency. Comparative treatments in these two studies had different results, in which symptom frequency drops came more quickly, but believability dropped more slowly or not at all. Furthermore, it was shown in the Bach study that great acceptance and reduction in symptom believability helped psychotic clients stay out of the hospital, even when psychotic symptoms continue to occur.

Based on these data, in a successful ACT intervention with Sandra we would hope to see the following:

1. A rapid decrease in the literal believability of negative self-evaluations, worrisome thoughts, and anxious constructions
2. An increase in emotional openness and experiential acceptance
3. The display of new and valued behaviors, especially when not specifically targeted in therapy, that require steps 1 and 2 to occur
4. A significant reduction of phobic avoidance
5. Significantly improved relationships.

CONCLUSION

Our culture is full of "feel good" advice, but persons with painful histories, such as Sandra, have no healthy way to produce a life that is dominated by positive feelings, at least not any time soon. Indeed, all of the quick avenues of that kind (e.g., drug abuse, pretense, avoidance, dissociation) are themselves forms of psychopathology. What dignifies human suffering is that it is about something. If Sandra is willing to have her life be about something, and if she is willing to carry her painful history with her, she can start really living, right now. For a long time she will not feel *better* by doing so. In all likelihood, because she will be pushing her own buttons, she will feel worse. But she will immediately *feel* better and *live* better. That is the painful but honorable and vital path ACT could help her take.

REFERENCES

Addis, M. E., & Carpenter, K. M. (1999). Why, why, why?: Reason-giving and rumination as predictors of response to activation- and insight-oriented treatment rationales. *Journal of Clinical Psychology, 55*, 881–894.

Addis, M. E., & Jacobson, N. S. (1996). Reasons for depression and the process and outcome of cognitive-behavioral psychotherapies. *Journal of Consulting and Clinical Psychology, 64*, 1417–1424.

Bach, P. (2000). *The use of acceptance and commitment therapy to prevent the rehospitalization of psychotic patients: A randomized controlled trial.* Unpublished doctoral dissertation, available from the University of Nevada, Reno.

Bloor, R. (1983). 'What do you mean by depression?'—A study of the relationship between antidepressive activity and personal concepts of depression. *Behaviour Research and Therapy, 21*, 43–50.

Bond, F. W., & Bunce, D. (2000). Mediators of change in emotion-focused and problem-focused worksite stress management interventions. *Journal of Occupational Health Psychology, 5*, 156–163.

Borkovec, T. D., Hazlett-Stevens, H., & Diaz, M. L. (1999). The role of positive beliefs about worry in generalized anxiety disorder and its treatment. *Clinical Psychology and Psychotherapy, 6*, 126–138.

Borkovec, T. D., & Roemer, L. (1995). Perceived functions of worry among generalized anxiety disorder subjects: Distraction from more emotionally distressing topics? *Journal of Behavior Therapy and Experimental Psychiatry, 26*, 25–30.

Cioffi, D., & Holloway, J. (1993). Delayed costs of suppressed pain. *Journal of Personality and Social Psychology, 64,* 274–282.

Dugas, M. J., Gagnon, F., Ladouceur, R., & Freeston, M. (1998). Generalized anxiety disorder: A preliminary test of a conceptual model. *Behaviour Research and Therapy, 36,* 215–226.

Hayes, S. C. (1987). A contextual approach to therapeutic change. In N. Jacobson (Ed.), *Psychotherapists in clinical practice: Cognitive and behavioral perspectives* (pp. 327–387). New York: Guilford.

Hayes, S. C., Barnes-Holmes, D., & Roche, B. (Eds.). (in press). *Relational frame theory: A post-Skinnerian account of human language and cognition.* New York: Academic Press.

Hayes, S. C., Bissett, R. T., Strosahl, K., Wilson, K., Pistorello, J., Toarmino, D., Polusny, M. A., Batten, S. V., Dykstra, T. A., Stewart, S. H., Zvolensky, M. J., Eifert, G. H., Bergan, J., & Follette, W. C. *Psychometric properties of the Acceptance and Action Questionnaire (AAQ).* Manuscript submitted for publication.

Hayes, S. C., & Hayes, L. J. (1992). Verbal relations and the evolution of behavior analysis. *American Psychologist, 47,* 1383–1395.

Hayes, S. C., Strosahl, K., & Wilson, K. G. (1999). *Acceptance and commitment therapy: An experiential approach to behavior change* New York: Guilford.

Hayes, S. C., Wilson, K. G., Gifford, E. V., Follette, V. M., & Strosahl, K. (1996). Experiential avoidance and behavioral disorders: A functional dimensional approach to diagnosis and treatment. *Journal of Consulting and Clinical Psychology, 64,* 1152–1168.

Orsillo, S., & Roemer, E. (in press). Expanding our conceptualization of and treatment for generalized anxiety disorder: Integrating mindfulness/acceptance-based approaches with existing cognitive-behavioral models. *Clinical Psychology: Science and Practice.*

Strosahl, K. D., Hayes, S. C., Bergan, J., & Romano, P. (1998). Assessing the field effectiveness of acceptance and commitment therapy: An example of the manipulated training research method. *Behavior Therapy, 29,* 35–64.

Suls, J., & Fletcher, B. (1985). The relative efficacy of avoidant and nonavoidant coping strategies: A meta-analysis. *Health Psychology, 4,* 288.

Wegner, D. M., Erber, R., & Zanakos, S. (1993). Ironic processes in the mental control of mood and mood-related thought. *Journal of Personality and Social Psychology, 65,* 1093–1104.

Wegner, D. M., & Zanakos, S. (1994). Chronic thought suppression. *Journal of Personality, 62,* 615–640.

Wells, A., & Papageorgio, C. (1995). Worry and the incubation of intrusive images following stress. *Behaviour Research and Therapy, 33,* 579–583.

Zettle, R. D., & Hayes, S. C. (1986). Dysfunctional control by client verbal behavior: The context of reason giving. *The Analysis of Verbal Behavior, 4,* 30–38.

6

Context-Centered Therapy

Jay S. Efran and Leonard C. Sitrin

THE TREATMENT MODEL

The Importance of Language

A central tenet of context-centered therapy is that words and symbols determine how people experience themselves and their world (Efran, Lukens, & Lukens, 1990). Language is the communal choreography that shapes people's self-definitions. Without language, people would not know who they were or where they were going. They would not know whether they were winners or losers, successes or failures. In other words, happiness and distress depend as much on self-talk as on actual accomplishments or visceral sensations. Similarly, the experience of pain is not simply a function of neural stimulation—it is a complex amalgam of neural response and linguistic interpretation (see Efran et al., 1989). Moreover, words and symbols are the ingredients that transform circumstances into problems. Problems and the solutions psychotherapists propose for dealing with them are fundamentally linguistic creations—a by-product of the contexts language makes possible.

It should be noted that language is never simply epiphenomenal; it is always and inevitably consequential. Just as the grooming behavior of chimps helps establish and sustain a social hierarchy, the linguistic meanings people exchange maintain their communal organization. People use language to arrange marriages, wage wars, play games, negotiate business contracts, and conduct psychotherapy. By using different words and symbols, people change how they view themselves and relate to one another.

Of course, words and practices are braided in an endless loop. If you intend to eat thymus glands you will probably call them sweetbreads. If you order horse meat from the Harvard faculty club menu, it will be presented as gourmet fare. Words both open up and close off options. As contextualist Theodore Sarbin (1968) explains, "Labels contain implicit and explicit connotations . . . [that] constrain implications for action" (p. 416).

Symptoms and Deficiencies

Because context-centered therapists are *sufficiency-oriented*, they do not consider clients defective organisms in need of repair work. Instead, they assume that clients are always behaving sensibly if one takes into account their biological structure and sociolinguistic setting. Other therapy approaches tend to rely heavily on what Goldiamond (1972) calls eliminative strategies—for instance, clients are taught to identify and eradicate maladaptive cognitions or to modify negative relationship patterns. By contrast, context-centered therapists show clients how to make better use of their natural proclivities. They recognize that it is generally easier for people to "ride the horse in the direction it is going." Thus, they make much use of the time-honored Zen concepts of acceptance and detachment.

Context-centered therapists also have a different take on symptoms: They view them as *high-cost operants*. In other words, symptoms are considered expensive solutions to pressing predicaments (Goldiamond, 1972). Freud, too, argued that symptoms are signs of an organism's desperate problem-solving efforts. Furthermore, as Goldiamond notes, symptoms reveal critical contingencies. After all, why would individuals pay a heavy price to achieve an outcome that was not of great importance to them?

Context-centered therapists assume that symptoms will tend to disappear automatically when lower-cost solutions become available. Think of it this way: Your old jalopy is a noisy, unreliable, oil-burning, gas-guzzling heap, yet it still gets you from one place to another. Therefore, you are willing to put up with its idiosyncrasies. You will be glad to ditch it, however, if and when you gain access to a more efficient model. Similarly, people are forced to make use of high-cost solutions until less pricey options come into view. Luckily, inefficient behavior often becomes obsolete as clients grasp the larger picture.

Orthogonality

The major therapeutic operation in context-centered therapy is *orthogonal interaction* (Maturana, 1993). The therapist interacts with the client in a way that elicits novel reactions and behaviors. The principle of orthogonality takes advantage of the fact that all of us are capable of a much larger range of behaviors than we typically enact. Because the therapist is outside the client's ordinary milieu, he or she can trigger responses that in other settings are unavailable, underused, suppressed, or prohibited. For instance, few of us consider the family dinner-table an appropriate place for discussing intimate sexual fantasies, whereas in therapy such topics are permitted and even encouraged. The "space" afforded by the consulting room encourages a conversational exchange that is not likely to arise elsewhere. An important implication of the principle of orthogonality is that when therapists are unsure about what to do, they ought at least to do something different from what other people in the client's life are already doing.

In effect, the client and therapist form a new, albeit temporary, club—a micro-society in which existing beliefs and behaviors can be reevaluated. In that environment, the effects of various role prescriptions and club conflicts often stand out in stark relief. Most teenagers, for example, behave one way at home and another way with peers, and it can be embarrassing for them to be seen shopping with their parents (Harris, 1998). If spotted by friends at the local mall, the teenager may have to engage in image control by walking a pace or two behind the rest of the family or by rolling the eyes in silent disdain at just the right moment.

Such awkward social situations create palpable but temporary stress. The teenager's cool is disrupted only momentarily, and various face-saving remedies (Goffman, 1959) are readily available. Not all role clashes are that obvious, temporary, or benign. Some individuals find themselves faced with more pervasive identity struggles. Being members of a variety of social organizations simultaneously—the family, the church, the firm, the community—they are compelled to hide bits and pieces of themselves from others (and sometimes from themselves as well). These role conflicts create "emotional contradictions" (Mendez, Coddou, & Maturana, 1988, p. 152) that often motivate people to seek treatment.

For example, a college student resisted telling his immigrant father how poorly he was doing in school (Efran & Cook, 1999). The father had sacrificed to send him to college, and the boy feared his father's reaction to discovering that he was missing assignments and cutting classes. For a while the son tried to convince himself that he had some sort of learning block or study-skills problem, a point of view endorsed for some time by his academic advisor. Finally, he admitted to himself that he lacked motivation and was only in school to please his family. A flagging interest in his courses was the source of his study problems, not vice versa. Actually, he wanted to be able to work in the family business, an option his father had previously dismissed derisively as amounting to nothing.

The advisor's suggestion that the student sign up for a study-skills workshop merely prolonged the agony. The boy finally met with a counselor who was able to grasp the larger picture. She arranged for a meeting with the family, and the son was able for the first time to discuss openly his intention to drop out of school. The father was disappointed, of course, but he realized that he could not keep his son in college through coercion. The son left school, worked in the family store, and agreed to reconsider college at a later point in time. The conversation with the counselor set the stage for giving voice to the unspeakable and thereby resolving what had been a troubling and persistent emotional contradiction.

From a context-centered viewpoint, therapy is a social influence process, more akin to education and politics than to science and medicine. In a sense, the therapist ferments small revolutions in the consulting room by engaging clients in orthogonal interaction. These encounters change the client's purview, allowing hidden assumptions about life to be aired. In guiding this process, the therapist listens carefully to the client's language, bringing to light inconsistencies, hazy descriptions, linguistic hypocrisies, and other instances of "disclaimed action" (Schafer, 1983). Such linguistic markers point to domains in which the client's context is narrow and limiting and which therefore present ideal opportunities for therapeutic intervention.

THE THERAPIST'S SKILLS AND ATTRIBUTES

The only special prerequisite for practicing context-centered therapy is a willingness to recognize the extent to which people's choices are linguistically grounded. The magic, so to speak, of the approach hinges on establishing a clear and workable client-therapist contract. In this regard, we concur with Thomas Szasz's (1973) portrayal of a therapist as a kind of court jester. In the Middle Ages, jesters were granted immunity from certain rules of court etiquette so that they could safely bring various painful truths to the attention of their clients—in this case, the royal couple. Jesters often possessed valuable information because they were frequently worldlier than other members of the court. Thus, they could expose potentially detrimental aspects of the court's provincialism.

Therapists, too, have a breadth of knowledge and experience that enables them to demonstrate to clients how they are being imprisoned by their own belief system and allegiances (Rabkin, 1970). In our terms, they are well positioned to generate orthogonal interaction. Of course, orthogonality is hampered when therapist and client affiliations overlap too completely. It is problematic if both client and therapist happen to be members of the same church, work group, family, or micro-community. Under such circumstances, the client and therapist both will be prone to mistake local ordinances for universal truths.

More than just a sympathetic listener, the context-centered therapist is a kind of linguistic detective, eternally curious about the ways in which people voice their problems and the suppositional structure their phrasings reveal. He or she adopts the role of an active, friendly research consultant who isn't afraid to offer concrete suggestions or propose small investigatory experiments clients might undertake in the outside world. The therapeutic conversation this produces is remarkably free of mental health jargon. The therapist neither pathologizes nor spends much time tracing the presumed childhood antecedents of current linguistic frameworks. In fact, context-centered therapists pride themselves on being direct, efficient, and straightforward as well as compassionate.

THE CASE OF SANDRA

Assessment

Context-centered therapy is two parts sleuthing and one part healing, yet we do not use any special tests or assessment devices. The premier diagnostic tool is a therapist willing to listen carefully to the client's rhetoric for clues about unexamined suppositions and linguistic evasions. Clients initially appear to describe their experience in straightforward, reasonable, and transparent terms. As in Sandra's case, however, closer examination reveals that such narratives contain a variety of half-truths, exaggerations, circular assumptions, and disclaimed actions. For example, Sandra's self-presentation is peppered with dramatic generalizations: She states that "all she hears" from her parents is criticism, that she lives in a "constant state of apprehension," and that she doesn't "trust anybody." Such statements convey the frustration she experiences and may be effective at justifying her actions and winning sympathy, yet they are not accurate depictions of reality. For instance, Sandra frequently reifies *fear*, claiming that it runs her life. On the contrary, from a context-centered perspective Sandra runs her own life and chooses her own actions. That doesn't mean she should or could choose differently. On the other hand, true empowerment begins with the recognition that a person is—as the existentialists have always argued—his or her choices. As we discuss in some detail later, most of what Sandra labels *fear* is actually a by-product of her tenacious fear-avoidant strategies—her discomfort is amplified by her chronic unwillingness to allow her experience to unfold.

A central context-centered assumption is that life works better when goals, beliefs, commitments, and responsibilities are accurately labeled. Couples, for instance, often describe themselves as unable to communicate when they simply mean they have strong disagreements that complicate living together. If they really could not communicate they would have more trouble role-playing each other's positions, a task they can often do with aplomb and without much coaching. Once it becomes clear that a couple's troubles stem from ordinary conflicts in expectations, values, and goals—not communication deficits—it becomes easier to help them handle their differences.

Therapeutic Goals

In this approach, therapists typically begin by inquiring into a client's treatment expectations. "What can I do for you?" is a valuable opening question because it reveals expectations and leads directly to a discussion of the client-therapist contract. In our experience, vague inquiries ("What brings you here?" "What seems to be the matter?" "What's bothering you?") are less useful. Although clients cannot always immediately articulate what they hope to accomplish in therapy, even a nebulous response can reveal misconceptions that would get in the way later if left unexplored.

For example, some clients think that consulting a therapist is similar to visiting a family physician or a medical specialist. However, as George Kelly (1955) observed years ago, medical model terms like "patient" are misleading; they imply that individuals should wait *patiently* (and passively) for the good doctor to prescribe a cure. Similarly, many clients arrive at the therapist's doorstep believing they have a mental disorder that can be excised or cured if duly diagnosed. Context-centered therapists do not share this view. From our perspective, clients are disordered only in the most metaphorical sense. Our aim is not to cure, but rather to initiate a specialized form of dialogue that—if all goes well—will lighten the client's life burdens and make interpersonal impasses seem less mysterious.

From our viewpoint, psychotherapists who imply that treatment will produce major characterological changes may be promising more than they can deliver. In our experience, therapy rarely modifies a person's basic personality traits. Moreover, when clients fail to achieve the goals they have been implicitly or explicitly promised, they not only become discouraged but they may become intropunitive as well. They assume they must be an exceptionally difficult case, that they did not work hard enough, or that they weren't careful about following the therapist's directions. To avoid such pitfalls, we are clear with clients from the outset that major personality alterations are both unlikely and unnecessary (Efran, Greene, & Gordon, 1998). We recall, for example, a painfully shy individual who struggled throughout years of therapy to change his basic style. Finally, he saw a context-centered therapist and came to the realization that he could succeed in life just by being himself. As he put it, "The second part of my life began when I really accepted that I was shy and withdrawn and that it was a waste of time and energy to pretend otherwise."

Consider Sandra's situation. She is undoubtedly blessed (and cursed) with a particularly reactive temperamental style (Efran & Greene, 2000). As context-centered therapists, we do not assume that such an individual can be transformed into a relaxed, easygoing, carefree person. As we suggest below, Sandra can gain increased life satisfaction without having to deny, ignore, or pathologize her basic personality attributes.

Timeline for Therapy

Context-centered therapy aims for efficiency, so we schedule meetings only when there are specific tasks to be accomplished. We have found it a detriment to follow the traditional therapy practice of automatically scheduling weekly sessions. Too often, these become routine meetings at which little is accomplished, or they occur at exactly the wrong moment. There are times when it is necessary to meet several days in a row, and other times when a month should be allowed to pass between meetings. Context-centered therapists also employ a decidedly unorthodox flexibility about the length of a given session. We have held sessions as short as 10 minutes and as long as 3 hours. Again, session length is a function of the job at hand, not the ticking of the clock. Sometimes it takes only a few minutes to become clear about the next step in the therapeutic process, and sometimes it takes considerably longer to reach completion on a given issue. We like to think of therapy as a bit like surgery. The surgeon estimates how long he or she will need to be in the operating room, yet unforeseen circumstances may arise that make it wise to complete a given procedure before adjourning.

In context-centered therapy, the therapist gets right down to business, and it is not unusual for cases to require only ten sessions or less. At the same time, the door is never closed—we don't believe in terminating clients. They are always welcome to call about an unexpected complication, to request a booster, or to discuss a new issue. The kind and frequency of contact is flexible and easily negotiated. If you contract the flu you may visit your internist several times in a row. When you are feeling better, you visit less often but you certainly do not consider yourself terminated.

Case Conceptualization

With some clients—and Sandra would be a prime example—it is important to clarify our position on various medical model concepts. For instance, it is a detriment to allow potentially confusing terms like "phobia" and "anxiety disorder" to be bandied about without comment. It should be remembered that historically, before anxiety became a disease category, it was considered a personality dimension, a secondary drive, a temperamental style, an explanatory scheme, and a normal state of apprehension. The word itself is a variant of the Middle English "anguish," a derivative of the French *anguisse*, meaning a painful choking sensation in the throat. It was introduced into the English language as part of the thirteenth-century religious reforms that emphasized internal affirmations over external rituals. In brief, the term is a metaphorical transformation of the literal experience of choking, and to this day we still talk about people choking up during high-stakes performances. As with so many of our mentalistic terms, the metaphorical roots of the concept have evaporated over time and the notion of anxiety has become increasingly reified.

The word anxiety began to appear in psychiatric textbooks in the 1930s. By that time Freud had already distinguished between realistic, moral, and neurotic anxiety, depending on whether the person was thought to be reacting to a realistic threat, a superego recrimination, or the potential resurfacing of a repressed thought (Rychlak, 1981). Harry Stack Sullivan (1953) had an entirely different idea. He reserved the term for the physical tensions that mothers (or "mothering ones") presumably transmitted directly to their infants through physical contact. He believed, but could not prove, that these tactile experiences formed the basis for all later interpersonal insecurities.

It was not until the third edition of the *Diagnostic and Statistical Manual of Mental Disorders* (*DSM-III, DSM-III-R*) (American Psychiatric Association, 1980, 1987) that anxiety became a stand-alone category. Whereas earlier it had been an adjective, a symptom, and an explanatory hypothesis, it was now accepted as the label for a particular set of syndromes. This completed anxiety's transformation from metaphor to disease entity.

From our perspective, it is unfortunate that laypersons and mental health professionals alike have now subscribed to the view that anxiety is an affliction rather than simply a subjective report of distress. As Kutchins and Kirk (1997) write, the basis on which the anxiety disorder classifications were established was "largely arbitrary, not scientific" (p. 27). Panels of experts were simply asked to vote about when "relatively common experiences such as anxiety . . . should be considered evidence of . . . [a] disorder" (Kutchins & Kirk, 1997, p. 27). Thus, diagnoses such as post-traumatic stress disorder, panic disorder, generalized anxiety disorder, and phobia are little more than social judgments masquerading as psychiatric discoveries.

Consider for a moment a client who arrives at a therapist's office reporting a fear of snakes, rats, or spiders. Such fears are common in the population and vary in intensity depending, of course, on the person's neurophysiology and learning history. Moreover, these fears are *biologically prepared*, an important and normal component of the species' survival equipment. Nevertheless, when clients report such fears to a therapist, they are automatically branded as phobic. This twist of language converts a survival mechanism into a mental health condition. Sociologists call this *languaging up*. An element of mystification is added to an otherwise simple set of facts. Of course, calling an experience a disorder justifies hunting for esoteric causes, usually by scrutinizing the person's upbringing. Yet most hypotheses about the causal relationship between early childhood events and current symptomatology have turned out to be false and misleading (Seligman, 1993). In any event, context-centered therapists have little interest in those explanations. Wherever possible, they prefer to translate psychiatric jargon back into the ordinary English from which it derived.

As we have implied, context-centered therapists presume that so-called symptoms generally reflect clashes between cultural expectations, role demands, and biological propensities. For instance, the stress experienced by the college student in our previous example was due mainly to the strain of being a sham student. Sandra's situation is perhaps a bit more complex. She is attempting to maintain an adult façade while struggling with the infantilizing effects of a hyperreactive biochemistry. As developmentalist Jerome Kagan (1994) reports, about 20% of infants are born with a physiology that causes them to be excessively responsive to new experiences or startling events. Many of these hypersensitive infants become fearful, cautious children and some—like Sandra—go on to become vulnerable, apprehensive adults.

Of course, Sandra's fear of being left alone and her desire to sleep in her parents' bedroom will strike observers as increasingly odd as she grows older. These are the sorts of childlike behaviors that adults are expected to outgrow. However, individuals like Sandra who have oversensitive temperaments tend to remain prisoners of their primitive survival mechanisms. Their behavior represents the system's legitimate attempt to reconcile juvenile vulnerabilities and grown-up responsibilities. Unfortunately, these clients frequently misunderstand and despise their own coping needs. To make matters worse, friends, family members, and mental health professionals often add to the burden by pathologizing clients' behavior and implying that it can be easily changed or eliminated. From our perspective, it is this very context of deficiency that turns an inconvenient temperamental circumstance into an unmanageable problem. The context-centered therapist is interested in identifying the ramifications of that context and pointing to alternative frameworks.

The Therapeutic Relationship

The Therapeutic Bond

In some forms of therapy, the clinician devotes the early stage of treatment to building an alliance. By contrast, the context-centered therapist goes right to work on the problem, expecting to produce discernible results even after one session. We assume that the best way to build an alliance is to demonstrate that our suggestions are on target and make a difference. In some ways, traditional approaches are a subtle form of bait and switch: The therapist is initially accepting and, for the *sake* of alliance-building, withholds more challenging interpretations until later. We operate differently. We are not shy about presenting reasonably bold (and occasionally unpopular) hypotheses from the outset. As explained earlier, we consider the generation of orthogonal interaction to be the prime therapeutic mandate, and this involves doing something novel. At the same time, like the court jester that Szasz describes, our demeanor communicates that we have the client's best interests at heart, and we are always willing to be proven wrong about any hypothesis we have entertained. Under such conditions, we find that the process of establishing a secure bond tends to take care of itself.

Roles in the Therapeutic Relationship

As we have indicated, we consider the generation of orthogonal interaction to be the therapist's prime mandate. In this approach, the therapist is quite active—asking questions, making suggestions, challenging inconsistencies, and pointing to hidden assumptions that serve to limit the client's options.

We should reiterate that context-centered encounters tend to be relatively transparent, that is, the therapist talks plainly and avoids jargon. Although we construe therapy as a collaborative venture, the job requires that client and therapist play different roles. In a nutshell, the client is allowed to be confused, and the therapist is continually permitted to ask for clarification. In some ways, the context-centered therapist plays the role of a probing research consultant, helping clients design and test life hypotheses and see beyond assumptions that they previously took for granted. For their part, clients are entitled to keep raising questions and objections until or unless the problems for which they sought assistance disappear.

Treatment Implications and Outcome

Techniques and Methods of Working

In Sandra's case and others like it, the context-centered therapist will almost surely begin by discussing the role of genetics, a core factor in many people's difficulties that other mental health professionals frequently seem to downplay or ignore. In this case, we believe there is ample evidence that Sandra's reactive temperament has genetic underpinnings. For instance, she is reported to have been fearful "for as long as she can remember," and her family labels her a constant "worry-wart." Her biological mother's schizophrenia lends some additional weight to the genetic hypothesis.

We know from the literature that people with Sandra's disposition continually overreact to stimuli (Kagan, 1994). When threatened, their systems shift rapidly into overdrive and are very slow to return to neutral, so situations that others take in stride are experienced as terrifying events. Such incidents often leave long-term psychological scars. Although the case history describes her childhood as turbulent, it is possible that Sandra would have grown up to be a fearful adult even if she had had a more mundane upbringing. As we have implied, the fight-flight mechanism of reactive individuals is easily triggered.

On the other hand, it should also be recognized that most people have trouble dealing with events such as house break-ins. The awareness that a prowler has been stalking the premises generates intense feelings of personal violation, making it difficult for individuals who have had such experiences to recover their equanimity. Those with sufficient resources—such as Jon-Benet Ramsey's family—often flee their surroundings, finding it easier to begin again than to adjust in the setting in which the traumatic event occurred

Early in therapy, a context-centered therapist would want Sandra to understand that we think she comes by her problems honestly. In other words, her distresses are understandable, given her reactive temperament and her past background, and it is unlikely that she is exaggerating her suffering. To a reactive individual, even minor perturbations can seem like life-and-death struggles, so if there are any secondary gains in this case, they are probably of minor significance. If anything, Sandra deserves much credit for having maintained a responsible job despite her personal encumbrances.

In therapy as well as in life, people give to get. They take risks when the payoff seems worthwhile. They reevaluate old beliefs when they glimpse the advantages of a new perspective. Part of the skill of the context-centered therapist is to broker a kind of conceptual exchange in which a client is willing to trade a familiar viewpoint for a novel perspective.

In Sandra's case, for instance, we would urge that she accept a genetic interpretation of her hypervigilance. In fact, this hypothesis is a double-edged sword. On the one hand, it reduces personal blame and guilt—Sandra's reactions (genetically speaking) are not her fault. Yet because inherited traits tend to be stable, the genetic connection raises doubts about whether Sandra can ever expect to be free of tension. Even pharmaceutical interventions may offer only limited relief.

Despite the potential downside of genetic explanations, we have found that clients seem to like them. In fact, they have usually harbored misgivings about various environmental interpretations of their symptoms that they have previously been offered. They know firsthand what it is like to be buffeted by temperamental forces they have never fully understood. They are relieved to find out about the biogenetic aspects of the puzzle. It feels right to them and helps set the stage for the acceptance strategy we then go on to propose.

The Zen Connection. In these kinds of cases, context-centered therapists have found value in citing a well-known Zen principle, namely, that *whatever you resist persists, and whatever you let be lets you be.* As everyone knows, trying to dodge unpleasant thoughts and feelings can intensify the very experiences one was hoping to avoid. In that sense, Sandra's avoidant strategies have been doubly ineffective. First, her attempts to skirt danger provide only momentary pockets of relief. Second, they limit her mobility, tarnish her reputation, and exhaust potential helpers. Instead of building self-confidence, they foster helplessness. Sadly, mastery and avoidance are at opposite ends of the spectrum for such individuals.

Students of Zen argue that the twin practices of acceptance and detachment can allow people to move toward mastery—to make better use of their strengths and to gracefully compensate for their weaknesses. For centuries, these practices have helped people cope with life crises and adjust to their personal idiosyncrasies. Moreover, because these Eastern notions sound foreign to Western ears, they generate orthogonality and help initiate fresh problem-solving approaches.

Note that in this context *acceptance* does not mean passive resignation, and *detachment* does not imply disinterest or lack of enthusiasm. In the East, in fact, acceptance and detachment are considered ideal tools for opening pathways to joyful satisfaction and vigorous participation. They help reduce the heaviness with which many of us characteristically troop through life.

In brief, the goal is to accept oneself nonjudgmentally and to be able to step back and observe one's own processes at work. As a metaphor, picture placing your hand, palm open, firmly against the front of your face. In that position, your hand would undoubtedly limit your view of the surroundings and cramp your style. If, however, you were to reposition your hand an inch or two away from your face, it would cease to be much of an obstacle. You would be able to see easily through your open fingertips. This inch of detachment makes all the difference. Observing oneself from a distance lessens hair-trigger reactions and increases flexibility. It enables people to take themselves and their reactions less seriously.

When people achieve a modicum of detachment they discover that although they *have* thoughts, *they* are bigger than those thoughts; although they *have* feelings, *they* are bigger than those feelings; although they *have* reactions, *they* are bigger than those reactions. Detachment has sometimes been described as recognizing that one is the motion-picture screen, not the film that happens to be showing at any particular moment. Envisioning oneself as the screen—the context—is empowering. Being overly attached to snippets of film—the content—is not.

In Japan, it is said that feelings and emotions are as changeable as the Japanese sky, that is, they come and they go. People who practice acceptance and detached observation begin to notice that their systems crank out an enormous range of *stuff*—a continuous flow of evaluations, judgements, beliefs, body sensations, warnings, predictions, and so on (Smothermon, 1979). Upon examination, many of these thoughts and reactions turn out to be illogical, transient, repetitive, trivial, small-minded, and inconsistent. There are false alarms and overly personal interpretations. The system insists on issuing an unending series of edicts and position papers that sound authoritative but are often of questionable quality and value. Very little that passes through the psychic apparatus actually requires immediate action. Very little requires drawing firm conclusions. As people practice detachment, they begin to understand the vagaries of their systems and are therefore less prone to overreact. For individuals with constitutionally hyperreactive systems, this is indeed a valuable lesson.

It is helpful to teach clients to call the products of their system "considerations." The term serves as a reminder that such reactions are a hodgepodge of raw sensations and perceptions that are not yet fully sorted or evaluated. Practicing detachment gives the person the space to consider how much attention to give to any particular response. The detached individual can make such judgments more easily on the basis of a set of fundamental commitments or declarations.

In this lexicon, a declaration is a statement of goal, purpose, principle, or direction. Declarations affirm a stand. For example, the Declaration of Independence asserts that all men are created equal. It represents an affirmation or commitment of that principle. Such statements are obviously not summaries of the research evidence. They are linguistic pronouncements that strengthen principles, point directions, and recommend operating guidelines. Declarations provide reliable road maps for dealing with the torrent of considerations that tumble out of systems, particularly during times of reactivity.

As Sandra becomes better acquainted with how her system operates, she will undoubtedly notice that her mind frequently races ahead of her intellect, concocting all kinds of scary, albeit improbable, scenarios. At threatening moments she may even experience her thought processes grinding to a complete halt, leaving her temporarily immobilized or in a state of panic. She will begin to recognize her system's tendency to dramatize even mildly threatening events.

Sandra may also come to realize that most of her defensive tactics are crude half-measures, symbols of safety rather than truly useful devices. For example, because intruders are most likely to strike after people are asleep, her insistence on going to bed before others provides no real increase in security. Sandra may not focus on the logical gaps in her protective rituals, but her context-centered therapist—in the role of court jester—may gently allude to them. Ordinarily, however, practicing detachment automatically puts people in touch with the paradoxes inherent in the way their systems function. Clients can begin to describe the limitations of their defensive maneuvers without having to wait for the therapist to point them out.

Something Sandra is not likely to notice is that she has always had a choice between two basic or broad operating modes—what we call *the context of survival* and *the context of living.* The first privileges safety and comfort over experience and opportunity. The second reverses those priorities. Sandra has usually operated in the first mode rather than the second, perhaps without ever realizing that she was making a choice. Like other reactive individuals, she also has probably labored under the false assumption that the context of survival helps keep fear in check, when just the opposite is the case. Constantly monitoring the environment for signs of danger is a bit like watching someone hold a sharp needle close to an inflated balloon. After a while, the anticipation of the balloon's bursting becomes far more noxious than the actual sound of the pop. Perhaps Shakespeare said it best when he wrote, "Cowards die many times before their deaths; the valiant never taste of death but once."

We have indicated that operating contexts determine how considerations are processed. Unfortunately, survival-oriented individuals tend to miscalculate the odds and overreact to minor perturbations. They confuse vigilance with safety. They lose perspective and along with it their sense of humor. They fail to take into consideration that all of life's pursuits, from mountain climbing to answering the telephone, entail risk. Without risk, there can be no participation. Without participation, there can be no satisfaction. Without satisfaction, there can be no peace of mind. In other words, declarations that place survival ahead of other goals virtually ensure a hellish existence.

On the other hand, contexts that focus on something larger than oneself can exert a steadying influence. Although firefighters have their anxieties, their behavior at a burning building is anchored by their precommitment to obeying orders and serving others. Nervous actors find solace in their solemn responsibility to the professional motto (probably invented by a producer) that the show must go on.

Sandra needs to know that at any point in time she can declare a shift from the context of survival to the context of living. She can become open to experience rather than continuing to defend against it. The therapist prepares her for this shift, but only Sandra—drawing on that orthogonal conversation—can finally make the choice. As an ancient Chinese proverb states, Teachers can open the door, but students must enter by themselves. Sandra's willingness to play by a new set of rules hinges on her awareness that (a) she is always making choices, (b) she is paying a heavy price for her present strategy, (c) her fear-avoidance methods do not actually work, and (d) the alarm cues that her system produces are capricious and unreliable.

Shifting contexts is an act of declaration. It does not require an increase in skill or the gathering of additional evidence. It can happen in the blink of an eye. By shifting contexts, Sandra agrees to allow and accept the very feelings that she has studiously avoided in the past. She needs to be willing to float with her feelings rather than fight them (Weekes, 1976).

Making It Real. Sandra's therapist would undoubtedly suggest projects and exercises that will help her see how her choices operate and how she can solidify her commitment. Some of these will superficially resemble exposure methods. However, their intent and rationale are different. The aim, for example, is not to alleviate fear, although fear will automatically diminish. As we said earlier, whatever you let be, lets you be. Instead, the emphasis is to allow thoughts, feelings, and reactions to visit freely, to come and go as they please.

The exact content of the exercises the therapist suggests is unimportant. They do not even have to relate directly to the client's primary complaints or symptoms. For example, we have occasionally invited reactive clients to join us at the local amusement park for a ride on the roller coaster or Ferris wheel. Thrill rides are wonderful laboratories for practicing detachment and testing commitments. They have been designed to evoke maximum reactivity in a context of minimum risk. Before getting on the roller coaster, clients can decide for themselves whether to float or fight, whether to ward off danger or welcome experience. After the ride, clients can assess whether they honored their declarations.

Make no mistake about it. People who choose the context of living—whether for a minute or a lifetime—still experience upsets. However, they are less likely to be derailed by them, and they need less time to recover. The solid footing provided by a commitment helps them regain their composure even when momentarily jarring events occur.

As therapy unfolds, Sandra's therapist might encourage her to experiment with traits other than her reactivity. For example, she could play with her perfectionistic tendencies. Is she willing to allow a gaffe to go uncorrected? Can she take charge of her perfectionism, or must it take charge of her? Woody Allen has been shy his entire life. Yet instead of letting his social inhibition slow him down, he has used it to his advantage, turning his distinctive timidity into a lucrative show-business trademark. As Alexis de Tocqueville noted long ago, "We succeed in enterprises which demand the positive qualities we possess, but we excel in those which can also make use of our defects."

Including the Family.   As context-centered therapists, we do not draw sharp distinctions between individual, couples, and family therapy. We see whoever needs to be seen, putting people together in different combinations for different purposes. In this case, the therapist might be tempted to broker a kind of quid pro quo between Sandra and her parents. Her parents would be urged to acknowledge the reality of her pain, and she in turn would forgive their past slights, wrongdoings, and transgressions. In point of fact, there is no actual evidence that her current predicament is at all connected to her biological mother's gloomy prognostications, her foster mother's criticisms, or her adoptive brothers' sexual advances. Recent research suggests that neither parenting practices nor early childhood experiences play a major role in determining adult mental health status (Efran & Greene, 2000; Efran et al., 1998; Harris, 1998).

This rapprochement might lower family tension, making it easier for Sandra to relate to her foster mother. Toward that end, it would be useful if Sandra were given an opportunity to reexamine a core contextual difference between children and adults. It is our opinion that adulthood is defined in terms of a person's willingness to accept full responsibility for his or her actions, attitudes, and attributes, even those with genetic precursors. Adults are defined as whole and complete. Their well-being is no longer centrally contingent on receiving parental approval. They can, if they like, stay up past their bedtime.

Adults are expected to derive satisfaction primarily through fulfilling their own commitments, not from winning external applause. In that context, approbation from others is simply the icing on the cake. As individuals mature, they are expected to find their own voice and create their own unique set of declarations and guideposts.

People (of any chronological age) keep themselves stuck in childhood by defining their worth solely in terms of what others think. In that context, no amount of praise proves sufficient. Feelings of inadequacy and insecurity persist. The person continues to feel like damaged goods and constantly hankers for approval. In terms of her past relationship with her mother, it sounds as if Sandra is caught in that kind of self-perpetuating trap. At any point in time, she can simultaneously strengthen her own sense of self and her relationship to her mother by beginning to embrace the role of adult.

In addition, when offspring mature they are expected to recognize that parents have their own issues. Parents, like children, have a history and a biology, and their responses reflect their own conditioned reality (Emery, 1978). It is no surprise then that some parents are temperamentally incapable of being demonstrative. Others—and this may include Sandra's foster mother—can only show their concern by voicing criticisms, giving unwanted advice, and dramatizing disappointments. Still others, like Sandra's biological mother, may be able to express affiliation only by issuing dire and frightening warnings of potential doom. Such affiliative gestures are awkward and difficult to accept, but they are not necessarily ill-intentioned.

Mature offspring learn to see past the forms that relationships take in order to grasp the larger meanings of human gestures. Again, operating from a broader context can help lighten life's burdens. As Kelly (1969) noted, "There is nothing so obvious that its appearance is not altered when it is seen in a different light" (p. 227).

If Sandra can move into the adult role, she will become less reactive to her mother's criticism and less desperate for her approval. She will be able to express her appreciation more freely for the support her mother has provided over the years (and continues to provide). Ironically and paradoxically, as the atmosphere improves, her mother may begin to respond more positively, allowing Sandra to experience more of the acceptance she previously craved.

At some point, Sandra may be ready to invite her boyfriend and her parents to discontinue the protective services they have been providing. This would represent a very satisfactory resolution to this potentially difficult case. In the process, Sandra would undoubtedly become more relaxed about sharing aspects of herself, including her foibles, with others. She will discover that when people accept themselves, others are more than happy to follow suit. In other words, people take their cue from how they see us treating ourselves.

Potential Pitfalls

It was Sandra's boyfriend who suggested that she seek therapy because he could see the heavy toll her fears were taking on her life. We suspect that his suggestion was also motivated by the toll her fears were taking on *his* life. Undoubtedly, Sandra has been a high-maintenance project. A possible pitfall to treatment is that Sandra sought therapy mainly to appease her boyfriend and forestall his leaving. Context-centered therapy emphasizes the value of personal choices and responsible behavior, or claimed action. It is a detriment when therapy is motivated primarily by someone else's distress rather than by the client's own intentionality.

Termination and Relapse Prevention

By insisting on a clear-cut termination date, therapists of other persuasions often create unnecessary and unproductive management problems. Human beings never do well with good-byes, and they resist abrupt shifts in routine. The human organism—like other systems—is, by its very nature, conservative. People strive to maintain the status quo. In other words, the concept of termination introduces an artificial punctuation that creates more problems than it solves, including the need to have special procedures in place to handle any so-called relapses. As we have already stated, we have no need or wish to terminate clients. We see ourselves like the dentist or family doctor who sees you when something hurts and meets with you less often when health has been restored. Like the dentist or family physician, we arrange contacts— phone conversations, sessions, postcards, and letters—as needed.

Mechanisms of Change

People live within a cocoon of partially self-perpetuating linguistic structures and often become prisoners of their own suppositions, unable to see beyond the boundaries of their belief systems. Because they have simultaneous obligations to various social groups, they experience role conflicts. They are also faced with the sometimes difficult job of negotiating varied social expectations equipped with a set of biological propensities that are good for some purposes and detrimental for others. As the psychological costs of keeping oneself and others happy escalates, psychotherapy becomes a more likely prospect. As we have argued, context-centered therapists are a bit like medieval court jesters. Because of their wider purview, they can help people break out of traditional boxes and contemplate new alternatives. This works because all of us are capable of a broader range of behaviors than we ordinarily employ. In other words, the orthogonal relationship of the consulting room taps underutilized resources.

CONCLUSION

People's self-definitions are shaped by how they converse with themselves and each other. From this perspective, therapy is simply a specialized form of conversation. Unlike most traditional approaches, context-centered therapists are sufficiency-oriented. In other words, they are not primarily interested in repair work—eliminating, fixing, or improving. Instead, they invite the client to ride the horse in the direction it is going. Using the twin Zen concepts of acceptance and detachment, clients find that even intense symptoms tend to disappear or fade into the background when recontextualized.

Early therapy methods focused on the *content* of the client's productions—the recounting of a dream, the report of a symptom, or the description of a complaint. Later methods changed the emphasis from content to *process;* for example, the therapist interpreted the client-therapist relationship. Context-centered therapists are interested in neither content or process. They want to move another step up the ladder of abstraction in order to call attention to the framework of assumptions that dictates how relationships will develop and how symptoms will be expressed and experienced. Because the contextual level is superordinate to the other levels, context-centered approaches can be rapid and powerful. In other words, as a person's context shifts, process and content are automatically modified. The major vehicle for accomplishing this kind of shift is orthogonal interaction. In the novel mini-society the client and therapist create, clients can see beyond their limited frame of reference and begin to notice how often they have confused local ordinances with universal principles. That realization opens up choices and opportunities they didn't previously know they had.

REFERENCES

American Psychiatric Association. (1980). *Diagnostic and statistical manual of mental disorders* (3rd ed.). Washington, DC: Author.

American Psychiatric Association. (1987). *Diagnostic and statistical manual of mental disorders* (3rd ed., rev.). Washington, DC: Author.

Efran, J. S., Chorney, R. L., Ascher, L. M., & Lukens, M. D. (1989). Coping styles, paradox, and the cold pressor task. *Journal of Behavioral Medicine, 12,* 91–103.

Efran, J. S., & Cook, P. F. (1999). Linguistic ambiguity as a diagnostic tool. In R. A. Neimeyer & J. D. Raskin (Eds.), *Constructions of disorder: Meaning-making frameworks for psychotherapy* (pp. 121–144). Washington, DC: APA Books.

Efran, J. S., & Greene, M. A. (2000). The limits of change: Heredity, temperament, and family influence. In W. C. Nichols, M. A. Pace-Nichols, D.

S. Becvar, & A. Y. Napier (Eds.), *Handbook of family development and intervention* (pp. 41–64). New York: Wiley & Sons.

Efran, J. S., Greene, M. A., & Gordon, D. E. (1998). Lessons of the new genetics. *The Family Therapy Networker, 22*(2), 26–32, 35–41.

Efran, J. S., Lukens, M. L., & Lukens, R. J. (1990). *Language, structure, and change: Frameworks of meaning in psychotherapy.* New York: W. W. Norton.

Emery, S. (1978). *Actualizations: You don't have to rehearse to be yourself.* Garden City, NY: Doubleday.

Fancher, R. T. (1995). *Cultures of healing: Correcting the image of American mental health care.* New York: W. H. Freeman.

Goffman, E. (1959). *The presentation of self in everyday life.* Garden City, NY: Doubleday.

Goldiamond, I. (1972). Toward a constructional approach to social problems: Ethical and constitutional issues raised by applied behavioral analysis. *Behaviorism, 2,* 1–84.

Harris, J. R. (1998). *The nurture assumption: Why children turn out the way they do: Parents matter less than you think and peers matter more.* New York: The Free Press.

Kagan, J. (1994). *Galen's prophecy: Temperament in human nature.* New York: Basic Books.

Kelly, G. (1955). *The psychology of personal constructs* (Vol. 1). New York: W. W. Norton.

Kelly, G. (1969). *Clinical psychology and personality: The selected papers of George Kelly* (B. Maher, Ed.). New York: J. Wiley & Sons.

Kutchins, H., & Kirk, S. A. (1997). *Making us crazy: DSM: The psychiatric bible and the creation of mental disorders.* New York: The Free Press.

Maturana, H. R. (1993, November). *The biology of knowing.* Paper presented at the Conference of the American Society of Cybernetics, Philadelphia, PA.

Mendez, C. L., Coddou, F., & Maturana, H. R. (1988). The bringing forth of pathology. *Irish Journal of Psychology, 9,* 144–172.

Rabkin, R. (1970). *Inner and outer space: Introduction to a theory of social psychiatry.* New York: W. W. Norton.

Rychlak, J. F. (1973). *Introduction to personality and psychotherapy* (2nd ed.). New York: Houghton Mifflin.

Sarbin, T. R. (1968). Ontology recapitulates philology: The mythic nature of anxiety. *American Psychologist, 23,* 411–418.

Schafer, R. (1983). *The analytic attitude.* New York: Basic Books.

Seligman, M. E. P. (1993). *What you can change and what you can't: The complete guide to successful self-improvement.* New York: Fawcett Columbine.

Smothermon, R. (1979). *Winning through enlightenment.* San Francisco: Context Publications.

Sullivan, H. S. (1953). *The interpersonal theory of psychiatry.* (H. S. Perry & M. L. Gawel, Eds.). New York: W. W. Norton.

Szasz, T. (1973). *The second sin.* Garden City, NY: Doubleday.

Weekes, C. (1976). *Simple, effective treatment of agoraphobia.* New York: Bantam Books.

7

Contextual Family Therapy

Morrie Olson and Bruce Lackie

TREATMENT MODEL

Contextual family therapy (CFT) is an integrative approach to psychotherapy that seeks to unify individually oriented methods of treatment with the larger system, which is comprised of all the person's family members as well as other nonrelated individuals who play a significant role in the persons psychological and emotional life. Comprehensively, this forms their relational context, the nucleus of which is the family of origin.

The unification of the totality of one's relationships and the ethics and loyalties inherent within those relationships are the central foci of the theoretical underpinnings of the contextual-family-therapy model. The belief in the inherent power to heal by positively utilizing the untapped synergistic potential of family loyalty, trust, and fairness is mobilized through the actions of the contextual-family therapist and the willing participation of those persons active in the therapy sessions. In keeping with other traditional forms of family therapy, contextual family therapy utilizes a three-generational (multigenerational) model as its scope of family information, which provides a perspective for understanding the larger picture of relationships of which the patient is a part. This more comprehensive view, which incorporates several generations of family members as well as friends and significant others, also takes into account the time, place, and ethnicity of those involved. This is considered to be the *context* within which a person's circumstances occur. The contextual perspective is nonreductive, allowing therapists and patients alike to consider how the passage of time and the influence of numerous factors have contributed to a given set of circumstance by learning about their progression. The information acquired has tremendous explanatory power.

In addition, the contextual-family-therapy orientation stresses the need for ethical consideration of all parties connected to the individual who is seeking treatment. The comprehensive nature of the approach to treatment is attended to within the following four dimensions: facts, psychology, transactions, and relational ethics. *Facts* are described as those determinants that exist for an individual independent of his or her perception, such as ethnicity, the state of health, or the circumstances of his or her living conditions.

In the *psychology* dimension, the mental and intrapsychic functioning of the individual and resultant attitudes and perceptions are considered. *Transactions* focus on patterns of relating and the nature of the parties' interactions with others. This may include dynamics by which a person consistently positions himself or herself to "be in control" or to draw attention to another individual in a distinctly positive or negative manner.

The fourth dimension, the bedrock of the contextual-family-therapy model, is called *relational ethics*, within which matters of "fairness" come into play. References to ethics are not a matter of concrete morals and judgements, but rather are a paradigm for determining equitability in a relational sense that is not centered on any one individual's perceptions or feelings. This allows for the establishment of a renewed understanding of the relating parties' willingness to reconstruct relationships in which each participant is entitled to be heard and understood. This is directly linked to the loyalty one has to family members or other individuals of meaningful significance, even if those feelings have led to negative consequences or have yet to be consciously acknowledged.

At the core of contextual family therapy and theory is the belief that the establishment of *fairness in relating* creates the most powerful and meaningful context for positive change to develop and persevere over time. It is from this core ideology that the term "contextual" is derived. The contextual-family-therapy orientation utilizes a set of terms that, once understood, serve to elucidate factors and determinants that are frequently overlooked by other approaches and attempts to understand

and interpret matters involving family loyalty. For instance, contextual family therapy and theory provides a basis for explaining and aiding people in coming to terms with their feelings of being owed or indebted as a result of being part of their family or being in a given role with a family member (i.e., daughter, husband, etc.).

Matters or circumstances as extreme as incest, or as routine as attending a family function to which both divorced parents would be present, serve as examples, where a child's loyalty or forced participation may have proved ultimately to be detrimental to his or her psychology and resultant emotional well-being.

Historically, contextual family therapy developed from the work of the psychiatrist Ivan Boszormenyi-Nagy, who in 1957 instituted at a program at Eastern Pennsylvania Psychiatric Institute while working with hospitalized patients who were psychotic. The treatments being utilized at the time were within a conjoint family model. This was gradually expanded to include a broader spectrum of patients and an increased number of family members. The field of family therapy continued to progress throughout the 1950s. In the following decade, family therapists began to explore the potential healing for families that might be possible by expanding the scope of *family*. Assuming a multigenerational perspective, it allowed for the possibility of understanding the context of the parents of children presently in treatment. It also allowed for the assessment of issues and dynamics between generations and for determining the extent to which they might still be operating in the present.

In the latter part of the 1960s, Boszormenyi-Nagy incorporated this enhanced multigenerational framework. This in turn expanded the possibilities of understanding ethical transactions and loyalty, which he believed were the core area of human interaction that had been virtually neglected in psychotherapy. This led to the publication of the book *Invisible Loyalties* (Boszormenyi-Nagy & Spark, 1973), which elucidated the underpinnings of what had become the contextual-family-therapy model.

Contextual-family theory conceptualizes the nuclear family as being disconnected from its multigenerational roots. Consequently, it is seen to be suffering a similar disenfranchisement as the individual who is left with little or no relational resources. This disconnectedness leaves families to function as islands within the social stream of time, separate from the inherent legacy and loyalty issues that are present within the broader context of relating. The expansion of the basic family model to the multigenerational context was the logical next step in the progression from individualized orientation and the nuclear family. This evolving view was summarized by Boszormenyi-Nagy and Ulrich (1981).

We submit that the family is trying to exist in a vacuum that was left when the connection between intergenerational rootedness broke down and the ethical implications of that aspect of loyalty and legacy could not be reduced to functions of the superego. Multilateral determination transcends the individual as part of relational reality (Boszormenyi-Nagy & Ulrich, 1981, p. 161). Having moved into new areas of relational understanding at the time of its inception (multigenerational approach and relational ethics), contextual-family-theory contains its own terminology to convey these concepts more succinctly.

A wholly relational construct, contextual-family theory is centered around the very nature of human interactive experience. Therefore, the experiences of giving and receiving on an emotional and existential level, especially between family members and across generations, necessitate a mechanism of expression. These experiences are referred to as *merit, entitlement* and *indebtedness* (Boszormenyi-Nagy & Spark, 1973).

In terms of relational ethics, *merit* is the unit that counts. Merit is "earned" when an individual's actions are towards the goal of attaining a balance of fairness for all parties involved around a given issue or interaction. Such movement towards a more trustable environment is referred to as being *rejunctive*; efforts to the contrary are termed *disjunctive*.

Entitlement, in the contextual sense, describes the emotional accrual of merit that one earns by one's genuine efforts of caring and consideration. The tally of one's merit over time is referred to as the *ledger of merits* (Boszormenyi-Nagy & Spark, 1973).

Entitlement within this context is not something about which a person has a sense, as it differs in that way from what is generally referred to as self-esteem. Entitlement does not alter due to subjective parameters of circumstance. This means that if one is truly entitled, it will be retained in all other relationships. In short, *entitlement,* as a contextual-family therapy term, attempts to capture the long-standing feeling that is derived when a person truly believes he or she has worth and holds value and meaning to others. It is the living essence of validation. This also holds true of the negative aspects of entitlement that can occur when one has been disadvantaged in a relationship and is, therefore, deemed *destructively entitled.* This is often seen in cases where children are abused or taken advantage of relationally and are then bearers of

unresolved and conflicted feelings of both loyalty and personal suffering. Situations such as these—regarding children, in particular—led
to one of most well noted of the terms of contextual-family theory:
parentification. Parentification describes an imbalance of relating,
wherein one of the relating parties, in many instances a child or children, are subjected to age-inappropriate responsibilities and thereby
are placed in relational circumstances in which their reserves of trust
are continuously depleted. This key dynamic within relationships, and
within families in particular, is central to maintaining a process of
dysfunctionality. The scope of the implications of the concept of parentification are vast and also encompass positive aspects that may result
from the role-reversed dynamic.

One of the most significant aspects identifying parentification and
its negative sequelae is that it provides the framework for identifying
the underlying potential for emotional suffering in relationships and
families that otherwise appear quite normal and well-functioning on
the surface. The filial aspect of parentification may be summarized as
follows: "The failures of parents to act responsibly and effectively within
the realm of transgenerational legacy has a 'malevolent domino-effect'
in which children are the most recent dominoes to fall" (Olson, 1993,
p. 199).

The nature of the similarly repetitive dysfunctional patterns illumi-
nated by the transgenerational family model is captured by the term
revolving slate (Boszormenyi-Nagy & Spark, 1973). The revolving slate
refers to the complexities of feelings and circumstances for the parent
in the middle generation who is trapped by feelings of guilt regarding
his or her children and disloyalty to his or her parent(s) for choosing
to be different.

Change as a means of healing through contextual-family therapy is
seen as a process of providing the space for a trustable environment
to be created in which relating parties can recommit to relating in the
present by freeing themselves of hidden loyalty bonds and binds. Once
free of dysfunctional patterns of both over- and under-giving, they can
truly form more clear and trustworthy relationships. The contextual-
family therapist is the catalyst for this multigenerational rejunction.

THE THERAPIST'S SKILLS AND ATTRIBUTES

The contextual-family therapist is best suited to facilitate healing in
family systems by having experienced and comprehensively understood

the power inherent in relationships, networks, and systems. Therefore, the greater the therapist's ability to continuously, if not overtly, understand and utilize a systems approach for and with the client, the greater are the opportunities for healing. In keeping with the systemic focus, the therapist is always planning and strategizing how best to move the client toward patterns of increasingly positive connectedness both within the therapeutic process as well in daily life. Ultimately, this serves to foster a basis for support and increasing connectedness for clients as they progress through the therapeutic process and eventually out of it. In this way, individuals begin to move toward freedom in their lives, functionally, as well as psychologically, as opposed to being bound to a person or process for their own health and well-being.

Therapists in this modality are encouraged to think methodologically and to begin to identify, as readily as possible, a motif for the therapeutic process, which is always flexible and open to modification. In the present case of Sandra, the contextual-family therapist would begin to look for themes or repeating sets of circumstances, which may be occurring within a family over the course of generations. The therapist will also ask questions about what is known and unknown. However, the therapist must be ready to abandon any given hypothesis if the facts fail to support even the most persuasive or likely possibilities. It is here that therapists may find themselves at risk to apply their own history of circumstances to their patients, if they are not clear and objective about them.

Hence, the family therapist is best served by having researched and dealt with their own family history and by having attempted to resolve any issues should that have been required. To accomplish this, individuals who think creatively yet maintain an organized and focused approach seem to be best suited. Therapists who can offer a truly empathic as well as motivational demeanor can oftentimes bring much-needed energy to systems that are often initially depleted and seemingly hopeless, cynical, and depressed. In conjunction with this, the appropriate use of humor is highly encouraged and further serves to solidify the therapeutic relationship and gain a deeper more humanistic insight into the client's personality. In order to facilitate relational connectedness, the therapist in this model is best served who can incorporate interventions and respond with an arsenal of skills that are most geared to moving the individuals to experience and reexperience themselves and their actions and interactions with others. As the process continues, responses to specific relationally based questions and interventions can be compared and either be openly used or held for a future time.

Psychotherapists utilizing this approach are best served by having been trained in contextual-family therapy and multigenerational psychodynamics, as well as by being versed in the concepts and theories assigned to various aspects of human adult developmental stages and change as they may relate to cognition and how that may differ from truly psychopathological manifestations.

THE CARE OF SANDRA

Assessment

A multigenerational-family-systems perspective requires a great depth of factual background about each of the client's biological and foster family members than we have regarding Sandra and her family. Facts become the basis of elucidating patterns of abuse, trauma, support, and abandonment, and even consistent forms of generational denial, as similar patterns regarding family members emerge or remain hidden across generations (i.e., nothing is known about the paternal grandmother over three generations). Patterns of past relationships are also reviewed to better understand the relational history of the parents portrayed in the case presented. The potential for understanding familial and possible genetic contributions to the presenting problems would also be enhanced if more data were available. The information provided also lacks relational and relevant medical, psychological, and psychiatric information on all but the client and her biological mother.

Positive aspects of interpersonal emotional resources that may have been present within the family system during the past generation are left untapped because of the minimal information provided. For example, during the course of Sandra's mother's 30 hospitalizations, what were Sandra's resources, if any? What were those first years like? Who was her caretaker? What was brought to bear in a positive yet invisible way for the client that she never saw or knew about? Did she ever sleep in the same bed as her birth parents? Did she experience night terrors? These are all contributions made on her behalf that she is unaware of. Therefore, she cannot draw upon this information in her attempts to understand her present life circumstances and her reactions to them. In most families, a part of parenting is invisible, because the child may have been too young to know about it, yet the child may come to learn about the efforts made on his or her behalf later.

However, in Sandra's situation the contributions of such *invisible parenting* remain unknown to her. The CFT model, as do other systems approaches, incorporates the genogram to assist in the assessment process. A genogram is a pictorial representation of relationships that has distinct markings to represent specific gender and relational determinants such as separation and divorce. This multigenerational family picture aids the family therapist in discerning trends and breaks and patterns in relating. These patterns act as a map for the trained practitioner, who can not only see what is present but identify what is missing. With the genogram as part of the patient's record, there is a constant reminder of the potential and power of the context of one's relatedness or the lack thereof. Although an individually oriented model may use various types of testing to learn more about the patient, the family therapist, while not discounting these findings, would also use the factual data in the genogram to understand the systemic context in which the individual's psychology was functioning.

By examining the context in which a person's behaviors, feelings, and attitudes exist, we can begin to understand circumstances that may have contributed to the person's overall development as well as how and why he or she is responding with a given set of behaviors in the present situation. It is important to note the extent to which individuals are capable of altering their set of responses to stressful circumstances or if they are stuck in having to rely on a few set of reactions. In some cases we can learn how past emotional and psychological injuries may leave people unable to grow and develop in various ways from that moment forward. Therefore, when we look at a genogram we can continue to embellish our contextual knowledge with questions that can piece together what we have learned verbally, by what we can hypothesize by visually seeing the network of relationships on paper. The therapist's hypotheses can then be reviewed for validation with the person or persons in treatment.

For example as we look at the genogram of Sandra, we may question whether the two older sisters were abused as well. We would begin to question the paradox between the ideals of the conservative Catholic family she was reared in and their acceptance of her sleeping at her boyfriend's apartment. We may also ask whether she is using birth control, and we would want to learn more about what her experience is like for her, given her past history of abuse.

Although we know that the client did not meet *DSM-IV* criteria for certain disorders, we do not know by how much she failed to meet such criteria. This is crucial, as in our experience multiple co-occurring disorders may act as confounds in meeting specific independent clinical criteria. In such cases the individual suffers from the underlying illness or illnesses, yet is deemed to fall short of definitive diagnostic parameters. In such cases, diagnostic cutoffs can further corrupt the presenting clinical picture.

From a family systems perspective, information about the biological mother and father (i.e., race, religion, ethnicity, relationships, etc.) is needed. Additional important information would include facts relating to drug or alcohol-related problems at the level of either abuse or dependence. Psychiatric diagnostic information relating to the parents and possibly the siblings would also be of importance, along with medical and health-related issues, ages at marriage, separations, as well as abortions and miscarriages. Other information about the families of the patient's parents and their parents would also be of consequence.

It would be useful for this particular patient to be assessed in order to rule out the probability of having a personality disorder or dissociative qualities. This would serve to further clarify and give perspective to some of the presenting symptomatology.

Therapeutic Goals

In Sandra's case, assistance in alleviating some of the negative symptomatology induced by her fears and their impact on her daily life is of primary importance. Therefore, it may be advantageous for her to have a psychiatric consult or evaluation for the purpose of affording her some immediate relief through the use of appropriately prescribed medication. Pharmacotherapy may assist her in functioning in a more flexible, relaxed fashion in her daily life, thereby achieving a less restrictive lifestyle, regardless of her psychological defenses. The issues that could be addressed pharmacologically would be her overriding fears, panic disorder symptoms, insomnia, anxiety, and possible depression or dysthymia. Amelioration of these symptoms may assist in paving the way for deeper insight and understanding. The attainment of a more stabilized emotional state could then be supplemented psychotherapeutically.

Once a degree of comfort was achieved, the psychotherapeutic work would be able to assist Sandra in developing a more individually differentiated life. This goal would be manifested by her ability to come and go at will and to be free of having to arrange her daily activities around the availability of others. To the extent that this change could not be attained by the use of medication alone, the underlying causative factors would need to be the focus of treatment. The work would then focus on her beginning to distance herself in a healthy way from her family and her reliance upon her boyfriend. These goals would be both the primary and long-term aims of treatment. The implications of Sandra's present behavior and the effect its changing might have upon others would also be addressed with Sandra and the affected significant others.

At present, Sandra's life is a patchwork of defenses and scheduling in a desperate attempt to cope in the real world. This patchwork assists her in maintaining her work life, which is currently the only area in which she is clearly succeeding. Through her work, she gains a form of pseudo-merit that she is craving from those more directly related to her basic sense of self. To this extent her boss and coworkers act as transferential entities. This further skews attempts at a positive balance of relating and in so doing makes her extremely vulnerable if her work life should falter.

In keeping with the way she is currently using her energy, important therapeutic steps would involve the clarification of her birth parent's role regarding her identity and the subsequent reenactment of abandonment in her foster family. Assistance in family sessions towards lessening any guilt or shame she may bear as a result of her molestations and family betrayal are also essential issues that need to be explored and overcome.

Timeline for Therapy

Oftentimes, stages or levels of this type of therapy depend upon the degree of commitment and tolerance to the stress of exploring the family themes. These stages could be further complicated by the willingness, availability, and ego strength needed to bring needed family members and significant others together. A brief therapy may not allow for this level of involvement to occur or for the underlying intergenerational themes to emerge to the fullest extent.

An interactional model of family therapy, focusing mainly on structural themes, would be briefer but might not exact as comprehensive a recovery, as deeper issues may be left untouched. With consistent involvement, a process such as this would require a minimum of 3 to 6 months of treatment, during which Sandra would attend sessions weekly or, minimally, biweekly. Some sessions would need to be longer than one full hour. Extended sessions are most generally planned when more than one person is in attendance and when the issues to be dealt with have never been truly addressed.

Case Conceptualization

Given her age, Sandra actually has very few deep emotional attachments, even taking into consideration the level of interaction with her boyfriend. Considering her biological mother's psychiatric illness, Sandra may be struggling with manifestations of a significant disorder of personality as there may be a genetic vulnerability in her situation. Given her parentified position in this family, she also appears prone to dissociation. Psychologically, she presents as insecure and empty. Her fears not only reflect her outward realities of the past but also her own internal void. She does not present as having an emotional and psychological center rooted in anything but fears of both the known and unknown.

Therefore, her ruminations and obsessions may act as cognitive avoidance of her own lack of a true self. Such fears and phobias further serve to promulgate an external focus for herself. Alternatively, they can be seen as a form of projection of her own psychology, the groundwork for which may have been laid by the word of her biological mother, who continuously made Sandra aware of the fears she had for her. However, these prophecies, may have been a conglomeration of the concerns of a more "healthy" mother, along with manifestation of her own mental illness. Sandra, whose life has been unsafe and filled with untrustworthy people, cannot help but hear the realistic aspect of her mother's concerns, but she is also unable to separate the fear from the reality, and is therefore left unsure and panic-stricken.

Sandra's basic male-female role concepts are split, in what appears to be an all-or-none fashion. In the words of one contextual-family therapist and theorist, "Split-loyalty is literally "split-self" (Hibbs, 1988, p. 29). Women such as Sandra's mother and stepmother are seen as ineffectual and therefore cannot be counted upon—clearly as a manifestation of untrustworthiness with regard to the mother-daughter relationship. Men, on the other hand, such as her stepfather and boyfriend, are effective, but disappointing and trust-depleting as well as exploitative; hence, her comment, "I don't trust anybody." Such preconceived ideas regarding how men and women function, predicated upon her own negative life experiences, can contribute to an overall feeling of loneliness and fear and, in the extreme, concern for her own physical well-being and even survival.

Her boyfriend is just a functional object to assist her in coping. Although his actions have earned him merit, Sandra does not yet have an internal basis of trust to allow her to fully acknowledge his contributions. She does not understand her utilitarian employment of him and therefore questions her feelings for him. Thus, she harbors fears that she will lose him and, in so doing, remains destructively loyal to her legacy of isolation and fear. This speaks directly to her internal emptiness and lack of trust, which are manifestations of her parentified status.

Sandra's fear of being killed represent the ultimate denial of the self. This is the culmination of her mother's projective fears and her internalized overall lack of trust in the world. Here, knowing more about the dismissal of her biological father in early adolescence would be key. Was there sexual abuse? Her fear of a nervous breakdown is in part a predictive measure of her waning abilities to sustain and maintain herself and an example of her destructive loyalty to her mother in wanting to join her in death, if not physically, then psychically. Her hypervigilance may be seen as a survival mechanism of constantly being on guard to what may befall her.

On the positive side, her hypervigilance also demonstrates her desire to be able to protect herself. This overattentiveness can be further attributed to the actions of her untrustworthy brothers, stepfather, and whoever else. Not surprisingly, she presents with many of the features of a trauma client. Overall, she is truly bound by her situation. She is trapped by her fears and loyalties to those people who have betrayed her and that she has, in turn, betrayed by telling what they have done to her. She has become a prisoner to their anger and her fears. Her success at work and school is her way of validating herself, perhaps the only way. She is certainly not free to play. By not prosecuting her adoptive family, she demonstrates her inability to separate and advocate for herself or in any way act in her own best interest, which perhaps assists her in bearing any guilt she may have, however unwarranted.

Sandra admitted rather than reported her abuse. She is truly objectified in virtually all her relationships, except perhaps by her boyfriend. Interestingly, she has virtually objectified him. Her stepfather's threat to kill himself places the value of another life over her own. Her fears, phobias, and other life-denying limitations have constricted her life in a way that has "deadened" her. Is she now just waiting for it to happen while fearing its eventuality? Sandra is lacking the entitlement to experience feeling suicidal! In a dynamic sense she has a great deal of power in her hands but she cannot act. She is powerful but disempowered.

The Therapeutic Relationship

The Therapeutic Bond

The therapeutic bond resembles all other generic therapeutic modalities in which there are variations in the posture of the therapist. In the more traditional forms of family therapy as well as in the contextual-family-therapy approach, the position of the therapist is one of catalyst and choreographer. The therapist guides, facilitates, and orchestrates the therapeutic setting in accordance with the needs of the client and the system in which he or she is involved. This is achieved by considering how all parties involved can benefit and serves to assist the clients with their progress by encountering less resistance with specific individuals and the system as a whole. Possibilities for this outcome to occur are optimized when all involved can be helped to feel that there is something positive to be gained by their participating. The greater the involvement of relating individuals, the greater the potential to minimize blaming and scapegoating.

This approach moves directly towards the building of trust. Naturally, this cannot always be accomplished in a brief period of time and in many ways is limited by the flexibility of character and attitudes toward change of each individual involved. The depth and extent of the emotional and psychological and sometimes physical injuries that have been sustained may also act as barriers to the trust-building process.

Roles in Therapeutic Relationship

The therapist in this model is a guide, who seeks to continuously gain the trust of those involved. These actions actively demonstrate the trust-building process to those who are being encouraged to follow. The therapist functions as a compass, reliably pointing the way toward a healthy, more open, and trustworthy future for all involved. Healing contextually is cultivated as part of the trust-building process. Forgiveness is mobilized to replace suffering, defensiveness, and unclear compensatory functioning.

Therefore, the therapist does not say, "You should or ought to be doing. . . . " Instead, the clinician might ask, "What can be done in this situation?" If the patient is stating that someone is being resistant or difficult, the therapist may ask, "What might be helpful here?" In this way, the individual being discussed is not "bad" but merely requires his or her own assistance.

The therapist investigates, learns, and catalogues the key issues and factors affecting both positive and negative loyalty dynamics. If the client or the system is not ready or able to confront or deal with a key issue, it is recycled for another more opportune time or is presented to another system member who may be strong enough to begin to deal with it. Allocating the issue to another member in the system must be carefully gauged so as not to burden or further parentify that seemingly "stronger" individual. However, once an issue or matter has been openly acknowledged by the parties involved, the therapist in this system can be quite active and direct in posing questions and intervening in general.

The relationship between the identified client and other members of the family system is the key to the therapeutic process in CFT. Of course as in all relationships, there are individual characteristics of both client and therapist that make them naturally like or take to the other. However, in this modality of treatment, establishing and maintaining trust is of primary importance. Because a primary goal is always to involve relevant individuals, it is imperative to proceed and communicate with significant others, only when the central client is ready and only to the extent that he or she agrees to continue. Adequate preparation must precede the inclusion of additional people. The topics for therapy and the depth to which they will be addressed with significant others must be done in such a fashion as to aid the primary client's trust and comfort level.

The inclusion of significant others in the therapeutic process can be a tremendous source of information about the relational and transactional patterns of the client. Situations such as these also allow the primary client to see firsthand that the therapist will "hold" to his or her word. This type of interaction also allows all parties to learn new and, one hopes, more successful methods of relating. Overall, this tends to be a very powerful means of enhancing the therapeutic bond.

Treatment Implementation and Outcome

Techniques and Methods of Working

The unification of the totality of one's relationships and the ethics and loyalties inherent within those relationships are the central focus of CFT. The belief in the inherent power to heal by positively utilizing the untapped synergistic potential of family loyalty, trust, and fairness is mobilized through the efforts of the contextually trained therapist. The hallmark of this training has been termed "multidirected partiality" (Boszormenyi-Nagy & Spark, 1973).

The multidirected approach depends on the family therapist's manifesting absolutely the ability to nonjudgementally hear and acknowledge each person's side equally and fairly, giving due consideration to all. By the addition of *constructive developmentalism* (Kegan, 1982), another level of understanding can be achieved. Constructivism challenges us not only to hear and be empathic to what one is saying, but also to completely know how one has formulated his or her perspective. By learning how each person forms a construct of meaning, therapists can greatly enhance their ability to catalyze mutually beneficial transactions, while simultaneously increasing trust. This trust-building and more salient interactions can be accomplished by assisting parties in moving beyond the dimension of interaction where one acknowledges *hearing* what the other person has said, to understanding how and why they have *thought* to state it at all. Once people begin to understand, an entirely new avenue of relating can be achieved and methods of problem-solving approached.

The failure to have attained this level of understanding with each other leads to such cliches as, "I've told you a million times and you just don't seem to get it," "You don't care how I feel," or "You say you love me but you keep doing the same old things."

Expanding the context of relating to include the dimension of *meaning* allows not only for new insights to be gained through multigenerational understanding, but also for one of multidimensional enlightenment. In the most basic perspective, differing generations have varied *cultures of meaning*. Both the contextual-family and the constructive-developmental therapists subscribe to the orientation that the utilization of the respective methods will prove to be effective agents of change.

Although the focus of this chapter has been a multigenerational, family-systems perspective, the necessity for individuals to be assisted in dealing with the specifics of their individual struggles is not negated. With this in mind, we recognize that Sandra may well require some unique measures to aid her in coping. In certain cases like the one presented here where she has apparently been traumatized by past experiences, eye movement desensitization reprocessing (EMDR) has been shown to be of assistance. Given the emphasis on communication in relational treatment, a technique such as EMDR can often help those individuals who are still struggling around issues for which they have not yet found the words. For Sandra, who has experienced a form of "sanctuary trauma" in which the place where she may have found refuge is where she has been betrayed, EMDR may be a first step towards allowing for the building of trust to begin again.

Medical and Nutritional Issues

Although mentioning that Sandra is underweight, the information provided in this particular case does not give us any further reason to believe that this is either the direct or indirect result of a medical or psychiatric illness. Therefore, though her medical and nutritional stability would not necessarily be called into question, some questioning regarding her weight would be undertaken. In light of the fact that Sandra does have fears and anxiety it would be of value to question how this may be effecting her diet and intake of food. The psychiatric consultation mentioned earlier would further serve as another opportunity to review by a medical doctor the possible physical problems induced by psychiatric diagnosis. In other cases, issues regarding medical and nutritional matters would be covered during the assessment process and referred for further follow-up by the appropriate practitioners should it be necessary. In such cases where nutrition and medical circumstances were present, the psychotherapeutic aspects would be examined in terms of the ramifications of these conditions.

Potential Pitfalls

In the administration of medication, the more powerful the drug, the greater the potential for side effects. To some extent, this is borne out in the utilization of family therapy. Given that more people may be involved in the treatment, the chances for a dynamic to be enacted are increased. Although it is understood that these patterns are operating regardless, they may also appear to be more visible deterrents to treatment. More obvious pitfalls would be Sandra's refusal to accept medication should it be needed, or unwanted adverse effects should she accept it. Any disorders of personality of either Sandra or another family member or significant other can also act as sabotaging elements in the treatment. The possibility of yet uncovered traumas emerging also cannot be ruled out for Sandra or another participant.

Termination and Relapse Prevention

Even though systemic psychotherapeutic approaches seek to eliminate or at least ameliorate the accrual of transference between patient and therapist, transference can and does still occur. In its absence, the termination of any relationship of value is often met with difficulty in the most healthy of circumstances. The prospect of the termination of the therapeutic relationship must be addressed with all members involved throughout the therapy, especially the primary patient. The contextual-family therapist also strives to reinforce the positive accomplishments made by all the parties involved in the therapeutic process, along with the primary patient. The ending of the relationship with the therapist is addressed as an accomplishment on behalf of any person involved with the process. The therapist credits the participants for their courage in facing the issues that may have prevailed within a family over more than one generation and attempts to make known how altering previously negative patterns of relating can offer more positive potential for both present and future generations of the same family. Termination can be tapered and the need for periodic updates can be predetermined.

Oftentimes it is helpful to have a session scheduled for an extended period post "official" termination if the person being treated has manifested high degrees of dependence on other relationships or the therapist. This approval, at times, may head off a full-blown relapse or regression. By affording individuals the opportunity to reengage the therapist if needed, the possibility can be avoided that some individuals will "stay away" in order to make it seem that "things are all better," when in fact they are not. It is not uncommon for parentified persons to attempt to carry the responsibility for the success of treatment for all the others who have participated, including the therapist. This is directly in keeping with the role they may have assumed as a once overly responsible child in their family of origin. Family therapy should include the summation with those individuals who have participated in a routine manner or who have been more deeply affected through the experience. The accomplishments of the primary patient and of all involved should be noted and duly credited by the therapist. Should the patient or patients be continuing with another clinician initially enlisted by the family therapist, the recognition can also be raised that continued progress can be monitored. The family therapist, being systemically oriented, sees to it that systemic relational networks are put into place to help safeguard the patient within her context. In keeping with this orientation, the practitioner also creates and mobilizes the needed professional to assist in bolstering and maintaining optimal functioning.

Mechanisms of Change

How and why people change is a complex topic. Therefore, it would be a vast overstatement to say concretely that any specific interventions of any one psychotherapeutic model, independent of the specific individuals that are participating, are the sole reason for positive change. However, when apparent improvements in the quality of people's lives appear to occur through the utilization of psychotherapy, we can begin to look at contextual-family theory and practice and to the belief that although the individual is central to all that pertains to him or her, we all are in fact dependant and interdependent upon those with whom we are continuously relating. How we understand our place in relationships is constantly subject to how we measure the impact of even subtle changes. The manner in which we weigh or place a positive or negative value (debts and credits) is the basis of our interpersonal *justice system*. The contextual-family therapist seeks to assist in the catalysis of change by having relating parties who are participating in the therapeutic process identify those aspects of their relationships that they have felt to be false and exploitative. This is more likely to occur as relating parties are authentic and a mutually understood reality can begin to emerge. A familial example of this is stated in *Invisible Loyalties* (Boszormenyi-Nagy & Spark, 1973).

> False filial respect can mask the taboos and injunctions against genuine exploration of the true relationship between one's self and one's parents. Yet learning about the struggles of the older generation could lead to a more genuine respect for them. The developing of dialogue of open and courageous question and answer between child and parent makes the latter more of a parent. (p. 35)

In this statement the authors refer to the potential for change that is possible when a true dialogue can be facilitated. Feelings of resentment, anger, and an overall lack of understanding about where someone "is coming from" can be more completely understood once we begin to understand their legacy and the trials and tribulations they have experienced; hence, the inclusion of information gathered across generations, which is inherent in this and numerous other forms of family therapy.

Once the causative factors are comprehensively understood, the factual determinants of each person's reality and the way they form their own justice system and ledger of merits can be more likely to change or grant a kind of *relational dispensation* for perceived past injustices. Such positive steps towards reworking injured relationships are what allow for the negative aspects of invisible loyalty to be brought to light and a potential ending for silent suffering made possible.

In essence, the key ingredient to change in contextual family therapy is genuine, knowledge-based dialogue, whereby all parties, with the assistance of a trained therapist, can begin to abandon long-standing or even lifelong roles in which one or more individuals have been perceived as relegated to imbalanced relational positions. Such imbalances in relating fall predominantly into two categories: being overly given to (infantilized); or being deprived of an age- or role-appropriate treatment or depleted in other ways that may have forced them into overly responsible roles too soon (parentified). The knowledge we are referring to derives from the information gained from both direct dialogue and through researching the past of one's own multigenerational family history.

CONCLUSION

Contextual family therapy is a multigenerational systems approach to treatment. Within this model each dimension of an individual's life is considered. The quality of one's relationships is viewed as a key determinant to one's balanced world view, a paradigm for evaluating and addressing the areas of loyalty, relational ethics, and trust. To this end, contextual family therapy prescribes a multidirected approach to its treatment of systemic, not symptomatic, problems. This focus, in turn, allows for all relating parties to be acknowledged for their individual betterment and the improvement of systemic functioning.

Although this chapter sought to view Sandra's situation from a family systems perspective, an adjunctive approach would be the use of eye movement desensitization and reprocessing (EMDR), which may help Sandra develop a better perspective on her situation and greater mastery. It is a trauma-focused approach and her history and present situation that speak to the need to address her unfinished business, especially in the areas where there are no words, where she becomes speechless. She has suffered a kind of "sanctuary trauma" in which the place where she might have reasonably expected refuge is the very place where her trust was betrayed. Though there is little chance that the family is going to change significantly—and could in fact decompensate in the face of her potential therapeutic gains should she make changes—an attempt would be made to engage them in support of her efforts. The secondary gains of her self-infantilization may act as deterrents to systemic change. If that should be the case, an individually oriented technique such as EMDR could prove useful.

In actuality, Sandra has accommodated to her situation in a relatively functional way, taking into account her present symptoms and possible genetic predispositions because of her biological mother's psychopathology. Sandra continues to function well in her job in spite of the restrictions she felt she needed to implement, the limited depth of the relationships she has formed, and limited support. Overall she has managed to keep a schedule that brings her a modicum of autonomy and accomplishment, especially within the work setting.

The long-term outcome of her treatment is contingent upon several variables: her ability to be compliant with medication and her tolerance for it, as well as general compliance with psychotherapy. The extent of any underlying correlates of personality and how they may play out within the confines of the therapeutic relationship are also of importance.

If no overtly restrictive issues of personality or compliance arose, this individual could very well achieve a significant amount of relief and make great strides toward a more balanced and normal lifestyle. The basis for this prognosis is her strong ability to do quite well in other areas of her life and to continue to be productive and function relatively well in the wake of the significant problems she faces on a daily basis. To her credit, she has the ability to have found solutions to her difficulties in functioning and to her fears, coupled with a willingness to adapt to those problems and still function in the workplace and maintain her family and romantic relationships.

REFERENCES

Boszormenyi-Nagy, I., & Spark, G. M. (1973). *Invisible loyalties.* New York: Brunner/Mazel.

Boszormenyi-Nagy, I., & Krasner, B. (1986). *Between give and take.* New York: Brunner/Mazel.

Boszormenyi-Nagy, I., & Ulrich, D. N. (1981). Contextual family therapy. In A. S. Gurman & D. P. Kniskern (Eds.), *Handbook of family therapy* (pp. 159–186). New York: Brunner/Mazel.

Hibbs, B. (1988). The context of growth: Relational ethics between parents and children. In L. Combrink-Grahman (Ed.), *Handbook of family therapy with children* (pp. ___). New York: Guilford Press.

Kegan, R. (1982). *The evolving self.* Cambridge, MA: Harvard University Press.

Olson, M., & Gariti, P. (1993). Symbolic loss in horizontal relating: Defining the role of parentification in addictive/destructive relationships. *Contemporary Family Therapy, 15,* 197–208.

8

Adlerian Therapy

Richard R. Kopp

TREATMENT MODEL

Alfred Adler's *individual psychology* views the individual as a holistic, self-consistent unity striving toward a subjectively conceived sense of significance and security within a social/interpersonal field. To understand an individual, the Adlerian therapist seeks to understand the individual's lifestyle or "law of movement," i.e., the subjective meaning (or *private logic*) unconsciously constructed by the individual and the unconscious lifestyle goal reflected in the behavioral movement of the person in the context of the person's social-relational systems. The lifestyle goal reflects the individual's unique way of striving for significance, security, completeness, and sense of power or efficacy.

Adler named his system "individual psychology" because the German meaning carries the connotation that the individual is an *indivisible* whole and must be understood as a self-consistent, indivisible unity. Unfortunately, this holistic meaning is lost in the English translation, which implies that individual psychology concerns the individual as a single, isolated entity. In fact, the opposite is true—individual psychology is fundamentally a social psychology.

I will use a case example to illustrate how the Adlerian treatment model may be employed in psychotherapy. John began his first session with me by stating that he was "interviewing therapists." He said that he didn't intend to be in therapy forever and wanted to know how long therapy would take. He sat rather stiffly while maintaining a tight hold on the arms of his chair.

An Adlerian clinician begins to formulate hypotheses about the client's lifestyle immediately, and then considers additional information and behavioral observations to see if they support the initial hypotheses. Based on John's verbal and nonverbal behavior in the first few minutes of the session, I hypothesized that John feels anxious, especially when faced with a new situation, and compensates for these feelings by striving toward feeling safe and secure. From the perspective of his lifestyle, this means attempting to create a feeling of being in control. For example, John attempts to structure the relationship with the therapist as one in which he is interviewing the therapist, that is, he is in control and he will choose. Another way that John appears to seek control is by gathering information in order to create a feeling of certainty and predictability. His stiff posture and tight hold on the arms of his chair are examples of what Adlerians refer to as behavioral movement with the goal of control, metaphorically trying to maintain a firm grasp of the situation.

Adlerians view resistance in therapy as a conflict of goals between the client and therapist. The therapist can resolve or avoid resistance by aligning the therapist's goal with the (unconscious, or, more precisely, nonconscious) goal of the client. A major organizing theme in John's lifestyle appears to be that of the "Controller/Organizer" (Kopp, 1986). Such individuals typically experience insecurity as feeling out of control and strive for a sense of significance and security through gaining a feeling of control, order, and organization. Other lifestyle themes frequently encountered in Adlerian psychotherapy include the "Victim-Martyr/Advocate" whose security revolves around issues of fairness; the "Getter/Harvester" who strives to get (attention, material things, etc.) in order to gain a feeling of significance; and the "Opposer/Individualist" who may oppose others and seek to establish their individuality and independence as a way of gaining a feeling of significance (Kopp, 1986).

My initial conceptualization of John's lifestyle as that of a controller/organizer suggested that by being organized and systematic in my approach while creating opportunities for John to experience feeling some control of the therapy, I could align my goals with his nonconscious psychological goal of security. I told John that I thought that interviewing therapists in order to choose one with whom he was most comfortable made sense to me. I suggested that if he would describe the issues he wanted to explore and what goals he wanted to achieve in therapy, we could come up with an estimate of how long it would take to achieve those goals.

After John described his issues and goals for therapy (which included reducing symptoms of anxiety and depression), I asked how long he thought it should take to see improvement with those issues. To my surprise, he said, "About a year to a year and a half." I told him that certainly seemed reasonable to me. I suggested that we meet for 6 weeks at which point we would discuss whether or not he (and I) felt we were making progress. This approach also reflects Adler's emphasis on creating and maintaining a therapeutic relationship of mutual respect and cooperation between equals who are neither superior nor inferior to each other. John stated at the end of the session that he felt comfortable with me and wouldn't need to interview any other therapists.

In contrast to my usual style, I took a very structured approach in the first few therapy sessions. However, John began our third session by asking if it would be okay to discuss something that occurred during the previous week. John started the fourth session by stating that he realized therapy was more indirect than he had initially thought, and that he would be comfortable just discussing his issues each week and seeing what emerged.

According to Adlerian theory, people tend to move toward a feeling of significance and power on either a vertical or horizontal plane (Sicher, 1955). Those who move along the vertical plane seek to overcome feelings of inferiority and inadequacy by seeking a position of superiority and power over others. In contrast, people who move along the horizontal plane regard others as equals and move in collaboration with them to overcome common challenges and difficulties. Horizontal movement expresses social interest and community feeling in which one feels a part of one's community and, ultimately, experiences an identification with, and a feeling of belonging within, the community of humankind. Vertical movement indicates dysfunction in individuals, relationships, or society, whereas horizontal movement indicates individual, interpersonal, and societal health. The initial session with John illustrates how the therapist can establish a cooperative, horizontal therapeutic alliance by quickly grasping and aligning with the client's unique law of movement and the dynamics and goal of the client's lifestyle.

Adlerian theory and methods are also relevant to improving social relationships between different groups, countries, and other entities. Adlerians have developed approaches for resolving conflict and promoting social equality between parents and children, in couples, families, organizations, and between social groups (Dreikurs, 1971; Kopp, 1997).

THE THERAPIST'S SKILLS AND ATTRIBUTES

Perhaps the most important attribute of an Adlerian therapist is the ability to model for, and stimulate in the client, the expression of social interest. Adler (Ansbacher & Ansbacher, 1964) often described social interest as the ability to see with the eyes of another, hear with the ears of another, and feel with the heart of another. Adlerian therapists seek to develop the ability to enter the client's subjective world and convey this deep empathy to the client.

Because Adlerians view therapy as an exercise in cooperation, the therapist must be able to create and maintain a therapeutic relationship based on mutual respect. Although the therapist may possess knowledge that the client does not have, this does not make the therapist superior to the client. To convey this message of mutual respect and interpersonal equality, Adler always conducted his sessions using chairs of equal height so that neither he nor the client would be above or below the other. Similarly, the therapist's goal is to strive for power, significance, and security in ways that seek to contribute to the welfare of others, in contrast to seeking power and significance by striving for power over others.

To Adler, most psychological and behavioral difficulties result from discouragement. Courage is the confidence in one's ability to meet the demands of life. The discouraged person lacks this confidence and may seek to avoid life's demands. Distortions in one's lifestyle beliefs and goals and the development of symptoms are viewed by Adlerian therapists as nonconscious strategies whose purpose is to avoid situations that one believes will result in revealing to the world one's inadequacies and feelings of being worthless. The origins of discouragement in childhood usually result from pampering, neglect, or abuse by the child's caretakers.

It follows that therapists must have the ability to encourage clients. Encouragement involves focusing on assets and strengths while building another's confidence and self-worth. Encouragement is the process of stimulating the courage to be imperfect: the acceptance of one's inevitable imperfections and failures (Dinkmeyer & Dreikurs, 1963) while responding to the needs of the situation with one's best effort. Space does not permit a full discussion of the concepts, methods, and impact of encouragement in therapy, parenting, and in human relationships. A fuller understanding of the theory and methods of encouragement may be found in *Encouraging Children to Learn* (Dinkmeyer & Dreikurs, 1963), *Leadership by Encouragement* (Dinkmeyer & Eckstein, 1993), *Children: The Challenge* (Dreikurs with Solz, 1964), and *Systematic Training for Effective Parenting* (Dinkmeyer & McKay, 1976).

An understanding of one's own biases and beliefs is an essential factor in conducting effective psychotherapy. Adlerian therapists often receive didactic therapy to increase their awareness of their own lifestyles and the potential impact on conducting therapy with different clients.

THE CASE OF SANDRA

Assessment, Conceptualization, and Treatment Planning

Assessment

Two methods Adlerian therapists use to determine the client's lifestyle and its origins are described below. We begin with a discussion of additional information that would be needed for a fuller understanding of the client.

Additional Information

1. Sandra was repeatedly fondled by her two brothers and forced to look at their genitals. How did she experience this? How did this experience contribute to her lack of trust, her fears, and other concerns?
2. Sandra's description of herself as "daddy's girl" is important. Why does she describe herself this way? What was her relationship with her adoptive father? In what ways were they close? Were there boundary violations in addition to those reported?
3. How does Sandra know whether her parents are asleep or not when she falls asleep? If they fall asleep first, why and how does that make a difference for her?
4. Sandra reports that she used to think the abuse was her fault, but not anymore. It would be important to ask how she changed

from thinking it was her fault to realizing it was not? Her answer could suggest ways to help Sandra change other distorted and maladaptive beliefs.
5. Post-traumatic stress disorder seems likely as a comorbid diagnosis. Additional information should be obtained to rule out PTSD. If confirmed, treating Sandra's PTSD could be incorporated into the middle phase of her therapy.

Specific Assessment Tools. There are two assessment procedures Adlerians typically use to identify a client's lifestyle: early recollections and the family constellation interview.

An early recollection (ER) is a specific, one-time incident that one remembers from childhood and that one can picture in the mind's eye like a scene. Adlerians use ERs to identify major lifestyle beliefs, expectations, and goals (Mosak, 1977b). The rationale for this approach is based on Adler's view that ERs are selective, subjective reconstructions of past events and thus express subjective, in contrast to literal, meaning. According to Adler, we remember from childhood only those incidents that support our current view of life. Adlerians often collect six to eight ERs at the outset of therapy as part of assessment of the client's life style (Shulman & Mosak, 1988).

The family constellation was first discussed by Adler (Adler, 1981; Ansbacher & Ansbacher, 1964) and further developed by others (Mosak, 1972; Shulman, 1962; Shulman & Mosak, 1988). The family constellation describes our early subjective experiences within the family system. This information helps the Adlerian therapist paint a picture of the circumstances within which clients' personal beliefs, meanings, and behavior patterns developed as they strove to find their place in the family, one's first social group. The main elements of the family constellation are the sibling constellation, family values, family atmosphere, parental behavior, and the family role played by each child (Shulman & Mosak, 1988).

Following Adler's view that individuals strive for a feeling of significance within a social context, the family constellation allows the Adlerian therapist to understand the subjective context, within which the lifestyle developed. This subjective context is seen in the child's behavior patterns, alliances and rivalries, areas of success and failure, subjective views, conformity or rebellion, and social roles the child developed while seeking to find a place in his or her family (Shulman & Mosak, 1988).

Therapeutic Goals

The Adlerian therapist's therapeutic goals for Sandra are presented next. These include encouraging hope, developing insight and awareness into her lifestyle dynamics, empathic mirroring, and stimulating social interest. Specifically, the Adlerian therapist would seek to achieve the following objectives:

1. To encourage hope that things can change and that Sandra's life can be better.

2. To help Sandra gain insight into her life style. This understanding includes how she came to develop the beliefs, expectations, unconscious organizing principles, and goals that characterize her lifestyle.

3. To help Sandra understand how she strives for significance and security in the world and the role that her fears, anxiety, and other symptoms play in her attempts to safeguard herself from what she perceives and experiences as a hostile, dangerous, and scary world.

4. To help Sandra understand how her actual experience of being victimized and betrayed as a child influenced the development of her current views of herself, others, and the world.

5. Through interpretation and empathic mirroring, help Sandra understand that her lifestyle conclusions were appropriate and adaptive during her childhood. Yet when used as assumptions about the present, those same conclusions tend to exaggerate the dangers in her current experience and lead to employing excessive degrees of control in an attempt to compensate for those exaggerated fears and anxieties.

6. To increase Sandra's awareness of cognitive style, that is, her perfectionistic expectations and her all-or-nothing thinking, by empathically confronting Sandra when she engages in these patterns. Also, to increase Sandra's understanding of the safeguarding purposes of these patterns.

7. To help Sandra understand the unconscious purposes of her dreams. More specifically, to help her understand how her nightmares serve to maintain her vigilance and her concern that some things in her current life are scary or threatening. The therapist could use metaphor, associations, or investigation of dream symbols to help Sandra explore the extent to which these concerns are real or imaginary.

8. To help Sandra understand the functions that her emotions (especially her fears and anxieties) serve in moving toward her subjective goal of safeguarding herself against anticipated danger.

9. For the therapist to remain aware of the potential for resistance and to keep the therapist's goals in alignment with Sandra's unconscious lifestyle movement and goals.

10. To increase Sandra's involvement with others and with her community. To help her experience a feeling of belonging in the world.

Though Sandra begins therapy with a very low level of trust and a significant degree of discouragement, Adlerians would anticipate that Sandra could achieve a relatively high level of coping. These coping skills include being able to reduce her fears and anxieties to a manageable level, develop mutually respectful relationships with others, experience a sense of satisfaction and gratification in her work, and, eventually, develop an emotionally rewarding intimate relationship.

Timeline for Therapy

The anticipated length of therapy would be 18 to 36 months. I would ask if Sandra would prefer to meet once or twice a week at the outset of therapy. The initial focus of therapy would be developing trust and overcoming potential resistance. Resistance would be assessed based on responses to interpretations and confrontations. The establishment of trust would be signaled by Sandra's willingness to explore her feelings and childhood hurts at a deeper level. Exploring the roots of her lifestyle, especially her experience of abuse and betrayal would be the focus of this middle phase of therapy. The final phase of therapy would focus on developing more constructive lifestyle beliefs and expectations and developing a more effective repertoire of behavioral coping strategies. It would be important to meet twice a week while doing this more intensive therapeutic work.

Case Conceptualization

Lifestyle. One's lifestyle beliefs and goals are conclusions one has reached about oneself, the world, and others based on one's subjective perception of experience, especially early childhood experience. Sandra's core beliefs or schema of apperception (Ansbacher & Ansbacher, 1964) and lifestyle goals may be summarized as follows (Shulman & Mosak, 1988):

> *Image of life and the world:* Life is hostile, dangerous, scary and threatening.

Image of self: I am vulnerable and victimized by others and by life. When I am alone, nowhere is safe.

Image of others: Others are untrustworthy, critical, treat me unfairly, and can hurt me at any time.

Therefore (goals): I must protect myself from situations that I believe may cause me harm.

Adlerians view behavior and emotions as nonconsciously created by the individual in order to safeguard the self. Sandra's anxiety and fears serve to keep her focus on potential dangers. Her behavioral responses to these fears also serve to keep her safe from anticipated harm.

Sandra also uses control as a mechanism (subgoal) for maintaining safety. Fear and anxiety are protective reactions stemming from her childhood experience of being doubly victimized. She was abused by her brother and blamed for destroying her mother's (and others') illusion of the family as perfect, an example of blaming the victim. She appears to have developed the lifestyle of a victim-martyr, using behaviors and fears in order to gain some feeling of control over hostile and hurtful forces, and to avoid being victimized again. Her convictions, feelings, and behaviors were realistic responses to her early childhood experience. In her current life, however, Sandra fears and control mechanisms appear exaggerated and unrealistic.

Sandra's attitude toward men is consistent with her overall lifestyle. She generates anger toward men (her father, men she supervises at work, her boyfriend). Her anger serves to keep her guard up while maintaining her view of herself as a victim.

Sandra's apparent mistaken belief that she must avoid mistakes at all costs is illustrated in her comments in the fourth session of therapy. Her therapist states, "So [mother] never recovered from the past. Is that it?" Sandra responds, "That's true and I've been paying for it ever since." She may have formed the belief that *One false move and you pay for it for the rest of your life. Therefore, I'd better not make any mistakes; I must strive to be perfect or I will pay.*

Developmental History and Family Constellation: Influences on the Development of Sandra's Lifestyle. The family constellation describes the social-interpersonal context of the client's first social group, and how, as a child, the client sought to find a place in the family group. In the Adlerian view, each child develops those qualities that he or she believes will allow him or her to achieve significance in the family structure (Shulman & Mosak, 1988). Note that these qualities of the lifestyle can sometimes be derived from objectively accurate events and experience. This is the case with many of Sandra's lifestyle convictions.

Sandra's biological mother is reported to have suffered from paranoid schizophrenia and had more than 30 psychiatric hospitalizations. Her mother also had strong fears concerning her daughter's safety. Thus, Sandra received early training (modeling) in developing irrational fears and exaggerating the dangers of life. Sandra *was* unfairly blamed for abuse in the family. In response to these and other discouraging childhood experiences, Sandra appears to have developed the expectation that others will criticize and blame her if she does something they don't like. In the present, Sandra continues to experience herself as a victim in her family. The family system apparently requires that she continue to play this role in order to maintain the family's homeostasis. For example, she reports in the fourth session that "All I hear from my family is criticism. It's like they gang up on me."

Sandra recalls slipping out of the house early on summer mornings with her siblings and spending the day playing outside the home (a strength). This suggests that she was able to have a pleasant time outside the home. She also slips out of the house now in the early morning. Perhaps this behavior is "over determined," serving multiple purposes at the same time. For example, slipping out of the house may now serve the purpose of avoiding contact and possible conflict with Sandra's family, while achieving the goal of avoiding being alone at work of which she is fearful.

Between the ages of 8 and 12, Sandra reports being repeatedly fondled by her two brothers and forced to look at their genitals. These events seem to have contributed to her developing the view that others (especially men) will invade and harm her; they can be malevolent, controlling, menacing, and not worthy of trust. This sexual abuse reinforced earlier experiences that led her to this conclusion and reinforced her self-image as a victim, grounded in the reality that she actually *was* a victim of abuse. Sandra's conclusion that men are not trustworthy and may desert and abandon her is also supported by her biological father's leaving soon after her birth. Sandra reports being abused by her adoptive mother, both physically (mother hitting Sandra and pulling her hair) and emotionally (mother threatening "If you don't behave, I'll send you back to the agency"). Sandra probably experienced this as additional evidence that she is unloved and, perhaps, even unlovable.

When she was 12, Sandra again became fearful of her 16-year-old brother, Brad, who reestablished his pattern of sexually fondling her.

This pattern is likely to have reinforced her view and experience of men: that their intrusion and attack might come at any time, and she is helpless to do anything to stop it. This belief seems related to her fear of an intruder breaking in at night. It seems likely that these earlier incidents occurred when it was dark.

Sandra reports that when she was 13 years old, her adoptive father engaged in an uncharacteristic drinking binge and made a sexual advance toward her, fondling her breasts and stopping when she became upset. Sandra's reaction was that the idealized image of her adoptive father was "shattered." She felt this incident was "devastating" and that it "ruined" her life. We can understand Sandra's feelings and conclusions based on this betrayal. Yet it also reflects Sandra's all-or-nothing thinking style. She appears to require that things (e.g., the behavior of others and herself) be error-free and believes that one event can ruin her life forever. Similarly, she is discouraged about being able to have a safe relationship with others.

It is reported that Sandra's mother accused her of lying when Sandra described the brother's sexual overtures in a letter. Sandra felt "completely abandoned" by her mother in her time of need. Indeed, she was abandoned. This example of blaming the victim underscores the fact that others in Sandra's life actually *have been* untrustworthy. Her lack of trust in others and her belief that others won't believe her and won't come to her aid are conclusions that are consistent with how she has been treated, especially by those in her biological and adoptive families. Thus, Sandra's healthy, appropriate emotional needs were not met. It seems likely that her physical needs were not consistently met either.

At age 19, Sandra finally found an advocate in her mother's friend, who took action against the priest and contacted the department of human services on her behalf. Despite this advocacy, Sandra was "damned if you do and damned if you don't": either she keeps quiet or she tells the truth and is blamed for smearing the family's reputation. Of course, it is the males in the family who are responsible for their inappropriate and abusive behavior. Their actions constituted the true betrayal and the disgrace. This experience served to strengthen Sandra's belief that any action she may take will "boomerang" and others who perpetrate the wrong will attempt to make her the perpetrator of the wrong. Put another way, Sandra received training in helplessness and hopelessness throughout her life. She also may have developed the assumption that she cannot solve her problems without creating more problems.

Sandra reports that she is "perfectionistic" and "constantly feels fearful that she may make a mistake or do a poor job." She feels she has to be "number one" in her boss's eyes and stated, "If I'm not, I'm nothing." Here again we see the expression of her lifestyle (and transference), this time in her approach to work. Her lifestyle belief may be stated as follows: "I must be perfect and avoid any mistakes, otherwise I will be attacked and helpless to defend myself." Sandra's all-or-nothing thinking is once again evident: "I must be number one or I am nothing."

Behavioral Movement and Goals.   Sandra has established a behavior pattern of arriving at 7 a.m. "precisely" when the security guard comes on duty so as to avoid being alone in the office. This pattern is a metaphor for her lifestyle movement and goal: to find, create, and arrange life so that she acts as her own security guard and safeguards herself from anticipated danger. Sandra's phobic symptoms also help her to strive for security and safety by attempting to control the perceived dangers in her life.

Adler suggested that neurosis is testimony to human creativity. Sandra's worrying behavior (others describe her as a worry-wort, she usually expects the worst to happen, she typically finds herself "jumping from one worry to another") and her worry about worrying are expressions of Sandra's creativity. She maintains a mental focus on worrying to support her belief and expectation that life is dangerous. From Sandra's subjective point of view, worrying is also a coping strategy—what Adlerians refer to as a safeguard mechanism—that serves the purpose of protecting Sandra by providing a sense of control. This psychological process may be stated as follows: If I constantly *think* about bad things that might happen, I have a better chance of preventing bad things from *actually* happening to me.

Dreams.   Adlerians view dreams as the "factory of the emotions" (Dreikurs, 1967). The dream's primary function is to generate an emotional stance in waking life (Gold, 1981; Shulman, 1973). Sandra reports that her nightmares often include people chasing her with weapons and that she has trouble getting away from them. A major purpose for Sandra's creation of this dream is to keep her afraid, maintain vigilance, and motivate her to get away from the perceived threat of physical harm.

Interpersonal Relationships.   Sandra is cautious in her interpersonal relationships and tends to remain aloof and wary of others. This stance, and her deep mistrust, serves the purpose of protecting her or at least keeping her alert to potential threats from others. It is as if she experiences herself as living in a hostile jungle. Thus, she feels she must be constantly alert to predators lurking in the bushes who prey on small and vulnerable mortals like herself. For example, Sandra reports that she cannot shower if no one is home with her. From the Adlerian view, Sandra sets conditions in order to control potential malevolent forces in the world. This is a generalization based on Sandra's actual experience of sexual abuse, intrusion, and betrayal.

Sandra's behavior of not going to church may serve one or more of the following purposes: to "drive [my] mom nuts," to gain some sense of influence and impact, to seek revenge for the injustice of mother's criticism and blame toward Sandra for "ruining" mother's false illusion of a perfect family, and to keep her distance from priests who may remind her of the priest who did not report Sandra's experience of abuse and thus failed to protect her.

Emotions and Their Purpose (Affective State). Emotions are nonconsciously generated by an individual based on the meaning the person attributes to a given situation in accordance with the individual's overall subjective organizing principle—their lifestyle. Like behaviors, emotions serve the purpose of safeguarding the self against perceived threats. Adlerians do not view affect as a *state* existing in a person, but as movement nonconsciously created by a person in the context of their social-interpersonal situation as perceived by that person.

Sandra generates her feelings of anxiety to create warning signals based on expectation of danger. Anxiety serves the purpose of alerting her to the need to create behavioral strategies designed to reduce the threat of danger.

Sandra states that fear rules her life. This metaphoric statement expresses her subjective view and experience: Fear is a controlling dictator and I am helpless to fight it. It is as if fear has power over her and her only option is to obey. Thus, Sandra's fears give her reasons and justification to keep herself safe by maintaining distance from others, sometimes telling others what they should or must do to protect her. For example, during a business trip Sandra "insisted that a coworker share her room so she would not have to be alone." Similarly, Sandra's tendency to remain emotionally aloof may be a way of keeping safe by maintaining distance from, and superiority in relation to, others. We might also guess that Sandra has concluded something like the following: *I had better base almost all of my decisions regarding what I do and don't do on my goal of anticipating and hopefully avoiding the bad things I believe and know will happen to me. Furthermore, because many bad things have actually happened to me in the past, I am justified in expecting the worst.* Sandra thus creates her fear to keep her safe from being traumatized again.

Following Adler's emphasis on dialectical thinking, Adlerian therapists focus on the implied but unstated opposite message to "I-can't" statements. Thus, Sandra's statement that she *can't* get the fear out of her mind, especially at night in the dark when she is alone, suggests an opposing message: I *can* keep my mental attention focused and riveted on my fear for long periods of time, especially when I am alone, when it is nighttime, and when it is dark. Her statements using the phrases "I don't" and "I have to" also indicate strategies that Sandra uses to quiet her fears.

Transference.   From the Adlerian point of view, transference is the expression of the client's lifestyle (beliefs, expectations and fears, behavioral tactics, and goals) in the relationship with the therapist (Mosak, 1977a). Sandra's lifestyle belief/expectation that others won't believe her suggests that she also may question whether the therapist believes her. It is anticipated that Sandra will want approval and acceptance from the therapist but may not let these feelings in because she also fears and expects that she won't get approval from others and that others (especially men) may not be trustworthy. I would guess that Sandra might experience a psychoanalytic approach that emphasizes therapist neutrality as rejection or lack of concern. On the other hand, Sandra may experience a therapist's using a directive style of therapy as controlling, arousing fears of not being in control of the therapy relationship and process.

Therapeutic contracts and outcome goals aimed at reducing Sandra's fears and anxiety may *reinforce and increase* Sandra's feeling of being out of control and thus be met with resistance due to the safeguarding function of these symptoms described earlier. The form of this resistance may be covert rather than overt. Sandra may agree to these goals and express a willingness to follow cognitive and behavioral change strategies with the hope that they might be helpful and as an expression of her desire to please the therapist. Paradoxically, any progress toward reducing her symptoms of fear and anxiety may cause an increase in anxiety if she feels that she is more vulnerable to the dangers, which her symptoms are unconsciously intended to ward off. Should this occur, the therapist may be able to overcome the resistance by realigning his or her goals with Sandra's unconscious lifestyle goals using reframing and empathic paradoxical strategies that are discussed later.

Strengths. Focusing on their clients' strengths is one of the ways Adlerian therapists offer encouragement and help build their clients' self-esteem. We also look for opportunities to reframe so-called weaknesses and problems, viewing them as strengths and attempts at problem solving. This is illustrated in the following discussion of Sandra's strengths.

Sandra acknowledges that not going to church drives her mom nuts. She shows insight into the purpose of this behavior when she reflects "Maybe that's why I do it." This is an encouraging sign and suggests that Sandra possesses the ability to develop insight and self-awareness of the dynamics behind her behavior.

Sandra is successful in the task of work. As a bank teller she earned several promotions and is currently a loan manager. She supervises 12 employees. She finds her job fulfilling yet stressful.

Sandra states that she ran way from home when she was 10 years old. In a metaphoric sense, she is still running (as symbolized in her dream), still trying to escape the menacing forces that she feels are chasing her but never being able to elude them. The dream indicates that Sandra is still trying to solve the problem of her fears. This is an indication of her persistence, determination, and a sign that, in spite of her discouragement, she has not given up hope.

Sandra's perfectionism, though exaggerated, does have a constructive side. Sandra seeks to perform well at work and strives to be "number one" in her boss's eyes. This suggests that she attempts to meet or even exceed the requirements of her job. In this way, Sandra's fear of making mistakes can serve to motivate her toward gaining a feeling of success.

That Sandra is seeking therapy is itself a positive sign. In addition, there are numerous examples that indicate Sandra is aware of her experience and the role that fear plays in her life. Sandra's ability to tune in to her inner experience and develop some insight are strengths that will serve her well in therapy.

It is impressive that Sandra finished in the top 25% of her high-school graduating class, given the abuse and turmoil she experienced in her youth. This accomplishment suggests that she can successfully distract herself and focus on mastering concepts and completing tasks. This is an excellent coping strategy. The therapist might employ this strength by offering interpretations that emphasize achieving insight and understanding. This approach might be especially helpful in the initial phase of therapy. The exploration of Sandra's feelings and their childhood origins could follow. To begin with an emotionally intensive approach might be too overwhelming for Sandra.

The Therapeutic Relationship

The Therapeutic Bond

The therapeutic bond in Adlerian therapy is characterized by cooperation, social equality and social interest. Although the therapist has certain knowledge and skills, this fact does not mean that the therapist is superior to the client. Thus, the Adlerian therapist demonstrates mutual respect in the therapeutic relationship at all times.

Roles in the Therapeutic Relationship

Adlerian therapists are active and interactive in the therapeutic relationship. Adlerians refer to four aspects of the therapeutic process (Dreikurs, 1967).

Developing the Therapeutic Alliance.   During the initial phase of therapy, the therapist develops rapport and a working alliance with the client by engaging the client in a collaborative process to identify the issues and problems the client wants to work on. The therapist seeks to understand the subjective experience of the client. The therapist models the expression of social interest, which Adler described, in part, as the ability to see with the eyes of another, hear with the ears of another, and feel with the heart of another.

Investigating Dynamics. A second aspect of psychotherapy— investigating dynamics—focuses on gaining an understanding of the client's lifestyle through interpretation of early recollections and family constellation discussed earlier. The therapist also seeks understanding of the client's movement and goals in the client's early and current relationships, including the client-therapist relationship. The result is the expression of deep empathy by the therapist and the client's feeling of being understood.

Developing Insight. In the third aspect of therapy, the development of insight is achieved through a variety of methods. As mentioned previously, Adlerian theory is both psychodynamic and cognitive. Those Adlerian therapists who emphasize the psychodynamic aspects of Adler's approach tend to prefer that clients generate their own insights. Guiding clients in exploring the metaphoric expressions of their lifestyle also emphasizes the therapist's role as facilitating a process within the client (Kopp, 1995, 1998, 1999). Adlerian therapists who emphasize the cognitive aspects of Adlerian therapy tend to offer interpretations of the beliefs and purposes of their client's behavior. Therapists using this approach tend to be more direct and confrontive (Shulman, 1971, 1972). Even so, most Adlerians offer interpretations using the phrase suggested by Rudolf Dreikurs (1967), "Could it be . . . ?" Thus, direct interpretation is not imposed on the client but offered for the client's consideration.

Reorientation: Stimulating Change. The fourth aspect of therapy, referred to as reorientation, involves changing one or more of the following: a client's unconscious organizing principles, beliefs and private logic, behaviors and symptoms, goals and purposes, and interpersonal functioning. To help stimulate change, Adlerians utilize an eclectic array of interventions drawn from psychodynamic, cognitive-behavioral, experiential-humanistic, and family-systems approaches. Special diagnoses such as alcoholism, PTSD, and phobias call for specialized techniques that are incorporated into Adlerian therapy, where appropriate. Some Adlerian therapists may emphasize techniques in which they have received special training such as hypnosis, psychodrama, couple therapy, or parent counseling.

Understanding and Dealing with Resistance. Although resistance may emerge at any point in Adlerian therapy, it is most likely to occur during the third and fourth phases of treatment. Kopp and Kivel (1990) describe an Adlerian model for understanding and resolving resistance in their article entitled "Traps and Escapes." They begin with the Adlerian distinction between stated movement, reflected in what the client says, and lifestyle movement, which is reflected in what the client does. It is not unusual for the client's stated movement to conflict with the client's actual movement, that is, the client's actions. When this occurs, the client is sending a paradoxical message. If the therapist accepts the stated message and proceeds to align the therapeutic goals with the client's stated movement, the therapist's goals become misaligned with the client's lifestyle movement and goals. The resulting therapeutic relationship is characterized by resistance, that is, a conflict of goals between the client and therapist.

Resolving the relational resistance requires that the therapist realign his or her therapeutic movement and goals with that of the client's lifestyle movement and goals. By doing so, the therapist is able to reestablish a cooperative relationship with the client (Kopp & Kivel, 1990; Mozdzierz, Macchitelli, & Lisiecki, 1976).

Note that the Adlerian conceptualization of resistance applies several key Adlerian concepts: that behavior is movement in a social (interpersonal) field, that behavior is nonconsciously created by the client for a purpose (usually also nonconscious), and that cooperation and goal alignment are the essence of a therapeutic relationship. Theories of psychotherapy that do not emphasize these constructs may limit understanding of the nonconscious, goal-directed, and relational dimensions of resistance and the importance of goal alignment in resolving resistance.

An Adlerian approach to understanding and dealing with Sandra's resistance is discussed later under "Potential Pitfalls."

Treatment Implementation and Outcomes

Techniques and Methods of Working

A variety of techniques and methods would be potentially helpful in working with Sandra. Some of these are listed below.

1. Sandra reported that when her biological mother sees Sandra she exclaims, "I thought you were dead!" It could be that Sandra's thoughts and fear of dying serve as ways of staying connected to her biological mother. The therapist might encourage Sandra to explore this by offering the following interpretation: "You mentioned that when your mother hasn't seen you for a period of time, she seems to assume you were dead. You also have fears of dying. Could it be that your own thoughts and fears of dying may be a way of staying connected with your mother?"

2. Sandra stated that "I also ruined her perfect world when I admitted the abuse in the past." The therapist might say, "Could it be that

you are still 'ruining it' by not going to church? I wonder if this is one way that you seek a sense of justice and fairness." Later the therapist may suggest that Sandra's private logic regarding her mother may go something like this: Since you won't give me the approval and acceptance I want from you no matter how much I do, then I am entitled to not do what you want me to do (e.g., not go to church).

3. Sandra stated that "I can't fall asleep at night. I have to fall asleep before my family does." The therapist might offer the following interpretation: "Could it be that your inability to fall asleep at night, your anxiety and fear that somebody might break into your house, and your fear of being alone each serve the purpose of creating a sense of security and safety by attempting to control the dangers in the world?"

4. Sandra says, "I can't even take a walk alone at night. I don't even watch the news. It scares me too much." The movement and purpose of these behaviors expresses the message, Look how bad things are for me—how much I am restricted by my fears and how victimized I am by them. The therapist might offer this as an interpretation, thereby aligning the therapist's goals with the lifestyle goals expressed in Sandra's behavior. For example, the therapist might say, "I can see the wisdom in your decision to not walk alone at night and not watch the news. It seems this would help you avoid exposing yourself to situations that you believe and expect will be threatening to your physical well-being. What do you think?"

5. Sandra's lifestyle movement is also reflected in the words "I can't," "I don't," and "I have to." Sandra feels compelled by her anxiety but doesn't realize the unconscious role she plays in generating her anxiety. Thus, the therapist might suggest, "Perhaps by remaining afraid you increase your chances of avoiding being mistreated or attacked in the real world. Better to maintain the fear then to let down your guard and be exposed to actual rather than anticipated dangers. Your anxiety symptoms may actually serve a creative function for you." This is typical of how Adlerians view anxiety disorders and symptoms (Ansbacher & Ansbacher, 1964; Dreikurs, 1967; Sperry & Carlson, 1993).

6. Sandra states that "No matter how hard I've tried [to win mother's love, protection and approval] it doesn't work." The therapist could empathically reflect this poignant statement, gently saying, "You yearn for your mother's love and approval and to be protected and supported by her, but no matter how hard you try she doesn't give it to you."

7. The following is an example of reframing a client's behavior as a strength. The purpose of such interventions is to offer encouragement

to the client. Thus, the therapist might say, "Sandra, your strategy for dealing with leaving work when it is dark shows creativity and planning. By parking under a light, running as fast as you can to your car, jumping into the car, and driving away as fast as you can, you minimize the threat of being attacked. This seems like a good example of how you serve as your own security guard. You are very skilled at devising strategies to keep you safe from the world and others."

8. It is noted that Sandra "has a difficult time controlling her worry." As an Adlerian, I hear this statement as "Sandra has a easy time creating anxiety." The psychodynamic reason that she has difficulty controlling her worry may be that her worry is generated as an attempt to *increase* her control of anticipated dangers. This conceptualization could be offered as an interpretation that might reframe her experience from worrying to focusing on her ability to brainstorm while looking for potential dangers and ways that things can go wrong. Further, the therapist could offer a gentle, empathic, supportive paradoxical intervention to establish an alignment of the therapist's therapeutic goals with Sandra's unconscious goal of worrying (Kopp & Kivel, 1990). For example, the therapist might say, "Could it be that your worrying may have a protective component? What do you think? How might worrying be a way that you try to protect yourself from danger?" Then later, "I wonder if it might be useful to notice when you are worrying and ask yourself how your worrying might serve the purpose of protecting you."

9. At some point I might consider a psychiatric referral to assess the need for medication to control anxiety. Antidepressive medication may be considered also if Sandra's level of depression increases as she gets in touch with the emotions associated with anger or rage, inner feelings of despair, and painful experiences in early childhood. I would also encourage Sandra to consider a referral to a molestation support group.

10. Sandra's success in school suggests that she might benefit from bibliotherapy in areas relevant to her symptoms, anxieties, and discouragenic beliefs.

11. I would use great caution assigning Sandra homework. This caution is based on the theoretical understanding that her current symptoms and beliefs serve to keep her safe. Any assignments designed to reduce Sandra's emotional and behavioral symptoms and cognitive distortions could, in fact, increase her anxiety and stimulate resistance. Should this occur, I would realign my goals with her resistance, using the techniques described under "Potential Pitfalls."

Medical and Nutrition Issues

I would want Sandra to have a complete physical at the beginning of treatment to identify any medical factors that may contribute to her symptoms and to rule out substance abuse.

Potential Pitfalls

Sandra doesn't feel able, and has had little or no experience of being able, to successfully prevent intrusion (her fear of someone "breaking in") and abuse from others. As a result, she may resist directive interventions designed to decrease her fears and anxiety because she maintains these symptoms as a way of keeping safe. If this occurs, Adlerians would shift to a paradoxical strategy that Adler referred to as "spitting in the patient's soup" (Ansbacher & Ansbacher, 1964; Kopp & Kivel, 1990; West, Main, & Zarski, 1986). This strategy involves respecting the client's symptoms as a coping strategy. Reframing the symptom as a coping strategy changes the client's relationship to the symptom.

For example, Sandra's statement that "fear rules my life" suggests that her subjective, metaphoric view and experience of fear is that of a dictator or tyrant (Kopp, 1995; Kopp & Craw, 1998). The therapist might reframe fear as a *benevolent* dictator, suggesting that it is a powerful friend, ally, and protector. This reframe would be followed with a suggestion that creates concordant alignment between the therapist's goal and the client's lifestyle goal reflected in the client's behavior (i.e., to continue to maintain the symptoms of fear and anxiety in the face of therapeutic interventions designed to decrease these symptoms). To achieve this alignment, the therapist might suggest the following:

> Because your fear serves to protect you, it makes sense that the thought of decreasing your fear and the protective behaviors it helps you generate would feel threatening to you and your sense of safety. Perhaps it would be better for us to drop our goal of reducing or eliminating the fear, at least for the present. Instead, it seems important that you continue to experience the fear and anxiety and continue to behave in ways that give you a feeling of safety. We can then discuss in greater detail how your fears and behaviors function so we can understand the dynamics behind them.

If the client agrees with this approach, the therapist might add, "So, it is important that you continue to experience fear and anxiety and come in next week ready to examine what you thought of, what you did, and how you felt whenever you experienced fear or anxiety."

Termination and Relapse Prevention

During termination, the client and therapist review and discuss their perspectives about the therapeutic work they have done together. In the Adlerian view, psychopathology and dysfunctional lifestyle beliefs, behaviors, and goals reflect a relatively low level of social interest, whereas healthy and constructive lifestyle beliefs, behaviors, and goals are characterized by a relatively high level of social interest. Thus, termination of Sandra's therapy would include an assessment of her present level of social interest expressed in the life tasks of work, love, and friendship (Adler, 1964).

Relapse will often be addressed during termination. I would discuss with Sandra the possible reoccurrence of her symptoms. I would suggest that the changes she has made in therapy are likely to mean that the intensity and duration of the symptoms may be diminished. I would add that should she feel stuck, she is always welcome to return for some additional work.

Mechanisms of Change

The following mechanisms of change in Adlerian therapy have the potential to contribute to constructive changes for Sandra. (Examples of these mechanisms were presented earlier in "Techniques and Methods of Working.") The relative importance of these mechanisms cannot be predetermined because they emerge out of the actual therapeutic work and include Sandra's subjective experience of the treatment.

1.   Developing a therapeutic relationship characterized by cooperation and mutual respect.

2.   Providing Sandra with the experience of being deeply understood by a fellow human being.

3.   Stimulating hope and encouragement in Sandra.

4.   Helping Sandra develop insight and awareness of her lifestyle and the purposes of her symptoms.

5.   Helping Sandra understand how her childhood experiences influenced her to develop (a) her current conclusions about herself, life, and others; and (b) the behaviors and symptoms that she believed would have the best chance of keeping her safe.

6.   Offering education regarding how people function (e.g., that we all strive for a feeling of security and significance and to overcome

feelings of inadequacy and insecurity, and that we create our emotions for the purpose of safeguarding the self from anticipated threat).

7.   Using reframing. For example, I would reframe Sandra's perceived weakness as strengths and her symptoms as coping mechanisms to keep herself safe.

8.   Using reframing as part of empathic paradox to resolve resistance by realigning my goal in therapy with Sandra's nonconscious lifestyle goal.

9.   Help Sandra develop her potential for expressing social interest, including increasing her involvement with others and her feeling of belonging to the human community.

CONCLUSION

Adler's holistic, social, teleological theory offers a unique synthesis of psychodynamic and cognitive approaches to psychotherapy that provides the Adlerian therapist with a conceptual base for employing a wide variety of interventions. Adlerian lifestyle theory and assessment methods facilitate rapid and deep understanding of the client's conscious and unconscious dynamics, subjective beliefs about self, life, and others, the meaning and purposiveness of behavior and symptoms, nature of discouragement, and the degree of social interest expressed in meeting the life tasks. The application of these concepts, assessment methods, and therapeutic interventions is illustrated in the case of Sandra.

REFERENCES

Adler, A. (1964). *Problems of neurosis.* New York: Harper.

Adler, A. (1981). Position in family constellation influences life style. In L. Baruth & D. Eckstein (Eds.), *Life-style: Theory, practice, and research* (2nd ed., pp. 15–23). Dubuque, IA: Kendall/Hunt.

Ansbacher, H., & Ansbacher, R. (1964). *The individual psychology of Alfred Adler: A systematic presentation in selections from his writings.* New York: Harper & Row.

Dinkmeyer, D., & Dreikurs, R. (1963). *Encouraging children to learn: The encouragement process.* Englewood Cliffs, NJ: Prentice-Hall.

Dinkmeyer, D., & Eckstein, D. (1993). *Leadership by encouragement.* Dubuque, IA: Kendall/Hunt.

Dinkmeyer, D., & McKay, G. (1976). *Systematic training for effective parenting.* Circle Pines, MN: American Guidance Service.

Dreikurs, R. (1967). *Psychodynamics, psychotherapy, and counseling.* Chicago: Alfred Adler Institute of Chicago.

Dreikurs, R. (1971). *Social equality: The challenge of today.* Chicago: Adler School of Professional Psychology.

Dreikurs, R., with Solz, V. (1964). *Children: The challenge.* New York: Hawthorn.

Gold, L. (1981). Life-style of dreams. In L. Baruth & D. Eckstein (Eds.), *Life-style: Theory, practice, and research* (2nd ed., pp. 24–30). Dubuque, IA: Kendall/Hunt.

Kopp, R. (1986). Styles of striving for significance with and without social interest: An Adlerian typology. *Individual Psychology, 42*(1), 17–24.

Kopp, R. (1995). *Metaphor therapy: Using client-generated metaphors in psychotherapy.* New York: Brunner/Mazel.

Kopp, R. (1997). Healing community: An Adlerian approach. *Individual Psychology, 53*(1), 23–32.

Kopp, R. (1998). Early recollections in Adlerian and metaphor therapy. *The Journal of Individual Psychology, 54,* 480–486.

Kopp, R. (1999). Metaphoric expressions of lifestyle: Exploring and transforming client-generated metaphors. *The Journal of Individual Psychology, 55,* 466–473.

Kopp, R., & Craw, M. (1998). Metaphoric language, metaphoric cognition, and cognitive therapy. *Psychotherapy, 35,* 306–311.

Kopp, R., & Kivel, C. (1990). Traps and escapes: An Adlerian approach to understanding resistance and resolving impasses in psychotherapy. *Individual Psychology, 46,* 139–147.

Mosak, H. (1972). Life style assessment: A demonstration focused on family constellation. *Journal of Individual Psychology, 28,* 232–247.

Mosak, H. (1977a). Predicting the relationship to the psychotherapist from early recollections. In H. Mosak (Ed.), *On purpose* (pp. 87–92). Chicago: Alfred Adler Institute of Chicago.

Mosak, H. (1977b). Early recollections as a projective technique. In H. Mosak (Ed.), *On purpose* (pp. 60–75). Chicago: Alfred Adler Institute of Chicago.

Mozdzierz, G., Macchitelli, F., & Lisiecki, J. (1976). The paradox in psychotherapy: An Adlerian perspective. *Journal of Individual Psychology, 32,* 169–183.

Shulman, B. (1962). The family constellation in personality diagnosis. *Journal of Individual Psychology, 18*(1), 35–47.

Shulman, B. (1971). Confrontation techniques in Adlerian psychotherapy. *Journal of Individual Psychology, 27,* 167–175.

Shulman, B. (1972). Confrontation techniques. *Journal of Individual Psychology, 28,* 177–183.

Shulman, B. (1973). An Adlerian theory of dreams. In B. Shulman (Ed.), *Contributions to individual psychology* (pp. 60–80). Chicago: Alfred Adler Institute of Chicago.

Shulman, B., & Mosak, H. (1988). *Manual for life style assessment.* Muncie, IN: Accelerated Development.

Sicher, L. (1955). Education for freedom. *The American Journal of Individual Psychology, 11*(2), 97–103.

Sperry, L., & Carlson, J. (1993). *Psychopathology and psychotherapy: From diagnosis to treatment.* Muncie, IN: Accelerated Development.

West, J., Main, F., & Zarski, J. (1986). The paradoxical prescription in individual psychology. *Individual Psychology, 42,* 214–224.

9

Interpersonal Psychotherapy

Reed D. Goldstein and Alan M. Gruenberg

TREATMENT MODEL

Interpersonal psychotherapy (IPT), a focused, time-limited research-based psychotherapy, was initially developed for the treatment of depression. IPT was extensively studied in the NIMH Collaborative Study of Psychotherapy of Depression (Elkin et al., 1989). To date, the efficacy of IPT for depression has been demonstrated in controlled clinical trials (Elkin et al., 1989). More recently, the IPT model for depression has been modified to treat other clinical presentations, including dysthymic disorder, bipolar disorder, depression related to medical illness, substance use disorders, and eating disorders. Research is currently underway to evaluate the efficacy of IPT in the treatment of social phobia, panic disorder, and post-traumatic stress disorder (for review see Weissman, Markowitz, & Klerman, 2000).

The IPT treatment model consists of five essential characteristics (Klerman et al., 1984). IPT is time-limited rather than long-term psychotherapy, focused rather than open-ended, and attends to the *current* life situation of the patient (i.e., here-and-now relationships). IPT also concentrates on the interpersonal realm as opposed to the intrapsychic or cognitive-behavioral. Although cognizant of the impact of personality on treatment response, the IPT therapist does not attempt to change enduring traits.

Proponents of the IPT approach acknowledge that characterologic traits or personality style shape an individual's response to a social interaction. IPT therapists also accept that psychiatric conditions, such as major depressive disorder or generalized anxiety disorder, and associated signs and symptoms involve both biological and psychological precipitants. However, the IPT model professes that a psychiatric disorder occurs within the context of interpersonal relationships. IPT is designed to alleviate symptoms, such as depression or anxiety, by specifically focusing upon the patient's current stressors in interpersonal relationships as well as the stress response associated with those relationships.

The IPT model incorporates three phases of treatment (Klerman et al., 1984). Phase 1 consists of approximately three sessions during which time the therapist performs a comprehensive diagnostic evaluation (including use of instruments/rating scales), completes a psychiatric history, and describes the framework for treatment. The therapist is expected to be thoroughly familiar with *DSM* criteria for disorders such as major depressive disorder and generalized anxiety disorder. This phase also permits evaluation of the role of medication in treatment. The therapist reviews the presenting symptoms, confirms that the patient has an illness, and describes the expected course of treatment. In this way, IPT assigns the "sick role" to the patient and emphasizes a medical model.

An important component of the psychiatric history, the *interpersonal inventory*, refers to an exhaustive review of the patient's social functioning and pattern of relationships at the time of treatment. The inventory draws attention to the association of current symptom onset, or maintenance of symptoms, and a change in an important current relationship (e.g., abandonment and onset of panic attack; death of a loved one and onset of depression; physical trauma and onset of social withdrawal or post-traumatic states). The association between symptoms and interpersonal change forms the foundation of the treatment framework: understanding the interpersonal context of symptoms such as anxiety or depression. During phase 1, the IPT therapist educates the patient about the association between symptom onset or maintenance of symptoms and current problematic interpersonal situations.

Consequently, the treatment formulation identifies four potential interpersonal problem areas: (a) grief or complicated bereavement, (b) interpersonal role disputes, (c) role transitions, and (d) interpersonal deficits. Complicated bereavement occurs when an episode of depression is associated with an abnormal grief reaction, such as when the individual does not negotiate the phases of the mourning process. Interpersonal role disputes occur between spouses or lovers and family members, including children or work associates and friends. In role transitions, relocation (e.g., to a new school, job, home) or change in economic or marital status are often identified as primary stressors. The patient's experience of loneliness or social isolation suggests a need to address his or her area of interpersonal deficits. The end of the first phase of IPT culminates in the formation of a treatment contract between therapist and patient to work on the relevant problem area.

During phase 2, the therapist establishes goals and uses specific strategies associated with the distinctive interpersonal problem area. Goals associated with alleviation of grief include facilitating the mourning process and establishing new relationships to replace those that have been lost. When a patient struggles with interpersonal role disputes, goals include the identification of the dispute, determination of a plan or course of action to resolve the dispute, and identification of faulty communications or expectations. Goals for difficulties with role transition include mourning the loss of the previous role and developing a positive view of the new role by improving mastery and self-esteem. IPT goals for the problem area of interpersonal deficits include a reduction in social isolation and the establishment of new relationships. The reader is referred to Weissman et al. (2000) for a detailed presentation of the various strategies associated with the goals for each of the four identified interpersonal problem areas.

Phase 3 is associated with the consolidation of gains made throughout the time-limited psychotherapy as well as a concentration on topics related to termination. During the termination phase, the IPT therapist and patient openly acknowledge the end of therapy, review ways to increase independent functioning of the patient, clarify the warning signs of anxiety or depression, review poor response to treatment (if relevant), and discuss the role of continuation or maintenance of treatment. Commonplace techniques associated with phase 3 include, but are not limited to, review of accomplishments, promotion of affect, and clarification.

To our knowledge, researchers have not modified IPT for the treatment of specific phobia and generalized anxiety disorder, the two diagnoses assigned to Sandra who is the subject of this book's case presentation. However, anxiety is noted to impact directly upon social situations and relationships in certain types of anxiety disorders. Sandra's anxiety certainly seems to impact on her interpersonal relationships (e.g., her fears of being alone). For example, social phobia involves mostly interpersonal symptomatology and thus presents an appropriate area in which to investigate the efficacy of IPT (Weissman et al., 2000). The goal in an IPT treatment of anxiety disorder is to decrease symptoms by improving social function. Weissman et al. (2000) review research asserting that issues such as rejection sensitivity, avoidance of conflict, and a passive orientation (e.g., difficulty with expression of anger or assertiveness) represent a focus in the modification of IPT applicable to social phobia and other anxiety disorders. These interpersonal difficulties are referred to as role insecurity. In another example, Weissman et al. (2000) maintain that disturbance in expectations about one's life (i.e., role transition) may be a consequence of panic symptoms and therefore may be amenable to a modified version of IPT.

In addition, the development of an IPT group format approach is underway for the treatment of post-traumatic stress disorder (PTSD) (Weissman et al., 2000). This group intervention highlights symptoms of PTSD in the context of current difficulties in interpersonal relationships. Emphasis is placed upon the four problem areas used in IPT for depression. IPT for PTSD centers upon the impact of trauma on relationships, specifically trust, clarification of cues for danger, and intimacy.

THE THERAPIST'S SKILLS AND ATTRIBUTES

The IPT therapist communicates warmth, is nonjudgmental, and advocates for patients. Notably, the IPT therapist explicitly assures the patient that the depression or anxiety symptom constellation is treatable. The therapist also instills hope for change (Weissman et al., 2000). In IPT, the therapeutic relationship is not formulated to emphasize transference. The therapeutic relationship is not considered to be a friendship. Typically, patient-therapist interactions are not explored. However, positive and negative transference reactions are addressed when a direct challenge to the treatment occurs (e.g., missed sessions or recurrent tardiness). When interpersonal deficits such as social isolation are identified, attention to the nuances of the patient-therapist relationship could help to identify similar difficulties in other relationships. The IPT therapist may also help the patient develop new approaches to interpersonal relationships. Though the therapist is active rather than passive, neither direct advice or reassurance are offered.

Training requirements for the IPT therapist are stipulated to include some type of advanced degree, including MD, PhD, MSW, or RN, in keeping with the multidisciplinary background of the originators of IPT. Experience in providing psychotherapy in general is necessary. The formal training program consists of four basic components (Weissman et al., 2000): (a) familiarity with the IPT manual, (b) participation in an IPT course, (c) use of videotaped cases during formal supervision, and (d) receipt of certification.

THE CASE OF SANDRA

Assessment, Conceptualization, and Treatemnt Planning

Assessment

The IPT approach requires a formal assessment of *DSM-IV* syndromes during the initial phase. The case indicates that its subject, Sandra, was administered various diagnostic instruments including the Anxiety Disorders Interview Schedule-Revised and Millon Clinical Multiaxial Inventory (MCMI-II). Sandra was noted to have met criteria for specific phobia and generalized anxiety disorder based upon the diagnostic instruments specified in the case. The MCMI-II has been criticized for the absence of a scale associated with post-traumatic stress disorder. However, the most recent version (MCMI-III; Millon, 1997) now includes a Post-traumatic Stress Disorder scale (scale T). Moreover, on the MCMI, the Anxiety Disorder scale (scale A), which presumably is elevated to a clinically significant degree consistent with Sandra's clinical presentation, is not necessarily specific to generalized anxiety disorder, particularly if the individual manifests specific phobia or has experienced trauma.

Therefore, in addition to mood rating instruments used to assess response to pharmacotherapy and psychotherapy (discussed later) and the third edition of the MCMI, we recommend the use of the Trauma Symptom Inventory (TSI) (Briere, 1995). The TSI consists of multiple questions that tap both acute and chronic post-traumatic symptomatology. The TSI is designed to assess responses or behavior consistent with current trauma as well as trauma from a distant time frame, that is, not necessarily the preceding 6 months. For Sandra, the administration of the TSI may be especially helpful given that she experienced early childhood loss and abuse years prior to the current treatment. Sandra's apparent degree of anxiety and avoidance as well as a history of schizophrenia in the family supports consideration of projective assessment techniques, although they are not required by the IPT approach. The Rorschach Inkblot Test, for example, may help to delineate the integrity of Sandra's ego function including level of reality testing, defensive function, and object relations. Sandra's capacity to think and perceive in a logical and reality-oriented fashion and her ability to tolerate significant stress without becoming transiently (or diffusely) disorganized are crucial to evaluate, especially in light of her family history of schizophrenia and her own pronounced avoidance and anxiety. The use of projective assessment techniques may clarify the extent, if any, of suspiciousness or overt paranoia. For example, Sandra is described as being "emotionally aloof . . . superficial . . . [having] a lack of trust seems to permeate all her relationships." Sandra herself stated, "I don't trust anybody."

Therapeutic Goals

For the present purpose, aspects of Sandra's clinical presentation may be amenable to intervention with IPT. The early sessions of IPT would focus on clarification of Sandra's symptoms and formal psychiatric diagnosis, the need for medication (see below), and assignment of the sick role. Rather than suggest that Sandra's symptoms are her fault, the therapist would inform Sandra that she has a medical illness (generalized anxiety disorder) with a favorable prognosis. Taking an interpersonal inventory is crucial during the early phase of treatment. The IPT therapist would need to understand fully the nature of Sandra's current relationships with her boyfriend, subordinates at work, and family before successfully identifying one of the four major problem areas that would become the focus of intervention. In addition, a comprehensive assessment of Sandra's interpersonal functioning may help to clarify the extent and pervasiveness of her long-standing vulnerability to anxiety and social isolation.

The IPT therapist and Sandra would work together in a collaborative manner to fully review her past and current important relationships in order to clarify the nature of her present interactions, maintenance of anxiety and social isolation, and acute exacerbations of symptoms when they occur. Weissman et al. (2000) describe the interpersonal inventory and recommend a systematic review of the patient's interactions with important individuals by clarifying the nature of:

1. interactions with the patient, including frequency of contact, activities shared, and so on;
2. the expectations of each party in the relationship, including some assessment of whether these expectations were or are fulfilled;
3. the satisfactory and unsatisfactory aspects of the relationship, with detailed examples of both kinds of interactions;
4. the ways the patient would like to change the relationship, whether through changing his or her own behavior or bringing about changes in the other person (p. 46).

Based on information presented in the case, two major problem areas can be identified in accordance with the IPT model. First, Sandra "is quick to snap at subordinates at work and her boyfriend has complained that she is overly irritable with him." Therefore, Sandra's behavior and symptoms might be conceptualized as representing the area of interpersonal role dispute. Accordingly, the goals of IPT would be to fully identify and understand the dispute (e.g., between Sandra and her boyfriend and Sandra and her subordinates), choose a plan of action, and bring about an acceptable resolution by modifying expectations or problematic communication style. Psychotherapeutic strategies may include (a) undertaking a review of Sandra's symptoms of anxiety; (b) defining the connection between the maintenance or acute exacerbation of anxiety with an overt or more subtle dispute between Sandra and a significant other; (c) specifying the nature of the dispute (e.g., impasse in relationship; difficulty in negotiations about important issues); (d) reviewing differences in communication style and in expectations; and (e) determining options as well as assessing available resources to promote change.

Notably, however, the case presentation underscores Sandra's chronic struggles with avoidance, dependency, emotional aloofness in the few interpersonal relationships she has sustained, an absence of strong feelings, and a lack of trust. These descriptions can be understood as symptoms associated with another major problem area identified in the IPT model: interpersonal deficits.

When interpersonal deficits are identified as the major problem area, the course of IPT helps to lessen the patient's loneliness and social isolation as well as develop new meaningful relationships. The interpersonal inventory clarifies the positive and negative features of important past and current relationships. Particular emphasis is placed on the identification of recurrent patterns. For example, in this case emphasis would be placed upon Sandra's ongoing experience of feeling invalidated. Attention to the patient-therapist relationship, necessary when interpersonal deficits are identified, provides information about how the patient is likely to interact with others (Weissman et al., 2000). Consequently, Sandra's feelings (whether positive or negative) about her relationship with the therapist would be reviewed and patterns would be identified.

In the IPT model, when interpersonal deficits are identified, a primary therapeutic goal would be for Sandra to recognize the association between problematic social skills and the maintenance of her anxiety as well as her experience of loneliness or social isolation. The identification of interpersonal deficits as the major problem area to be addressed by IPT requires the use of strategies in order to accomplish two specific goals: reduction of Sandra's social isolation, and support or encouragement around development of new relationships.

Timeline for Therapy

During the early phase of IPT, the therapist and Sandra would arrive at the primary psychiatric diagnosis and review the need for medication. Also, Sandra and her therapist would contract for weekly psychotherapy sessions to last for 12 to 16 weeks, in accordance with the focused and time-limited nature of IPT.

Case Conceptualization

Sandra is described as having "lived her life in a constant state of apprehension and fear ... [and being] trapped in her phobic world and paralyzed by avoidances." However, in the context of disabling symptoms and interpersonal difficulties, Sandra exhibits many strengths that she may be able to use during her treatment. For example, the case describes Sandra as "capable, attractive [and] professional." She is young and distressed. Although Sandra seeks treatment at the urging of her boyfriend, she may be motivated for change. Sandra struggles in her social interactions but has sustained a 5-year relationship with her boyfriend. The case suggests that Sandra achieved success in an academic setting (above-average student in high school; graduated in the upper 25% of her class). She is portrayed as being a "committed employee," having earned promotions, and as having "worked hard to achieve a sense of satisfaction in her life."

However, we maintain that in young adulthood, at age 26, the prominence of Sandra's anxiety, fear, and avoidance raise significant concern about the extent of her detachment, disconnectedness, and possible depersonalization. Often, these phenomena are associated with PTSD in general. Post-traumatic experiences are associated with unremitting panic and fearfulness. These experiences may even appear as severe psychiatric disturbance, such as vulnerability to psychosis.

The extent to which Sandra is capable of negotiating the breadth and severity of her multiple traumas (e.g., parental loss, parental rejection, overt transgression of body, more general violation of sexual boundaries, as well as the intruder breaking into her house) without developing post-traumatic symptomatology is an essential diagnostic question in this case. Moreover, Sandra's mother is identified as having paranoid schizophrenia. The genetic vulnerability and family environmental trauma would lead the treating clinician, in a carefully conducted longitudinal assessment, to follow Sandra's propensity for the development of psychosis. We recommend that the therapist maintain an open and flexible approach to revising the diagnostic formulation and provision of treatment to Sandra.

The Therapeutic Relationship

The Therapeutic Bond

Sandra has suffered through recurrent experiences of being invalidated. She has been emotionally, physically, and sexually abused. These feelings and experiences may impact upon her ability to trust in psychotherapy and underscore the importance of developing a therapeutic bond.

The authors have reviewed important therapist skills and attributes in an earlier section of this chapter. In the IPT model, a therapeutic bond would be more likely to occur when the therapist is nonjudgmental, communicates warmth, and instills hope for change by providing diagnostic clarification, education, and reassurance that Sandra's symptoms are treatable. The IPT therapist is called upon to actively convey acceptance, respect, and trust. In many respects, Sandra is unable to feel secure and develop trust in the context of important social relationships. The IPT therapist would strive to help Sandra contain her intense anxiety and dependent strivings. For example, it would be crucial for the therapist to form and maintain appropriate therapeutic boundaries, especially in the context of Sandra's history of abuse.

Roles in the Therapeutic Relationship

The therapeutic relationship in IPT is not formulated to emphasize transference or to more generally focus upon the patient-therapist relationship. However, Weissman et al. (2000) review the importance of the patient-therapist relationship when the issue of interpersonal deficits, including social isolation, is the identified major problem area. In the context of long-standing anxiety and social isolation, the relationship between Sandra and her therapist is likely to offer meaningful information about her interpersonal functioning. The nature of the interactions between Sandra and her therapist would provide a context in which the clinician could model appropriate social skills such as trust and intimacy. Consequently, Sandra would be encouraged to discuss any positive or negative feelings she harbored pertaining to the therapist or treatment. Weissman et al. (2000) underscore that the therapist-patient relationship serves as a model for learning how to resolve uncomfortable feelings within an interpersonal context. For example, the IPT therapist must work with Sandra to prevent a premature termination of treatment, thereby diminishing the likelihood of Sandra once again experiencing feelings of loneliness and a sense of invalidation.

Treatment Implementation and Outcome

Techniques and Methods of Working

IPT and Pharmacotherapy. The IPT treatment formulation includes a role for combined pharmacotherapy and IPT. Antianxiety medications, either alone or in combination with psychotherapy, have demonstrated efficacy in multiple anxiety disorders (Ballenger, 1999). Evaluation of the role of medication would occur during the early phase of Sandra's IPT treatment through a psychiatric consultation.

A clinical psychiatrist trained in IPT could effectively integrate the appropriate pharmacotherapy and psychotherapy. Alternatively, a collaborative model could be used by a nonphysician therapist and psychiatrist as long as they adhered to a well-defined collaborative treatment model.

In this case, the initial step in psychiatric consultation would focus on a complete working diagnostic understanding and an evolution of a diagnostic formulation communicated to Sandra in a straightforward, compassionate manner. Sandra experienced significant early trauma and currently struggles with prominent anxiety, fear, and avoidance. The severity of early and persistent symptoms of panic, generalized anxiety, phobic avoidance, and depression often cluster when there is co-occurring post-traumatic symptomatology.

Specific medical recommendations involve education of the patient toward self-monitoring of symptoms of anxiety and depression using standardized instruments for self-assessment. We customarily administer the Hamilton Depression scale (Hamilton, 1960) and Anxiety (Hamilton, 1959) Rating scale or Beck Depression (Beck et al., 1961) and Anxiety (Beck et al., 1988) Inventories to each patient in order to educate about the signs and symptoms that would be the target of treatment. In addition, we provide patients with daily mood rating instruments in order to assess response to pharmacotherapy and psychotherapy. For Sandra, the hallmark of pharmacotherapy includes adequate high-potency benzodiazepine treatment to bring remission and recovery from anxious symptomtalogy, including palpitations, sweating, muscle restlessness, and muscle tension. The standard anti-panic anti-anxiety treatment usually involves use of a longer acting high-potency medication such as clonazepam (Klonopin) to bring resolution of acute symptomatology.

Specifically, standard antianxiety treatment would include careful introduction of clonazepam (Klonopin), 0.5 mg up to 1.5 mg daily in the initial 2 to 3 weeks of treatment. If the persistent syndrome remained generalized anxiety disorder, then venlafaxine extended release (Effexor XR), beginning 37.5 mg daily up to 75 mg daily, would represent an appropriate initial dosing. The clinician would carefully monitor treatment response over the next 6 weeks. If there was remission of the symptoms, then ongoing pharmacotherapy would be continued during the next 12 months. A subsequent decision regarding maintenance pharmacotherapy would follow, depending on the overall response to combined pharmacotherapy and psychotherapy.

The initial antianxiety response to clonazepam occurs between 5 and 10 days. The choice to introduce antianxiety antidepressant pharmacotherapy is based on a model of heightened cortisol and neurotransmitter dysregulation that is seen in most anxiety states. These biological changes occur in childhood and adolescence in response to exposure to environmental trauma (Yehuda, 2000).

Following the introduction of clonazepam, acute resolution of anxious symptoms allows for more deliberate decision-making regarding the indication for antianxiety antidepressant medications. We monitor carefully for the evolution of persistent depressive symptomatology upon resolution of overt anxious symptoms.

The choices of antidepressant pharmacotherapy include standard selective serotonin reuptake inhibitors (SSRI) that have been approved for use in major depressive disorder, panic disorder, obsessive compulsive disorder, and PTSD, such as sertraline (Zoloft). In addition, venlafaxine extended release has been approved by the FDA in the treatment of generalized anxiety disorder.

The ongoing assessment following resolution of Sandra's overt anxious symptoms would guide the choice of a first-line antidepressant. If the predominant symptomatology was consistent with generalized anxiety disorder, a broader spectrum antidepressant such as venlafaxine would be indicated. If the persistent symptomatology was consistent with PTSD then the SSRI sertraline (Zoloft) would be a first-line choice, given its recent approval by the FDA for the treatment of PTSD.

In summary, Sandra would benefit from standard assessment of anxiety and depressive symptomatology in a carefully monitored pharmacotherapy, which is completely consistent with provision of the sick role, use of the medical model, and more general principles of IPT.

IPT Components. The case presents information suggesting that Sandra encounters role disputes and struggles with a lack of social skills. Weissman et al. (2000) advocate focusing on the interpersonal problem area (e.g., role dispute) instead of interpersonal deficits when the two problem areas coexist. Individuals who evidence impaired social skills and have interpersonal deficits are found to be more psychiatrically disturbed.

However, in our opinion, Sandra's long-standing social isolation, lack of meaningful relationships, and chronic and disabling symptoms of anxiety override transient role disputes such as irritable behavior toward her boss and boyfriend. Rather than a dispute with her boss or boyfriend, it is Sandra's chronic struggles with isolation, avoidance, and emotional aloofness that interfere directly with the development of relationships, and this compels the IPT therapist to identify interpersonal deficits as the major problem area. A diagnostic evaluation, review of medication issues, use of the interpersonal inventory, and establishment of a treatment contract would unfold during the early phase of IPT. Weissman et al. (2000) recommend asking these important questions:

- Do you have close relationships? With whom?
- Tell me about your current friends, your close family. What do you enjoy with them? What problems do you have with them?
- Do you find it hard to make friends?
- Is it hard for you to keep close relationships once you make them?
- Is getting close to people something you enjoy or would like to do? What about it makes you uncomfortable?
- How can you find friends and activities now that you used to enjoy in the past? (p. 105)

In the middle phase, Sandra would be encouraged to address the negative and positive aspects of important past and current relationships. Also, the patient-therapist relationship is more critical during IPT with the individual who is socially isolated relative to those with different problem areas. Sandra will be encouraged to solve problems rather than enter into an impasse with the therapist, with the hope of establishing a template or model to be used in interpersonal situations outside the therapy relationship.

Two specific techniques are recommended during the middle phase of IPT with the individual who has social-skills deficits and significant isolation: communication analysis and role-playing. In Sandra's case, the goal of communication analysis would be to help her communicate more effectively by reviewing exchanges between herself and significant others as well as through the identification of long-standing patterns. For example, Sandra can be encouraged to communicate in an explicit, direct fashion instead of in an indirect or nonverbal manner. Sandra's assumptions about what has been communicated or understood can be explored in the context of her relationship with her boyfriend, family, subordinates at work, or in the therapy itself. Patients who are isolated or unable to feel comfortable in relationships tend to express themselves indirectly, silently, or remove themselves from the interaction (e.g., premature treatment termination). Consequently, Sandra's attention would be drawn to her faulty communication patterns (e.g., communication based on lack of trust or strong feelings; assumptions made in the context of snapping at subordinates or irritability expressed toward boyfriend).

In IPT, Sandra may benefit from role-playing anxiety-producing situations, a technique found to be especially helpful in the treatment of those with interpersonal deficits. For example, the IPT therapist would take on the role of an important person in Sandra's life (her boyfriend, subordinate at work, or family member). In IPT, role-playing provides the patient with an opportunity to clarify his or her feelings and manner of communication style. Role-playing permits a review or practice of healthier ways to relate to others as well. In Sandra's treatment, the IPT therapist might play the role of the boyfriend in order to further clarify the specific nature of Sandra's irritability. Furthermore, the therapist could encourage Sandra to pretend she is entering her family's house or an office filled with her work subordinates. Sandra would be encouraged to discuss how she might initiate conversation in each of those situations.

Medical and Nutritional Issues

The standard consultation also involves a comprehensive laboratory evaluation of the patient that includes complete blood count with differential, metabolic profile with evaluation of renal and liver function, thyroid evaluation, and broad-based screening for infectious or inflammatory diseases. Careful attention to appropriate general medical hygiene includes adequate hydration (eight 8 oz. glasses of water daily and three regular meals). Sandra may be particularly focused on the overt symptoms of generalized anxiety and fear and may neglect basic principles of good medical hygiene. She will require careful attention to her allergy-related upper respiratory problems.

Potential Pitfalls

Whereas Sandra exhibits many strengths, which have been discussed, and is identified as having specific phobia and generalized anxiety disorder (two relatively treatable conditions), potential pitfalls could be envisioned during the course of IPT. The evolution of Sandra's anxiety disorder into comorbid major depressive disorder or post-traumatic stress disorder must be entertained, even though those symptoms are not overtly identified in the case presentation. Furthermore, given Sandra's family history, the possibility of underlying vulnerability to psychosis must be monitored as well as her probable identification with her mother (anxiety around need to feel safe; fearing that some day she will have a nervous breakdown like her mother). The evolution of Sandra's symptoms into PTSD, major depressive disorder, or a primary psychotic disorder represents a potential pitfall, and the therapist is encouraged to remain open and flexible regarding the diagnostic formulation.

Regardless of *DSM-IV* diagnosis, Sandra's struggles with dependency, inability to trust, avoidance, and superficiality may impact upon her ability to settle comfortably into a safe and collaborative working relationship. The therapist is called upon to establish and monitor appropriate boundaries and working environment, necessary factors in any therapeutic relationship, but especially in the context of Sandra's history of emotional, physical, and sexual abuse. More generally, Sandra has likely struggled with a recurrent experience of being invalidated. These feelings may impact upon her ability to tolerate distress or success in treatment.

Termination and Relapse Prevention

Issues pertaining to termination, such as mourning the end of treatment and bolstering the patient's sense of competence and independence, would be addressed during the final 2 to 4 sessions of IPT. Often, patients with personality disorder or interpersonal deficits are identified as being in need of long-term treatment. In Sandra's case, the IPT therapist would be encouraged to refer her elsewhere upon completion of the 12 to 16 week course of treatment. Another alternative is for the Sandra and the IPT therapist to develop a new treatment contract that will emphasize a different focus.

Mechanisms of Change

Information obtained during a systematic review of Sandra's current relationships and life events will clarify that she struggles with interpersonal deficits and could possess a vulnerability to post-traumatic symptomatology as well as psychosis. Consequently, promotion of the sick role, use of the interpersonal inventory, and identification of Sandra's social isolation and lack of meaningful relationships are crucial. The establishment of a treatment contract, as well as specific interventions such as communication analysis and role-playing, will instill hope for symptom reduction and positive change.

It is hoped that the experience of combined IPT and pharmacotherapy will not serve as another opportunity for Sandra to feel invalidated.

Rather, the therapist's adherence to boundaries and attention to Sandra's dependency, avoidance, and inability to trust will offer her a chance to feel validated as well as to tolerate distress and success.

CONCLUSION

The authors have reviewed the IPT model and the case of Sandra, a 26-year-old professional who was assigned the diagnoses of specific phobia and generalized anxiety disorder. To our knowledge, researchers have not modified IPT for the treatment of those specific diagnoses. Nevertheless, interpersonal role dispute and interpersonal deficit are identified as potential major problem areas upon which IPT can focus. The choice of interpersonal deficit is made in light of Sandra's long-standing social isolation, marked anxiety, and difficulties with social skills.

The therapist, regardless of orientation to treatment, is encouraged to maintain an open and flexible approach to revising the diagnostic formulation and provision of treatment to Sandra, given her vulnerability to post-traumatic symptomatology and possibly the development of psychosis. The use of medication is encouraged as well.

In IPT, specific techniques such as communication analysis, roleplaying and the use of the patient-therapist relationship are recommended when an individual is identified as having interpersonal deficit. Sandra has many strengths although her struggles with dependency, inability to trust, avoidance, and superficiality may impact upon her ability to enter into a collaborative therapeutic relationship, contain feelings of distress, or succeed in treatment. The IPT therapist is called upon to adhere to appropriate boundaries and will most likely focus upon Sandra's recurrent experience of not being valued or supported. Upon completion of the focused and time-limited treatment, the IPT therapist can refer Sandra elsewhere or develop a new treatment contract.

REFERENCES

Ballenger, J. C. (1999). Current treatments of the anxiety disorders in adults. *Biological Psychiatry, 46,* 1579–1594.

Beck, A. T., Ward, C., Mendelson, M., Mock, J., & Erbaugh, J. (1961). An inventory for measuring depression. *Archives of General Psychiatry, 4,* 53–63.

Beck, A. T., Epstein, N., Brown, G., & Steer, R. A. (1988). An inventory for measuring clinical anxiety: Psychometric properties. *Journal of Consulting and Clinical Psychology, 56,* 893–897.

Briere, J. (1995). *Trauma symptom inventory professional manual.* Odessa, FL: Psychological Assessment Resources.

Elkin, I., Shea, M. T., Watkins, J. T., Imber, S. D., Sotsky, S. M., Collins, J. F., Glass, D. R., Pilkonis, P. A., Leber, W. R., Docherty, J. P., Fiester, S. J., & Parloff, M. B. (1989). National Institute of Mental Health Treatment of Depression Collaborative Research Program: General effectiveness of treatments. *Archives of General Psychiatry, 46,* 971–982.

Hamilton, M. (1959). The assessment of anxiety states by rating. *British Journal of Medical Psychology, 32,* 50–55.

Hamilton, M. (1960). A rating scale for depression. *Journal of Neurology, Neurosurgery and Psychiatry, 23,* 5–61.

Klerman, G. L., Weissman, M. M., Rounsaville, B. J., & Chevron, E. S. (1984). *Interpersonal psychotherapy of depression.* New York: Basic Books.

Millon, T. (1997). *Millon Clinical Multiaxial Inventory-III manual* (2nd ed.). Minneapolis, MN: National Computer Systems.

Weissman, M. M., Markowitz, M. D., & Klerman, G. L. (2000). *Comprehensive guide to interpersonal psychotherapy.* New York: Basic Books.

Yehuda, R. (2000). Biology of posttraumatic stress disorder. *Journal of Clinical Psychiatry, 61*(Suppl. 7), 14–21.

10

Person-Centered Therapy

Stacey A. Williams

TREATMENT MODEL

Carl R. Rogers (1902–1987) introduced the client-centered treatment model of psychotherapy in 1940. This form of psychotherapy "has been buttressed by more empirical studies than any other therapeutic approach" (Kirschenbaum & Henderson, 1989). As the theory expanded and demonstrated effectiveness with wider populations, it was renamed person-centered psychotherapy in 1986. Person-centered psychotherapy is a nondirective approach to personality restructuring that is deeply rooted in Rogers' theory of personality development. Briefly summarized, Rogers' theory postulates that all people have within themselves the desire and the capacity to evolve into fully functioning, self-actualized individuals. This means that they can guide their lives in a manner that is personally satisfying and socially constructive.

Unfortunately, this natural internal guiding system is often skewed by the external judgements and conditions of worth placed on children by parents, other significant adults, and institutions in their lives during development. When conforming to another's value system, children fail to nurture their own value system, and they tend to split that off as bad or unacceptable to their significant adults. Instead they take in the thoughts and opinions of significant others as though they experienced these realities themselves. This process of introjection is an ineffective way to experience life, because the experiences have not been experienced by the child. They are, therefore, not fully formed ideas or experiences and cannot be fully effective vehicles for the person to use as a true basis of an evaluation system. In addition, it prevents the growth of the child's own internal evaluation system. This clash between what the child innately feels and what the child's parents reinforce him/her to believe creates difficulties.

This state leaves the person in conflict, which comes from *believing* one thing about oneself and the world and *feeling* a whole other set of things about oneself and the world. This state of internal confusion is called incongruence. There is a real self and an ideal self, and the two are in conflict: One self makes choices based on the introjections of others and receives constant reinforcement for that, while the other self makes choices that feel good, but receives no reinforcement and possibly experiences rejection for those choices. This is the root of psychopathology.

Psychological maladjustment is a result of incongruence between what individuals experience firsthand—viscerally, emotionally, and intellectually—and how they want to believe they are in the world, which is their *self concept*. The firsthand experience is rejected in favor of the self concept, which is reinforced by years of praise and valuing from external sources (parents, teachers, friends). This conflict is often expressed as incongruence between real self and ideal self. The client is unable to engage in behaviors that support, enhance, and maintain the self and to actualize, when they are behaving and thinking and feeling in ways that are inconsistent and at cross-purposes with their natural self-enhancing tendencies. The person-centered therapist listens as the individual attempts to express how he or she feels thwarted in being able to achieve what they want to do in life, and in some cases to stop doing.

The person-centered theoretical framework hinges on whether or not individuals are able to recognize value and put into practice their internal locus of evaluation. The particular type of helping relationship offered in person-centered psychotherapy frees individuals to find their inner locus of evaluation and begin making healthy choices based on this internal or organismic valuing system. Once that is in place, the discord once felt because of the incongruence dissipates, along with distorted perceptions of social interactions, subsequent immature behavior, and inappropriate life choices.

The person-centered relationship provides the necessary and sufficient conditions that allow a person to grow psychotherapeutically and make lifelong changes in their thoughts, feelings, and behaviors. This philosophy of therapy underscores the importance of a therapeutic relationship based on the respect and valuing of the individual and his or her thoughts, perceptions, and ability to grow, which leads to the ultimate restructuring of his or her personality.

The unique difference between the person-centered approach and numerous other psychotherapies and organizations within American society in general is the essential trust in individuals to set their own goals and make progress towards them without homework, examinations, inspections, or threats of periodic evaluations (Kirschenbaum & Henderson, 1989). This approach offers trust in the individual to continue to grow into a fully formed complete person. The person-centered approach to treatment only needs to offer individuals the atmosphere in which to work through their development in an atmosphere of acceptance.

The person-centered treatment approach encompasses the creation of a climate that offers the client unconditional positive regard, empathy, and congruence (sometimes referred to as genuineness). These components are some of the necessary and sufficient conditions for change. Current research has shown that a positive, nonjudgmental, accepting stance of the therapist towards the client while he or she expresses emotions significantly impacts the development of a therapeutic rapport and positively correlates with outcome (Asay & Lambert, 2002). Therapist's empathy, defined as the ability to understand fully the client's feelings, is highly correlated with positive therapeutic outcome (Miller, Taylor, & West, 1980). Finally, congruence, also called genuineness, was considered by Rogers the most basic of the attitudinal conditions that foster therapeutic growth (Rogers & Sanford, 1985) because it is demonstrating for the client that hiding behind the title of teacher, analyst, or doctor is unhealthy and puts an unnecessary barrier between therapist and client. Genuinely expressing to a patient the honest feeling that the therapist is experiencing enhances the therapeutic connection.

By experiencing warm, empathic, accepting attitudes within a therapeutic situation, clients are able to express their feelings of incongruence and identify how they recognize the same dynamic in their daily interactions and choices. The therapist reflects these feelings back to the client, along with what he or she perceives the client to be experiencing on a more intense emotional level. The client evaluates this feedback to be accurate or not. This process allows clients to evaluate themselves at that moment in an accepting environment, while being encouraged to express their feelings in a way that is based purely on their own internal valuing system. They are free of the introjected values and conditions of worth placed on them by others in order to be acceptable. They learn to accept themselves by being accepted and to value themselves by being valued. This situation releases the need to act and think in ways that are counterintuitive to their internal desire. This allows them to establish congruence because they now accept their real self and all of their sensory experiences without the internal noise of the "oughts and shoulds" of their loved ones, which created their ideal self. The freedom to make choices based on their own internal organismic valuing system also represents freedom from psychological symptomatology that developed because of the incongruence of rejecting their own thoughts and valuing another's.

THE THERAPIST'S SKILLS AND ATTRIBUTES

A person-centered therapist is most effective when he or she has had the opportunity to know and accept himself or herself through the guided hand of an experienced clinician. A solid therapist of any theoretical background can certainly benefit from this type of emotional congruence, but it is particularly key for a person-centered therapist to have a deep and conscious level of self-acceptance to draw upon readily. Providing unconditional positive regard for all issues that clients reveal can challenge the limits of many people's sensibilities, despite their desire to help a client. For example a young therapist who has small children at home may have some difficulty unconditionally prizing a child molester as a client. Thus, a therapeutic approach that relies so heavily on unconditional positive regard as a mechanism of change requires a clinician who is solidly grounded in his or her belief in the utility of that construct.

Other aspects of personality that lend themselves to effective person-centered therapy are patience and genuineness. It is vital that a person-centered therapist be able to convey warmth, acceptance, and nonjudgmental respect and caring for the client. The client has to trust in the therapist and the therapy process in order to grow from the therapy experience. A clinician who is interested in quick behavior change and rapid symptom reduction will fare much better implementing other methods of treatment. Truly allowing therapy to progress as fast or as slowly as the client is willing requires a great deal of patience from the therapist. Finally, genuineness is the most basic of all attitudinal conditions in practicing person-centered therapy. The therapist is practicing genuineness when he or she is fully aware of all the feelings and thoughts that the person evokes in him or her. The desire to hide those feelings behind a mask of professionalism is a great temptation. In person-centered therapy, expressing the persistent feelings that a person brings to mind in the clinician makes the relationship more intimate and less artificial. This type of genuine feedback is helpful to patients as they struggle in the growth process. A therapist who is capable of offering these attributes to patients will likely be very effective at fostering change.

THE CASE OF SANDRA

Assessment, Conceptualization, and Treatment Planning

Assessment

A person-centered therapist wants to get within the client's phenomenal field and thus would seek more information about Sandra's understanding of her biological parents' conditions and the genetic predisposition that could potentially be affecting her. How does she put that together? How did she learn about it? How does that make her feel about herself and what role, if any, does that play in her relationships? Exploring those factors allows the therapist and Sandra to better understand Sandra's level of comprehension of the complexities of events and relationships and how they got stored (or symbolized) within her as a child. I would want to know more about Sandra's level of self-acceptance and if she understands this concept and its importance to healthy ego development. For example, it is clear that she put her energy into achievement to gain acceptance in school. Even now, unless she is number one in her boss's eyes, she feels like nothing. Sandra was beaten when she tried to fight for her right to be physically safe at home, so she took that anger and used it as fuel to fight for herself in academic challenges. On some level, she knew that it was incongruent and characterizes herself quite negatively (an angry, vicious person) when she reflects upon that. Yet it is only natural for the ego to fight to be maintained, enhanced, and actualized. Understanding the affect behind

Sandra's statement about being nothing unless the boss values her work that day is fundamental in determining her level of awareness of her core conflict. Again, how she introjects values into her understanding of herself is key for the therapist to know. Performance-based, conditional relationships reduce the individual to the position of a dependent, helpless child. She does not realize how she is now re-creating her relationship with her adoptive family with her boss—who appears to be using her to do his work, just as her adoptive family took unfair advantage of her—further examination of these relationships is essential. Inquiring how she feels about this relationship and that with her boyfriend and assessing if Sandra reports a difference allows the therapist to know her level of insight. Her aloofness with the very people that make it possible for her to function on a daily basis is so incongruent that it would have to be explored in some detail. This type of genuine, open curiosity about each of her relationships with loved ones in her life is central to understanding Sandra's perceptual field and ultimately her reality.

I would not give a battery of standardized tests and was curious about why a MAST was given to a person who claims not to use drugs or alcohol and does not engage in risk-taking behavior by history and collateral support by her boyfriend of 5 years. (Many clinics use a standard battery not tailored to the individual and that may have been the case here.) The reason a person-centered clinician does not rely on standardized assessment tools is simply to maintain the status of the person as healthy enough to relate his or her history from his or her perspective. It is important to avoid putting the therapist in a role of having the answers (to the test) and putting the client in a position of being judged or evaluated by the therapist. Standardized psychological assessment may be construed as proof of a power differential in the minds of clients. Diagnostic labels take away from the person of the client; assuming a professional posture takes away from the person of the therapist (Raskin & Rogers, 1995). The person-centered approach strives to keep therapist and client on an even playing field where trust and openness flow between one another freely. Psychological testing may create an atmosphere of stiff procedure and professionalism, which disrupts that free-flowing process. It is essential to be mindful of this dynamic and how it fits with the person-centered philosophy: that a client is a person struggling on the road of life and the therapist is another person who is taking that journey with the client to help clarify and identify difficult parts. As Rogers has stated,

The therapist must lay aside his preoccupation with diagnosis and his diagnostic shrewdness, must discard this tendency to make professional evaluations, must cease his endeavors to formulate an accurate prognosis, must give up the temptation to subtly guide the individual and, must concentrate on one purpose only; that of providing deep understanding and acceptance of the attitudes consciously held at this moment by the client as he explores step-by-step into the dangerous areas which he has been denying to consciousness (Rogers, 1946, p. 420).

With reference to Sandra, she demonstrates a pattern of competing against people seen as more powerful than she is. She then feels rejected by these people because she does not know what they want from her and cannot figure out how to connect with them to get her needs met and be accepted by them. One would want to be very careful not to set oneself up as another controlling person taking data from her.

Therapeutic Goals

The ultimate therapeutic goal for Sandra is an increase in her self-acceptance. This will decrease the need to depend on the presence of another adult in order to shower, walk to her car, enter work, and stay home alone. By becoming a fully functional self-reliant adult, she will no longer need to have these external symbols of adulthood around her in order to function. Anything that she desires to do with her relationships after accepting herself will be driven from the innate desire to maintain, enhance, and actualize her self. For example, she may decide to confront her adoptive parents about the miserable job they did in parenting her. Or she can accept what they did and failed to do and simply move out and maintain her relationship with them, armed with the new knowledge that healthy parents don't do that, but they did the best they could with their emotional limitations. The goal of self-acceptance is rooted in personality reconstruction, and not simply symptom reduction or external behavioral control. Breaking erroneously formed bonds and misperceptions from childhood allows a person to form new connections and symbolizations of what is acceptable to them. These connections are now based on how clients internally value the issue, which is based on their own life experience and not on symbolized ideas introjected from their parents. Because they no longer have distorted or poorly formed introjections from parents guiding their reality, they are thinking for themselves and the thoughts are congruent with their own organismic valuing system, which will maintain, enhance, and actualize the self.

There seems to be an ideal self-image of a "perfect" employee, who is competent and hard-working; at home she is the good daughter who dutifully goes to Mass, is home before dark, is respectful of her adoptive mother's wishes, and visits her chronically ill biological mother.

In order to realize the ultimate goal, the primary goal of identifying incongruence in her life is essential. Secondary to this goal is identifying what her natural inclinations would be in the situations that have caused her the most incongruence. Finally, a tertiary goal would be to educate her on the realities of human nature. It is important that she understand she lives in a culture that devalues women and exploits them in the media as "Playboy bunnies" and objects of sexual satisfaction. Thus any woman, no matter how confident or accomplished, may fall prey to forcible rape (as she nearly experienced at the hand of her 16-year-old brother). It is important for her to realize that there was nothing in her behavior, words, or attitude that prompted that particular attack or her father's sexual assault. Recognition of those external beliefs in our society is helpful in supporting victims of sexual assault, who are racked by guilt because they buy into the societal myth that they must have done something to cause the assault (O'Hara, 1996).

Timeline for Therapy

Timelines in person-centered therapy vary because its foundation is comprised of each individual's level of comfort, intelligence, and awareness of their feelings. Initial weekly contact for traditional 50-minute sessions is ideal to establish rapport and become a place in the person's daily life. Insurance plans and finances can hinder that ideal situation. The beauty of the person-centered approach is that it is not locked into a stepwise progression of homework assignments or rigid treatment-planning, where the first session may be the last session in which the person benefits from the warmth, caring, and acceptance offered by the therapist. This good experience with therapists in general paves the way for the client to seek therapy in the future, having experienced it as positive.

Case Conceptualization

Sandra's personality is anxious and fearful at its core, based in early abandonment by her biological mother and father, which led to an unhealthy attachment to her adoptive parental figures. Her relationship with them is characterized as *enmeshed*. She still seeks her mother's basic level of approval and acceptance despite being an adult who no longer needs to rely on adults to guide her. She is also intellectually aware that she disapproves of her adoptive mother and father because they neglected and abused her and allowed others to violate her sense of safety in her own home. She is immature and counterdependent, which leads her to make choices based on imagined fears of danger. She does not have a healthy, mature relationship with others. Her behavior outwardly appears dependent on others to manage her fears, but she does not trust them, so her interpersonal relationships are more complicated. Sandra has a poorly formed sense of self, based on distorted introjections from her biological mother, who is chronically psychotic, her "very emotional, religious, and controlling" adoptive mother, and child-molesting adoptive father. These life events have left Sandra with a very low sense of self-efficacy and a belief that everyone will ultimately let her down. This long-standing belief, coupled with intermittent actual physical assaults, has led to her current anxiety disorder and hypervigiliance. Despite her complaints about her parents, if she holds on to the "fear" of being alone at home, she can remain attached to them and have them take care of her.

The Therapeutic Relationship

The Therapeutic Bond

One very important consideration in the development of a therapeutic bond with a person-centered therapist is the level of trust that the client can achieve with the therapist. Clients will test the waters slowly as they discuss their chief complaint and watch the therapist for his or her response. The person-centered therapist is attentively listening and clarifying feelings and meanings, all the while sending the message of unconditional positive regard. The better the therapist is at conveying a nonjudgmental attitude, the greater the chances that the client will receive this unconditional acceptance and the bond of trust will begin to take root. The development of a therapeutic bond with Sandra may take longer than it might for another client, because broken trust is at the core of her psychopathology. When she has given her trust to people, they have failed her and abused that trust. Significant events in her history, such as the damage to her initial bonds of trust with her biological parents and then subsequent violations of trust by her stepfather whom she trusted above all others, were major events in her life.

Rogers discussed transference in two ways. First, there are the feelings that arise within the client that are understandable responses to what the therapist is showing the client. An example of this is feelings of positive regard for the therapist because the therapist is unconditionally providing the same for the client. Second, there are the projections of feelings transferred onto the therapist from the client that have no origins in, nor relationship to, the therapist's behavior towards the client. The person-centered therapist is mindful of a client's need to relate in the therapeutic relationship in a manner that is as comfortable to them as a friendship or a consultation with a teacher or mentor. This creates expectations and transferential feelings from the client towards the therapist that the person-centered therapist does not encourage or explore any differently than any other type of feelings. It is important to stay in the here and now and within the current reality in therapy. An excerpt from a case example previously published, which eloquently illustrates this technique is offered below. In this example, Carl Rogers is working with a single woman in her 30s.

[From ninth interview]
S: I've never told anyone they were the most wonderful person I've ever known, but I've told you that. It's not just sex. It's more than that.
C: You really feel very deeply attached to me.

[From tenth interview]
S: I think emotionally I'm dying for sexual intercourse but I don't do anything about it . . . The thing I want is to have sexual intercourse with you. I don't dare ask you, 'cause I'm afraid you'd be nondirective.
C: You have this awful tension, and want so much to have relations with me.
S: [Goes on in this vein. Finally,] Can't we do something about it? This tension is awful! Will you relieve the tension . . . Can you give me a direct answer? I think it might help both of us.
C: (Gently.) The answer would be no. I can understand how *desperately* you feel, but I would not be willing to do that.
S: (Pause. Sigh of relief.) I think that helps me. It's only when I'm upset that I'm like this. You have strength, and it gives me strength. (Kirshenbaum & Henderson, 1989, p. 131)

As can be seen in this example, to allow or encourage a transference distorts the therapeutic relationship and sets up an unrealistic power differential that is harmful to the development of an egalitarian relationship of mutual respect and trust. The person-centered therapist maintains healthy boundaries and sets realistic limits on the therapeutic relationship. He or she discloses enough to the client that will allow the client to comfortably develop a therapeutic connection with the therapist without spending time fantasizing about the therapist or being frustrated by thwarted questions to the therapist. Setting an hourly appointment, fee schedule, office rules, and limits of confidentiality of that work setting are all openly discussed with the patient.

Roles in the Therapeutic Relationship

Rogers stressed a nondirective approach to psychotherapy. The role of the therapist is that of a caring listener and the role of the patient is that of a courageous explorer. The quiet patience of the therapist helps to create the atmosphere of acceptance and permission to express himself or herself about emotional turmoil. There is a varying degree of activity on the part of the therapist. Although it may appear that the person-centered therapist is inactive, he or she is quite actively listening and empathizing with the client. Person-centered therapists never set themselves up as experts. They are humbly aware that they cannot possibly be experts on the life of anyone they are just meeting. Rather, they respectfully embark on the journey of self-exploration with the client, as a fellow traveler and helpful participant, not as an expert. To pretend to be an expert is to don a mask of disingenuousness, which creates distance between the therapist and client. This is the antithesis of a central mechanism of change used in person-centered therapy. Therapy is collaborative because the process moves along at the pace of the client and the therapist does all that he or she can to support and enhance the client's level of self-acceptance throughout that process.

Treatment Implementation and Outcome

Techniques and Methods of Working

Working strictly in the traditional person-centered psychotherapy framework would be sufficient in treating Sandra's anxiety. After establishing a solid rapport with her and developing her internal evaluation system, it would be appropriate to invite her boyfriend of 5 years into the session to address issues that arise that are specific to that relationship. Helping her to deal with some of these concerns within the therapy context can serve to support Sandra as she learns to express herself in a mature congruent manner. This relationship is different from the one she has with her parents or siblings. Those interactions of her past and distorted anticipation of her future interactions with them will not become the major focus in therapy. However, the interactions of her current romantic relationship are appropriate to consider. As she changes from a person who is emotionally dependent, incapable of valuing herself, and reliant on the evaluations of others, the romantic relationship will also change. Person-centered psychotherapy focuses on the feelings and experiences of the here and now and this current relationship may be salvaged.

Medical and Nutritional Issues

If medical and or nutritional issues arose during treatment, a referral to a medical doctor would be made. Support for the client would be given on a consistent basis by following through on these referrals. Learning to care for oneself in a consistent and congruent manner is in accord with the person-centered therapy. Clients become fully functional, independent individuals when they take care of themselves physically and mentally.

Potential Pitfalls

It would be expected that making a psychological connection with Sandra would be very difficult. Her lack of trust in people, particularly men, may become a serious barrier to treatment. Sandra may also have trouble accepting the conditions the therapist offers her. Unconditional positive regard, genuineness, and empathy are not emotions that Sandra has experienced in her life, and she has learned to be suspicious of those who are kind to her (the clergy, her stepfather). Because the acceptance of the therapist's attitudes towards the client in this type of therapy is the most powerful change mechanism, it is imperative that the client be able to receive them. In Sandra's life her internal evaluation system has been disregarded; therefore it can be anticipated that she will be resistant to taking on this responsibility in her life. Extra patience and particular attention to clarify and make sure that the therapist is comprehending her perceptions is crucial to effective person-centered psychotherapy. On a positive note, Sandra appears ready to make a change in her life as evidenced by her frustration about the limitations she experiences at home, at work, and within her romantic relationship. This energy to explore and change behavior is an excellent catalyst to establish psychological contact.

Termination and Relapse Prevention

Discussing the growth that Sandra has experienced throughout her treatment and the changes she was able to make is helpful in the beginning of the termination process. Reinforcing her internal valuing system and the level of congruence achieved thus far are also important. Clients decide when they are ready to terminate therapy and if they may want to seek therapy in the future, so the person-centered therapist continues to offer unconditional acceptance for the client's ability to make these choices. By the end of the termination process, the client will tell the therapist what he or she can do to prevent relapsing into old habits and behaviors. Within person-centered psychotherapy, relapse is not a major issue of consideration. Once the clients accept themselves, and thus their behaviors, are congruent with their thoughts, feelings and interval evaluation system, there really is no inner pressure to revert to old patterns because these are no longer valued. An example might be that once a child learns to walk there is little need to prevent them from crawling again. There is no longer an internal desire to be less capable and dependent.

Mechanisms of Change

There are three major mechanism of change that I hope to see for this client. They are (a) the development of an internal evaluation system, (b) a decrease in incongruence, and (c) an increase in self-acceptance. The development of an internal evaluation system and the rejection of the poorly formed introjected valuing system would include Sandra's decreasing her reliance on the opinions of others and her dependence on the presence of others in order to function in daily tasks. The decrease in incongruence that she experiences will occur as she explores each area of internal conflict and receives acceptance for her natural set of feelings and opinions and desired behaviors about that issue. Acceptance of her self and the changes in her relationships come about as a result of the changes in her behaviors, because they are now driven by her internal evaluation system. These three major mechanisms of change will restructure Sandra's personality such that she will be a fully functioning, independent, emotionally stable individual.

CONCLUSION

The person-centered approach would be efficacious in treating Sandra. Specifically, her issues with mistrust and low self-esteem would respond well to an atmosphere of unconditional positive regard as she expresses her perceptions; to empathy for the experiences that have caused her to doubt herself; and to genuineness, particularly because she is just waiting for the therapist to betray her (as her stepfather did) and start making demands on her to change and do things his or her way. Because the necessary and sufficient conditions for change are not used as only initial techniques to establish a therapeutic rapport, there is never a switch to a different mode of interaction. Sandra can finally trust what this relationship has to offer her from the beginning to its natural end.

This style of therapy will be especially curative for a woman who has experienced sexual assault. These women need to tell their stories and receive validation for *their* perception of what happened to them. The person-centered approach offers that consistently throughout the relationship. Sandra would likely respond very well to this mode of psychotherapy.

REFERENCES

Asay, T., & Lambert, M. (2002). Research on therapist relational variables. In D. Caine (Ed.), *Humanistic psychotherapies: Handbook of research and practice* (pp. 531–557). Washington, DC: American Psychological Association.

Kirschenbaum, H., & Henderson, V. (1989). *The Carl Rogers reader* (p. 131). Boston: Houghton Mifflin.

Miller, W. R., Taylor, C. A., & West, J. C. (1980). Focused versus broad-spectrum behavior therapy for problem drinkers. *Journal of Consulting and Clinical Psychology, 48,* 590–601.

O'Hara, M. (1996). Rogers and Sylvia, a feminist analysis. In B. Farber, D. Brink, & P. Raskin (Eds.), *The psychotherapy of Carl Rogers, cases and commentary* (pp. 284–300). New York: Guilford.

Raskin, M. J., & Rogers, C. R. (1995). Person-centered therapy. In R. J. Corsini & D. Wedding (Eds.), *Current psychotherapies* (5th ed., p. 150). Itasca, IL: F. E. Peacock.

Rogers, C. R. (1946). Significant aspects of person-centered therapy. *American Psychologist, 1,* 415–422.

Rogers, C. R., & Sanford, R. C. (1985). Person-centered psychotherapy. In H. I. Kaplan, B. J. Sadock, & A. M. Friedman (Eds.), *Comprehensive textbook of psychiatry* (4th ed., pp. 1374–1388). Baltimore: Williams & Wilkins.

11

Supportive-Expressive Psychotherapy

Alan L. Schwartz and
Katherine Crits-Christoph

TREATMENT MODEL

Supportive-expressive psychotherapy is grounded in the principles of psychodynamic change as initially presented by Freud (1924), though it has been progressively transformed and codified by a number of psychoanalytic theorists, clinicians, and researchers. Over the course of the 20th century, supportive-expressive psychotherapy emerged as a psychoanalytically informed psychotherapy that addressed some of the limitations perceived in classical psychoanalysis. These included the needs of a more diverse patient population, the technical restraints of classical psychoanalysis, the huge investment of time and money, and the proposed length of treatment. The seminal works on supportive-expressive psychotherapy were developed at the Menninger Foundation (Wallerstein et al., 1956) and were subsequently manualized by Lester Luborsky (1984). Although supportive-expressive psychotherapy may be conducted on an open-ended basis with a wide range of patient populations, it has also been utilized in short-term, time-limited formats with success (Luborsky, Barber, & Crits-Christoph, 1990). An active program of research on supportive-expressive psychotherapy continues at numerous sites including the Center for Psychotherapy Research at the University of Pennsylvania.

The nomenclature of supportive-expressive psychotherapy derives from the two key components of the treatment process. The term *supportive* refers to improving the patient's ego functioning, adaptive abilities, and self-esteem (Rockland, 1989). This occurs through the structural apparatus of the treatment as well as aspects of the therapeutic relationship that reinforce the patient's functioning (Luborsky & Mark, 1991). In terms of the former, the regularity of appointments, consistency of time and place boundaries, and identification of and progress toward goals are among the inherent supportive aspects of psychotherapy identified by Luborsky (1984). With regard to the latter, the development of a positive therapeutic alliance with the therapist being seen as a helpful, encouraging figure is an important supportive element. Supportive components of the therapeutic alliance also include the therapist's and patient's coming to an agreement on the goals of treatment and the process of achieving those goals (Bordin, 1979). These components—likely elements of all good therapists—should not be downplayed as the therapeutic alliance alone appears to have a substantial independent effect on outcome (Horvath & Symonds, 1991).

The expressive aspects of the supportive-expressive model are those that promote patients' understanding about their thoughts, feelings, and conflicts, which are often out of their conscious awareness. Through the use of well-known psychoanalytic techniques such as empathic listening, clarification, and interpretation, the patient comes to a greater understanding of his or her behavior. This is particularly important with respect to insight into their patterns of interpersonal relationships.

Supportive-expressive psychotherapy views psychological dysfunction and change through the lens of interpersonal relationships. The focus is on symptoms in the context of relational patterns. These are clarified through the patient's narration of significant interpersonal interactions, enabling the clinician to understand interpersonal patterns similar in concept to psychoanalytic transference. In supportive-expressive psychotherapy, the most prevalent and frequent pattern evidenced in the patient's interpersonal interactions is described as the core conflictual relationship theme (CCRT). The CCRT is a template of self and other responses formed from early and subsequent relational experiences that an individual frequently reenacts in various life relationships (Luborsky & Mark, 1991), including the therapeutic relationship. The CCRT consists of a refined understanding of an individual's central relational wish or need from others (termed the *wish*), the typical response that others provide to the wish (*response of the object*—RO), and the resulting response of the individual (*response of the self*—RS). Symptoms viewed as RSs are those that emerge out of conflicts in their relational themes. For example, a client experiencing marital difficulties may enter therapy due to a desire to be protected and cared for (wish), but she is ignored by her husband (RO), thus engendering feelings of depression and helplessness in the patient (RS). A therapist's use of the CCRT method involves eliciting and attending to the narratives of a patient's interplay with others, from which the components of the CCRT can be derived.

More specifically, with the use of the CCRT, the mechanism of therapeutic change in supportive-expressive psychotherapy occurs in three ways through three particular means (Luborsky, 1984). First, the patients gain increased understanding into symptoms and their relationships to important people in their life. By attending to the emotional insights into past and present relationships, an understanding of an individual's relational world (with conflicting wishes, expected responses from others, and typical symptom patterns) can be gained. The use of the current therapeutic relationship facilitates this process through an understanding of transference and assisting the patient in exercising more adaptive ways of relating. Supportive-expressive psychotherapy assists patients in developing a sense of mastery such that while the central CCRT may not markedly change over time, their ability to achieve their wish, moderate their object choices, and more successfully adapt will improve their quality of life. (Luborsky et al., 1988).

Second, therapeutic change is facilitated by the patient's experiencing the therapist as a helping and supportive ally in the treatment process. The therapeutic or helping alliance is crucial to the survival of therapy as the patient encounters successive manifestations of difficult, anachronistic relationships from the past in the present. The joint struggle of working collaboratively appears to be an integral aspect of positive therapeutic outcome (Luborsky et al., 1988), no matter what the theoretical orientation. Luborsky (1984) has even suggested that the therapeutic relationship may be even more important to outcome than insight and understanding.

Third, for change to be more than ephemeral it must be incorporated into the patient's psychological functioning, often through the process of internalization. Maintaining therapeutic gains becomes particularly salient in discussions around the meaning of terminating therapy. Acknowledging the many feelings that ending a treatment relationship engenders (including sadness, anger, and fear) provides an opportunity to negotiate an important separation process. Patients often become concerned about the persistence of gains after treatment ends with the absence of the therapist. Reviewing the patients' goals, their investment in the process, and the progress they have made reinforces the gains made.

THE THERAPIST'S SKILLS AND ATTRIBUTES

Because supportive-expressive psychotherapy is essentially a form of psychoanalytic psychotherapy, the most basic skills required are rooted in attending to the various elements of the therapeutic relationship. Although many of these skills are attributes common to most successful therapists, supportive-expressive therapy makes their centrality explicit. Many of these critical clinical and personal skills are delineated in Luborsky's (1984) manual for supportive-expressive treatment. Primarily, therapists must attend carefully to the building of a positive therapeutic alliance to facilitate and enable the subsequent tasks of therapy. The therapist must be sensitive to cultivate an atmosphere of trust, collaboration, respect, and responsiveness with the patient who has entered treatment in distress. Supportive-expressive therapists must possess the capacity to empathically involve themselves in their relationship with their patients because their role as a supportive and helpful figure is paramount in the mechanism of change. Although the therapist is certainly viewed as a professional and expert to some degree, the therapist must communicate to the patient that they are involved in a joint venture of working toward the patient's goals of relieving his or her emotional pain.

Two of the key skill elements to this end are the capacity for listening and understanding (Luborsky, 1984). Rather than injecting one's a priori conjectures regarding the context of a patient's difficulties, the supportive-expressive therapist must listen in an attentive, yet unbiased and open manner. Allowing oneself to be receptive to the material offered by the patient allows for subsequent analysis of its meaning. Patience is required to be freely receptive to the patient's narrative: "If you are not sure what is happening and what your next response should be, listen more" (Luborsky, 1984, p. 91). Because of the relational focus of supportive-expressive psychotherapy, the therapist must be active in eliciting specific and detailed interpersonal interactions between the patient and other individuals in the present and past. An active involvement by the therapist is required to generate the elements of these interactions including the setting of the interactions (context), what was said (content), how it was said (affect), and the outcome. These rich, interpersonal interactions are called relationship episodes (RE). By listening to these REs, aspects of the patient's relational world and central CCRT pattern will emerge. As in most psychodynamically rooted psychotherapies, the therapist must also develop a keen attention to the vicissitudes of their relationship with the patient. At times, this requires asking the patient specifically about the status of the relationship as well as reflecting upon long-standing patterns that are emerging in the present. Thus, the therapist must listen for, and be prepared to address, transference issues.

Eventually, such listening and patience will lead to an understanding to which the therapist can respond. *Understanding* refers to knowledge gained about patients' symptoms in the context of their relationships, allowing the therapist to formulate the key relationship issues of the CCRT. With a modicum of understanding of the CCRT, the therapist responds to the patient to promote their understanding. The technical manner of this response is not as important as being able to convey the information to the patient in a way they can understand it and which reflects that they are being heard (Luborsky, 1984). To this end, the therapist tries as much as possible to use the patient's own words to describe the various components of the CCRT and to reflect back to the patient his or her central wish.

Listening freshly and understanding the patient's concerns will enable the clarification of the patient's presenting problems so that clear, agreed upon goals can be set, prioritized, and worked toward. Therapists must develop a vigilance in revisiting the patient's goals. This occurs for a number of reasons: It conveys that the patient's concerns and goals are important, that notable progress is expected and achievable, and that if progress is not forthcoming, a change in the course of the work is required.

THE CASE OF SANDRA

Assessment, Conceptualization, and Treatment Planning

Assessment

The evaluation processes presented thus far in Sandra's case are not inconsistent with an evaluative process at the initiation of supportive-expressive psychotherapy; that is, understanding a developmental outline of a patient's history, current presenting symptoms, medical problems, and *DSM-IV* diagnoses is important. The standardized assessment data gathered appear sufficient and will assist the therapist and patient in monitoring progress over time. Although no further formalized assessment is required, an evaluation utilizing diagnostic psychological testing is a productive adjunct to supportive-expressive psychotherapy (Luborsky, 1984). A particularly useful battery will include projective measures such as the Rorschach Inkblot Test and Thematic Apperception Test (TAT) from which finer distinction of a patient's psychology can be enunciated. Treatment planning strategies for the individual (e.g., Exner, 1994) and a preemptive understanding of a patient's subjective interpersonal world can facilitate the treatment process.

To further understand and structure Sandra's treatment, additional information from Sandra's history would be useful. The initial evaluation delineated a number of people in the patient's present and past relational network (biological and adoptive parents and grandparents, two brothers, a boyfriend, and coworkers). However, a more thorough explication of these relationships in the evaluation phase of treatment, including REs and specific interactions, are an important precursor to developing work on the CCRT. In research settings, an interview tool called the Subjective Understanding of Interpersonal Relationships Interview (SUIP) is used to this end (Connolly et al., 1999). The information can be gathered as well by focused exploration of the patient's experiences in the various important relationships cited, if the information is not naturally forthcoming (Mark & Faude, 1997). Questions that might be asked about REs are designed to focus on the narrative between the patient and the other person: What did you say? What did he say? How did you respond? In addition to conducting a more detailed exploration of Sandra's relationships than has already been provided, there are some key relationships about which we have little or no information. These include other significant intimate relationships (her first boyfriend, for example, who is alluded to but not mentioned), close friends from the past and present, as well as any other individuals Sandra considers important in her life. It is useful to understand why important people who were in her life at one time (e.g., friends) are no longer involved. The circumstances around these ruptures in relationships are likely to provide more data for understanding the CCRT.

From an assessment perspective, we might better understand Sandra's approach to therapy by learning about previous treatment experiences. We learn briefly in the evaluation that Sandra participated in a short-lived term of therapy around the age of 10 after forced sexual activity by her two brothers. It would be enlightening to hear Sandra's perspective on psychotherapy in order to listen for any potential roadblocks to the current treatment. She is likely to feel that her experience in psychotherapy was less than satisfying and positive. Although she does not appear to have engaged in any other psychotherapy since that time, her experience with her mother's psychosis and more than 30 hospitalizations is likely to have influenced her feelings about mental health and treatment. Acknowledging any negative attitudes toward the treatment process as early as possible can aid in forestalling resistance and obstacles to developing a positive working alliance. It is also unclear at this time if there have been any recent events that precipitated Sandra's seeking therapy at this time. We know she has sought therapy "at the behest of her boyfriend" but do not know anything more about the context of this request. Given that she has suffered for the majority of her life, the answer to the question "why now?" will be helpful in understanding the motivation of the patient as well as aspects of her relationship with her boyfriend.

The assessment process should be extended further to include Sandra's ideas regarding the nature of her symptoms and her perspective as to what contributes or maintains their presence. This is important as it speaks to the patient's ability to understand the nature of change and participate in the therapeutic process of supportive-expressive psychotherapy. That is, if Sandra strongly believes that biological or chemical factors are primary in contributing to her symptoms, much initial work will be required to help her understand the nature of the role of relationship issues in maintaining her symptoms. We should also be attentive to Sandra's statement in the session excerpt that she has recovered from the incidents of her past: "I've accepted it and moved forward." Although this suggests a certain resilience regarding very difficult issues, the therapist should be alert to assess Sandra's willingness or reluctance to discuss these issues and the extent to which her defenses may fuel her resistance.

Therapeutic Goals

Setting therapeutic goals for this patient would require of course a collaborative discussion with the patient and agreement on specific, achievable targets for treatment (Luborsky, 1984). In line with the tenets of supportive-expressive treatment, we would endeavor to identify the symptoms the patient is presenting in the interpersonal context. Thus, the primary goals of treatment for Sandra are for her to increase her understanding of her distressing symptoms—pervasive anxiety, fear of personal injury and attack, avoidance of perceived danger situations—by examining how they relate to conflicts in her core sense of interpersonal relationships. In supportive-expressive psychotherapy, symptoms are viewed as expressions of core conflictual relationships. As she gains understanding about how her symptoms are expressed, she will begin to exert a sense of control and mastery over their expression. Certainly, Sandra would see among her primary goals her ability to experience less anxiety and worry, to feel less fearful of her surroundings, less avoidant of typical daily activities, as well as to have less of a need to rely obsessively on a rigid timetable of activities to manage her anxiety. In supportive-expressive psychotherapy, the reduction of these symptoms as goals is concomitant with goals attending to her patterns of relationships. The expression of Sandra's symptoms is seen to be related to conflicts in her prototypical view of relationships. Thus, the relational goals that would address her core issues appear to involve her ability to experience relationships as reliable, safe, and worthy of her trust. Another goal for Sandra would be to experience a deeper, more affective connection with others with whom she relates. She seems to view her current relationships as tenuous and superficial. Despite this proclivity, she seems to desire a greater sense of independence from others, yet is persistently thwarted by her own internal and interpersonal obstacles. We can begin to understand a conflict between Sandra's desire for protection and closeness and a concomitant need to be independent from others. An important eventual goal for Sandra would be for her to feel a more adaptive sense of control and autonomy in relationships where she has for most of her life felt unacknowledged, exploited, and abused. A fuller description of these treatment goals follows in the conceptualization of Sandra's CCRT.

Despite Sandra's tumultuous life experiences, she has managed a number of relative accomplishments that speak to her resiliency. She is a sufficiently bright woman as evidenced by school performance. Her persistence in beginning her career as a bank teller and working her way up to loan manager provides some evidence about Sandra's determination, suggesting that her eventual level of adaptation and functioning could be higher with a successful outcome to her treatment. Although we do not have a great deal of information at this time about her boyfriend of 5 years, current information suggests that he has been supportive and that this is a positive relationship. This, one hopes, speaks well of Sandra's burgeoning capacity to engage in an interpersonal treatment and to benefit from it. In a concrete manner, we would endeavor to assist Sandra in sufficiently reducing her symptoms and understanding her relationships to the extent that she felt able to make clearer decisions about her life. One can imagine, for example, that through the course of treatment Sandra would move toward a less phobic existence to the point where she felt comfortable living outside the realm of her parents, relating in a more intimate way with significant others, and more easily managing day-to-day tasks without debilitating fear.

Timeline for Therapy

The timeline for supportive-expressive therapy is dependent upon the goals, needs, and wishes of the patient. Therapy can proceed in a time-open-ended (TO) or time-limited (TL) manner, the latter of which is also referred to as short-term supportive-expressive psychotherapy (Luborsky & Mark, 1991). Time-limited therapy typically involves a planned treatment length of 6 to 24 sessions with time-unlimited (open-ended) running from months to years (Luborsky, 1984). Although there is evidence to support the benefit of time-limited therapy (e.g., Woody et al., 1983), the complexity and longitudinal nature of Sandra's problems suggest a time-open-ended model of treatment. It should be noted, however, that the vigorous setting of goals and attention to progress toward those goals does not necessitate a "time-interminable" length of treatment.

Regardless of the length of treatment, the focus of the early psychotherapy sessions (i.e., the first and second sessions) involves efforts to develop the therapeutic alliance, gather the patient's perspective on their presenting issues, and establish preliminary goals. Some modicum of agreement between the therapist and the patient is required for each of these areas at the beginning stage of therapy in order for progress to be made. It is difficult, if not impossible, to predict the course of therapy; however, once goals have been mutually agreed upon, the subsequent work with Sandra would involve helping her express and understand aspects of the CCRT and how they relate to her symptoms. This is the primary work of therapy and is subject to reformulations, clarifications, and eventually "working through" (Freud, 1914/1958). Once goals have been met, the therapist and patient would mutually decide upon continuing to work by setting new goals or proceed with the process of termination, wherein the gains made in treatment are reinforced.

Supportive-expressive therapy typically involves weekly sessions though in some cases twice weekly or biweekly meetings are indicated, depending on the acuity of the patient, the phase of the therapy, and the judgement of the therapist. For Sandra, weekly sessions seem to be indicated. Sessions of 50 minutes are standard (Luborsky, 1984), though individual clinicians may range from 45 to 60 minutes based on personal preference.

Case Conceptualization

As highlighted earlier, one of the key tasks of supportive-expressive psychotherapy involves the elucidation of relationship patterns through the use of the CCRT method (Luborsky & Crits-Christoph, 1990). The following conceptualization follows the CCRT process as we have described it. It should be noted that in an actual evaluation the CCRT, a much more detailed description of a patient's narratives and REs are required. The components of the CCRT are usually expressed in a first-person statement of the wish, response from others, and response from the self (Luborsky, 1984). From the information and narratives we have, we can construct a number of REs as examples of this approach.

In Sandra's relationship with her adoptive parents, she expressed the desire (wish) to be accepted by them and to experience a sense of safety in her new family. However, after her father's inebriated sexual advances (RO), Sandra felt "devastated" (RS). Thus, Sandra might describe her RE with her father as follows: *I wanted to be protected and accepted by him, but when he tried to fondle me, I was devastated.* A similar wish seemed operative with her adoptive mother. Yet her mother's responses to her (RO) typically were rage, physical abuse, and threats of abandonment. Sandra's reactions to her mother (RS) were to both avoid her and attempt to escape the house and to experience intense anger toward her. The RE with Sandra's mother might be described this way: *I wanted to be protected and accepted by her, but she responded by abusing and threatening me, so I tried to avoid her and run away.* Through the early sessions with Sandra, we would endeavor to gather additional narratives about her relationships. Her current descriptions about past and present relationship might be outlined as follows:

Biological mother:
(W) I want to be cared for.
(RO) Psychotic concern for safety ("I thought you were dead").
(RS) I'm anxious and disturbed.

Boyfriend:
(W) I want to depend on him.
(RO) Encourages her to receive help.
(RS) I'm not sure he loves me.

Boss:
(W) I want to be seen as competent.
(RO) Lets her do his work as well as her own (i.e., he exploits her).
(RS) I'm fearful of making mistakes and not being seen as number one.

Brothers:
(W) I want to be part of the family.
(RO) Teasing and sexual abuse.
(RS) I ran away, became cautious and vigilant.

Biological father:
(W) I want to be cared for.
(RO) Disinterest.
(RS) I disowned him.

Adoptive mother:
(W) I want to be safe, protected, cared about.
(RO) Neglect, ignoring, rage, abuse, threats of abandonment.
(RS) I was angry, tried to escape, and felt abandoned.

Adoptive father:
(W) I want to be safe, protected, cared about.
(RO) Sexual advances.
(RS) I was devastated, angry.

Sandra's brief description of her history and relationships apparently suggests a core wish with two related components: to be cared for and protected, and to be valued and appreciated. First, she seems to wish desperately to be cared for, protected, and to feel safe in relationships. The wish to be cared for can be seen emerging from her numerous experiences when she was not protected as a child and her physical and emotional needs were violated. Beginning with her parents' divorce when she was very young, we see the progression of her biological mother's illness in a woman who voiced a disturbed concern herself for Sandra's safety. The physical and emotional rage of her adoptive mother and abuse by her brothers and eventually her adoptive father appear to have culminated in Sandra's feeling that the world is an unsafe place and wishing for safety, protection, and comfort. Thus, Sandra's wish can be expressed as, *I wish to be cared for and protected.* An elaboration of her desire to be cared for is Sandra's wish to be able to trust and depend upon important others. The relationships that typically serve those functions (i.e., her biological parents, her adoptive parents, and her siblings) sadly all consistently failed to provide a trusting and dependable holding environment. Even adjunctive relationships, such as with the parish priest who did not report her abuse to the authorities, contributed to Sandra's questioning her ability to trust. Her wish here is, *I wish to be able to trust and depend upon others.* Though not as related to problematic symptom responses, Sandra seems to have a secondary wish: *I wish to be valued and appreciated.* This theme emerges primarily in the context of her work relationships where she functions in a hyper-responsible and driven manner to the end of being highly valued by her boss. In addition, this was evidenced as a positive RO before the advances of her father disheartened Sandra.

In the CCRT formulation, given the relational wishes derived from the patient's narratives or REs, we next examine how Sandra feels others typically respond to her wishes. Though Sandra desires to be safe and protected in relationships (based on early troubling experiences), the response that she expects from others (RO) is to be abused and punished. Most of Sandra's key developmental experiences with primary objects were met with these consequences. In addition to the RO of abuse, Sandra also appears to see others as reacting to her wishes with threatened or actual abandonment, as seen in the threats of her adoptive mother to return her to the foster agency. She also feared revealing the abuse in her family for a similar reason. We can also identify a pattern of others reacting to Sandra with neglect and disinterest by simply ignoring her needs.

When Sandra's wishes are typically met with abuse, abandonment, and neglect, she has a number of prototypical reactions. She experiences a deep sense of feeling unsafe, fearful, and terrified of her surroundings. Thus, she has developed a resulting, complex constellation of symptoms. She lives in constant fear and is crippled by her rigid sequence of avoidance patterns, choreographed precisely to protect her from her terror. She responds to the usual demands of everyday life with hypervigilance, always alert to potential attacks from others. Her fears and lack of security stemming from a pattern of abusive relationships (and a related childhood incident) have consummated in the intense fear of being killed by a male attacker. Sandra concomitantly responds to others with mistrust, likely a result of her wish to be protected that was decimated through years of abuse and abandonment. In addition, with others responding to her with disinterest and neglect, Sandra feels negated and disconnected from others. A summarization of the elements of Sandra's CCRT is as follows:

Wish: To be safe and protected, to trust and depend upon others, to be appreciated and valued
Response of object (RO): Abuse, punishment, abandonment, disinterest
Response of self (RS): Anxiety, anger, fear, loneliness, and disconnection

Clearly, these relationship patterns have an integral role in generating and escalating Sandra's symptom patterns. Where once particular relationships provided her with responses to be feared, she has generalized this response to the world at large. Though she desires closeness with others and appears to have an opportunity to work toward an intimate relationship with her current boyfriend, she expects the response of others to be so toxic that she herself responds with an emotionless connection. This protects her from extending herself emotionally too far with objects. In many ways, Sandra's insufficient defenses in making herself feel safe renders others in her life literally objects that perform the function of being present to ward off her catastrophic fears. She subsequently becomes dependent on her object world for a facade of safety and protection—her wish—yet can never truly trust in their security. Her ambivalent reliance on this object world comes at the price of her autonomy. This is cogently expressed in the image of the adult Sandra, appearing as regressed as a young child, crippled by her fears, and needing to sleep on the floor of her parent's bedroom. Though she had looked to them for safety and protection that did not materialize, she was rather violated and struggles with her terror about the world. It is sadly ironic that despite her experience with her parents (both as internalized objects and real objects) she sees few options other than to retreat to them for support. She needs others for safety and protection yet also for bolstering any positive feelings about herself. For example, though likely motivated by her strengths and desires, Sandra's success in her career is perpetuated by her fear of failing in the eyes of her boss, subsumed under her core wish to be appreciated. Sandra's sense of self is a tenuous one. She appears to feel that if left to her own devices she cannot survive in a harsh and threatening world.

Sandra's personality style can best be characterized as dependent. Yet here we see an interesting and key element of core conflictual wishes. She depends monumentally upon others to protect her from a terrifying world, yet cannot become too close for fear of the emotional connection. One can speculate that this is exactly the conflict she experiences with her boyfriend. She questions his feelings toward her as a function of her fears of closeness. Although she did not meet the diagnostic criteria at this point, Sandra presents with many of the clinical features of an individual with a chronic, posttraumatic adjustment to a trauma. For Sandra, the world is a threatening place to be protected from and much of the stimuli present in everyday life have become potential threats to be avoided.

The Therapeutic Relationship

The Therapeutic Bond

As suggested earlier, the quality and nature of the therapeutic relationship and the patient's experience of the relationship as a helping one is a cornerstone of supportive-expressive psychotherapy. In addition to its important supportive role, the therapeutic alliance has been shown to predict subsequent outcome (Gaston et al., 1991). The salience of a positive working alliance or transference of course dates back to Freud, who saw it as the primary curative factor in psychotherapy (Stolorow, 1988). Thus there are numerous considerations when discussing the therapeutic relationship. The therapist must initially and persistently present himself or herself as a trustworthy and reliable professional. Genuine concern and attentiveness for the patient must be communicated through listening and empathic responding. The patient should know that the therapist truly wants to be helpful. In addition, portraying oneself as a positive agent of change who can convey that the patient will show improvement sets the groundwork for a fruitful course of treatment. The therapeutic relationship in supportive-expressive psychotherapy is a collaborative one. The work of therapy is a joint task of the patient and the therapist—which is a powerful and critical communication that is required to the patient. This communication is not only done in explicit ways (e.g., "We will be working together to explore some of the problems we talked about tonight"), but also in more subtle ways. For example, when speaking about the treatment Luborsky (1984) suggests language that includes the terms "we" or "let's" (let us) several times per session to highlight the collaborative nature of the treatment. Referring to "our work together" relieves the person of some of the huge burden of change that has eluded them, while also encouraging some responsibility in the tasks of therapy as work.

Roles in the Therapeutic Relationship

The respective roles of the therapist and patient are defined by and for both parties very early on in therapy. This is done initially through an introduction of the therapy, often referred to as a socialization to therapy (Luborsky, 1984). The information conveyed delimits the roles and responsibilities of the patient and therapist and sets the tasks and structure for therapy. Among the relevant information, patients are encouraged that their role in the collaboration is to be open and forthcoming with their thoughts and feelings. Unlike classical psychoanalysis, revealing everything through free association (Freud, 1924) is not as rigidly applied. Patients are encouraged to say what is on their minds to the extent that, if issues are forgotten or omitted, these may become the topic of exploration. Patients are told that they will be doing most of the talking and that the role of the therapist is one of a collaborative professional. The patient is told that the therapist will be helping them solve problems through listening and understanding, not by giving advice. The therapist will be assisting the patient is making them aware of aspects of their emotional life that they may not have been aware of. Patients are educated about the role of the unconscious and relationship patterns. The therapist should communicate to the patient that sometimes change is difficult and that things may worsen before they improve. An important concept to convey is that patients may have negative feelings at times about the treatment or the therapist and this may influence them in some way to avoid coming. It is at these times that talking about these issues and coming to therapy is most crucial. The therapist's role is also to comment on the patients' progress, making them aware of their movement toward goals.

In terms of the level of activity of supportive-expressive therapists, they are likely to fall somewhere in the vast gulf between the stereotypical inactivity of a psychoanalyst and the high level of activity of cognitive or cognitive-behavioral therapists. The therapist must direct a great deal of attention to empathic listening in order to gain understanding. This involves not only focused attention but also posing questions to the patient for clarification and the production of more material. However, the therapist must also be quite active in elucidating the elements of the CCRT, refining them and helping the patient understand. Therapists working in short-term supportive-expressive therapy are encouraged to be considerably more active, given the limited time available (Barber & Crits-Christoph, 1991). Supportive-expressive therapists, unlike their cognitive-behavioral counterparts, are typically not directive with respect to providing specific instruction. As in other dynamic psychotherapies, the role of the therapist is to assist patients in gaining understanding through their own methods of exploration. Rather than being directed to the tasks or the process of therapy, one might say they are invited to them. In this regard, assigned tasks or homework are generally less likely in supportive-expressive psychotherapy than they are in cognitive-behavioral work. With a patient such as Sandra, homework could tend to engender a perception of imbalance in the therapeutic relationship and unnecessarily raise negative transferences. This is not to say that supportive-expressive therapists do not encourage patients to engage in activities outside of therapy sessions. When insights are gained or patients come to new understandings about relationship issues, the therapist might suggest attempting a new way of responding in the ensuing week, as in the following example:

Sandra: In some ways I guess I do trust my boyfriend, but I can't tell him about this or he'll just ignore it.

Therapist: We've talked about how you have come to expect that reaction, but I wonder what would happen if you did tell him, if you could talk to him in a way that would help you feel less afraid.

The respective therapist and patient roles in supportive-expressive psychotherapy will be a highly important element to consider in Sandra's treatment. She has not been in any kind of ongoing or long-term psychotherapy previously. It is even doubtful that she has experienced more than a few (if any) relationships that were collaborative and positive. This is an area where the formulation of the CCRT can be helpful in understanding some of the likely reactions—transference reactions—that the patient will have with respect to her role in therapy. Given what we know about Sandra's CCRT, personality style, and methods of coping, she is likely to have great difficulty developing trust, as this was not forthcoming in her emotional development. The task of sharing her thoughts has led her in the past to ROs of abuse and abandonment and it will require her to feel an unfamiliar sense of safety and trust to begin to work in therapy. One may even speculate that with her wish to be protected and cared for and her driven perfectionism to be seen as competent in the eyes of others, participating in a collaborative struggle would be new and difficult territory for her. Thus, we may see Sandra vacillate between an overly controlling and overly dependent role in the course of the treatment. In fact, progressing to the point in the therapeutic relationship where a joint struggle is occurring may be a worthy goal in and of itself.

The tenor of the therapeutic alliance also depends to a large extent upon the level of interest and motivation present in the patient. Patients who are otherwise distracted from the task of change for external reasons (e.g., secondary gains) or internal reasons (e.g., not interested in changing, not interested in treatment) must be carefully assessed. Some concerns about Sandra's involvement in treatment at the behest of her boyfriend should be raised. Optimally, these potential pitfalls could be addressed with the patient either pretreatment or very early on. Patients should feel they are ready to take some progressive action to address their distress rather than simply contemplating making changes (Prochaska & DiClemente, 1984).

Treatment Implementation and Outcome

Techniques and Methods of Working

The specific techniques utilized in supportive-expressive therapy are appropriate for use with Sandra. As noted previously, the keystone of the supportive-expressive treatment is the formulation and use of the

CCRT. The therapist's task is to determine which aspects of the CCRT are amenable to change by the patient. This typically involves linking the distressing symptom presentation with the patient's relational themes. The more the CCRT can be identified in different contexts and with different relationships, the better likelihood that generalization of learning can occur (Luborsky & Mark, 1991). For Sandra, we see that an important aspect of her significant anxiety and avoidance relates to the fact that her wish to be protected is met with abuse and neglect, and thus the world is a terrifying place from which to hide. Communicating this formulation to the patient, linking her symptoms and CCRT might be presented in this manner:

> *Therapist:* Sandra, you seem to truly want to trust people and be protected by them. Yet when you have trusted people—your family in particular—that has resulted in your being taken advantage of. So now, rather than relying on people or reaching out to them, you pull back and avoid them. And you respond to them and the world around you as if there is a threat out there, even when you intellectually know there isn't. What do think about that?

The CCRT becomes most salient and useful when it can be interpreted in the context of the therapeutic relationship. With Sandra, we may see her enactment of behaviors that can be viewed as subtle signs of treatment resistance, but they can be understood as her CCRT functioning in the therapeutic relationship. Sandra may show resistance in many ways. One scenario is likely to involve her tendency to want to be seen as highly functional and competent (her wish to be valued and appreciated) in the eyes of the therapist, despite evidence to the contrary. The therapist might proceed as follows:

> *Therapist:* Sandra, I noticed right now and several times in our session today that you seem to be very close to crying but you hold yourself back.
> *Sandra:* It has been a little upsetting this week, but I'm okay.
> *Therapist:* This reminds me a little of how you described what it is like with your family and your boss. Really needing them but not wanting to let your guard down. I'm wondering if that is happening in here, with me, in our work together.

The therapist must walk a fine line in interpreting the CCRT and transference with Sandra. She tends to expect others to be harsh and punishing and may even experience the focus on the relationship as critical. Sandra is likely to slowly test the waters of the therapeutic relationship, as emotional safety is extremely important to her. Fortunately, if communicated in a caring manner, accurate interpretations of the CCRT are often experienced by the patient as supportive, engendering a bolstering of the therapeutic alliance. Accurate CCRT interpretations have also been found to be related to outcome (Crits-Christoph, Cooper, & Luborsky, 1988).

Supportive-expressive psychotherapy betrays its roots in classical psychoanalytic therapy in that it is essentially an individual psychotherapy whereby knowledge is gained through the therapeutic relationship and applied by the patient in their other relationships (Luborsky, 1984). However, because of the importance placed on interpersonal relationships, including family members in the treatment process—either in joint sessions or via information gathering in person or by phone—is not contraindicated. It is often helpful to observe the actual interactions between the patient and significant others as a way of increasing understanding of the CCRT and the therapeutic relationship. Involving significant others in Sandra's treatment would seem to be indicated, though likely at a later stage in the treatment. It would be very important for Sandra to develop a trusting and robust treatment alliance to meet some initial therapeutic goals first (e.g., symptom reduction). This would provide a sufficient holding environment for more intense work to be attempted. From a supportive-expressive standpoint, if Sandra was amenable to introducing significant others into the treatment process it may be helpful to address issues in her relationship with her boyfriend as an initial foray. This relationship seems to be the most stable and healthy at this point. Given the severity of Sandra's early experiences and the state of her relationships with her adoptive parents, a family-therapist colleague could be helpful in providing family systems treatment conjointly with Sandra's individual therapy.

Medical and Nutritional Issues

Sandra does not appear to have any current significant medical or nutritional issues about which to be concerned. Issues that arise should be considered first in the context of their relationship to Sandra's psychological functioning as well as her relational matrix (CCRT). To be cautious, and recognizing that treatment is likely to precipitate a temporary exacerbation in symptoms, we should be attentive to any changes in her vegetative functioning. An increase or decrease in sleep, appetite, energy, or libido may signal a burgeoning depression.

An important element in Sandra's treatment is the consideration of whether she requires an evaluation by a psychiatrist and perhaps medication to address some of her symptoms. This should be a collaborative decision between Sandra and her therapist. There is no inherent theoretical contraindication to the use of medication in supportive-expressive psychotherapy. In fact, there is research to suggest that patients will do better with a combination of medication and psychotherapy than with either alone (e.g., Smith, Glass, & Miller, 1980). The severity of Sandra's symptoms suggests that her therapist would be prudent in raising the need for a medication evaluation. A reduction in her symptom severity would not only be beneficial for Sandra, but would afford the treatment a more adaptive, functional participant. Medical issues that potentially would arise would be managed by referral to an appropriate physician consultant.

Potential Pitfalls

Sandra presents a number of potential areas of difficulty and resistance. As mentioned earlier, information from Sandra's CCRT suggests that developing a trusting therapeutic relationship may be initially difficult for her. Sandra is likely to be a patient with whom a very supportive approach should be used in the early phase of therapy to encourage her attachment to the therapist. We should be alert to signs that Sandra could drop out of therapy prematurely, fearing that the prospects of the therapy would be potentially even more distressing than her symptoms. We might also wonder how her fears ("I'm so afraid something bad will happen to me") might manifest in psychotherapy with respect to avoiding salient yet painful issues. We should similarly be concerned about Sandra's ability to learn new ways of managing her problems, both because of their chronicity and her obsessive and avoidant style. Developing new interactional patterns and behaviors is likely to be a terrifying experience for her initially. In addition to bolstering the therapeutic alliance, Sandra must be assisted in identifying her own reasons for involvement in therapy. When she confronts her overwhelming anxiety, her boyfriend's encouragement to continue with the process may not be enough to sustain her investment in treatment. Supportive-expressive therapists often have to assess the patient's need for more or less supportiveness, erring on the side of more, to support a patient's self-esteem and aid them in managing anxiety (Luborsky, 1984). Many of these concerns about Sandra's participation in therapy would require an increasing level of supportiveness and a parallel reduction in expressive techniques. It should be recalled that patients' symptoms, while certainly targets for treatment, serve an important homeostatic function in the psyche. Supportive-expressive therapy attempts to build the alliance so that expressive techniques can be utilized, rather than confronting and disabling defenses (Barber & Crits-Christoph, 1991).

One further consideration relates to the effects of positive change in Sandra's symptoms and relationships. We have come to understand that her symptoms serve the function of expressing areas of conflict in her relationships, as formulated through the CCRT. Through the supportive-expressive process of understanding, insight, and mastery of these issues, symptom change will occur. Sandra's symptoms appear to be of such intensity and have such a constricting impact on her and her family's life that the recession of these symptoms will change her life tremendously. Although these changes will be mostly positive, Sandra may need to be prepared for how her relationships might change and how others may view her. At the very least, we might imagine that when Sandra experiences a reduction in her fear and anxiety, she will be more able to be independent and thus require less of her family and boyfriend in certain respects.

She may also require *more* in other respects. This is likely to be a substantial family system change and may precipitate other than supportive responses from the system.

Termination and Relapse Prevention

The process of termination in psychoanalytic psychotherapies, including supportive-expressive psychotherapy, is of the utmost importance to the whole of treatment. Termination facilitates a review of the entire treatment process, endeavors to assist the patient in maintaining the gains made in treatment, and works toward helping the patient understand separation (Luborsky, 1984). A discussion of termination should begin at the outset of treatment when decisions are made regarding treatment length. In open-ended supportive-expressive psychotherapy, termination issues tend to arise when a patient feels they have achieved the goals they have set or when the therapist observes a patient's satisfaction through a reduction of symptoms. This does not necessarily mean that the patient has achieved all of his or her goals but rather has a sense of having better control over them (Luborsky, 1984). If new goals are not decided upon, proceeding with the process of termination attempts to help the patient reinforce the goals achieved and separate from the therapist. This latter process becomes the focus of the end stage of treatment. Patients will often raise issues regarding being able to function on their own without the support of the therapist. Symptoms may arise again in this context; helping the patient understand their meaning in the context of the therapeutic relationship and separation can facilitate the termination process and closure. Patients are not dissuaded from contacting the therapist after termination, particularly to inform the therapist of progress. Keeping the door open allows for the patient to return to a helpful relationship at some point, whether or not further treatment is required.

If Sandra makes the long journey through treatment in supportive-expressive psychotherapy, the process of termination will likely be rather arduous for her. If we imagine that she successfully forged a positive working alliance with her therapist (in light of her CCRT concerns regarding trust and safety), separation from this important person will be extremely difficult. One hopes that Sandra would make gains throughout the treatment in solidifying her sense of self and independence, which she could then call on to manage termination. Sandra's tendency to become dependent on others as well as her fears and anxieties are likely to reappear in ending the treatment. Here, the therapist must revisit the gains made with the patient and reinforce her understanding of the CCRT and its relation to her symptoms.

Mechanisms of Change

As discussed earlier, the mechanism of change in supportive-expressive psychotherapy occurs in three ways. For Sandra, the most salient agent of change would appear to be that she gain an understanding of her terrifying and fearful responses and need for protection as they relate to her past and present relationship patterns, that is, the CCRT. With a more complete and insightful perspective on her world, Sandra may be better attuned to her own wishes and needs, which would assist her in adapting better to the world around her. The therapeutic relationship serves an important role in the process of changes and thus a key component of Sandra's improvement will be her ability to benefit from the establishment of a positive working alliance with the therapist. In and of itself, the experience of collaborating within a safe holding environment as she pursues a journey of self-exploration and change will serve a powerful function for Sandra. Finally, assuming the previous mechanisms of change have been satisfactorily accomplished, one would hope that Sandra would internalize the gains made and be able to process the myriad thoughts and emotions that arise during termination.

CONCLUSION

Supportive-expressive psychotherapy carries on the intellectual tradition of psychoanalytic practice initiated by Freud. The manualization of the model by Luborsky (1984) and others has allowed the complex and enigmatic process of a dynamic psychotherapy to be scientifically validated, researched, and communicated to others. This case discussion of Sandra highlights the use of a time-open-ended supportive-expressive psychotherapy for a young women in significant acute and chronic distress. Supportive-expressive psychotherapy emphasized the importance of the therapeutic alliance and the focus on interpersonal relationships as the conduit to understanding symptoms and relational patterns.

REFERENCES

Barber, J. P., & Crits-Christoph, P. (1991). Comparison of the brief dynamic therapies. In J. P. Barber & P. Crits-Christoph (Eds.), *Handbook of short-term dynamic psychotherapy* (pp. 323–355). New York: Basic Books.

Bordin, E. S. (1979). The generalizability of the psychoanalytic concept of the working alliance. *Psychotherapy: Theory, Research and Practice, 16,* 252–260.

Connolly, M. B., Crits-Christoph, P., Shelton, R. C., Hollon, S., Barber, J. P., Butler, S. F., Baker, S., & Thase, M. E. (1999). The reliability and validity of a measure of self-understanding of interpersonal patterns. *Journal of Counseling Psychology, 46*(4), 472–482.

Crits-Christoph, P., Cooper, A., & Luborsky, L. (1988). The accuracy of therapists' interpretations and the outcome of dynamic psychotherapy. *Journal of Consulting and Clinical Psychology, 56,* 490–495.

Exner, J. E. (1994). Rorschach and the study of the individual. In I. B. Weiner (Ed.), *Rorschachiana: Yearbook of the International Rorschach Society* (Vol. 19, pp. 7–23). Seattle, WA: Hogrefe & Huber.

Freud, S. (1924). *A general introduction to psychoanalysis.* New York: Washington Square Press.

Freud, S. (1958). Remembering, repeating and working through: Further recommendations on the technique of psychoanalysis. In J. Strachey (Ed. and Trans.), *The standard edition of the complete psychological works of Sigmund Freud* (Vol. 12, pp. 145–156). London: Hogarth Press. (Original work published 1914)

Gaston, L., Marmar, C. R., Gallagher, D., & Thompson, L. W. (1991). Alliance prediction of outcome beyond in-treatment symptomatic change as psychotherapy progresses. *Psychotherapy Research, 1,* 104–113.

Horvath, A. O., & Symonds, B. D. (1991). Relation between working alliance and outcome in psychotherapy: A meta-analysis. *Journal of Counseling Psychology, 38*(2), 139–149.

Luborsky, L. (1984). *Principles of psychoanalytic psychotherapy: A manual for supportive-expressive treatment.* New York: Basic Books.

Luborsky, L., Barber, J. P., & Crits-Christoph, P. (1990). Advent of objective measures of the transference concept. *Journal of Consulting and Clinical Psychology, 54,* 39–47.

Luborsky, L., & Crits-Christoph, P. (1990). *Understanding transference: The CCRT method.* New York: Basic Books.

Luborsky, L., Crits-Christoph, P., Mintz, J., & Auerbach, A. (1988). *Who will benefit from psychotherapy? Predicting therapeutic outcomes.* New York: Basic Books.

Luborsky, L., & Mark, D. (1991). Short-term supportive-expressive psychoanalytic psychotherapy. In J. P. Barber & P. Crits-Christoph (Eds.), *Handbook of short-term dynamic psychotherapy* (pp. 110–136). New York: Basic Books.

Mark, D., & Faude, J. (1997). Supportive-expressive therapy of cocaine abuse. In J. P. Barber & P. Crits-Christoph (Eds.), *Dynamic therapies for psychiatric disorders: (Axis I)* (pp. 294–331). New York: Basic Books.

Prochaska, J. O., & DiClemente, C. C. (1984). Self change processes, self-efficacy and decisional balance across five stages of smoking cessation. *Progress in Clinical and Biological Research, 156,* 131–140.

Rockland, L. H. (1989). *Supportive therapy: A psychodynamic approach.* New York: Basic Books.

Smith, M., Glass, G., & Miller, T. (1980). *The benefits of psychotherapy.* Baltimore: Johns Hopkins Press.

Stolorow, R. (1988). Transference and the therapeutic process. *The Psychoanalytic Review, 75*(2), 245–254.

Wallerstein, R., Robbins, L., Sargent, H., & Luborsky, L. (1956). The psychotherapy research project of the Menninger Foundation. Rationale, method and sample use. *Bulletin of the Menninger Clinic, 20,* 221–280.

Woody, G., Luborsky, L., McLellan, A. T., O'Brien, C., Beck, A. T., Blaine, J., Herman, I., & Hole, A. V. (1983). Psychotherapy for opiate addicts: Does it help? *Archives of General Psychiatry, 40,* 639–645.

12

Psychodynamic Psychotherapy

Paul M. Lerner

TREATMENT MODEL

Psychoanalytic theory has always been in a state of flux and evolution. From an early concern with an identification of the instincts and their vicissitudes (drive theory) and a subsequent emphasis on studying the ego (structural theory), the focus—especially during the past several decades—has shifted to a greater interest in the early mother-child relationship and its impact on the development of the self (self psychology) and the quality of later interpersonal relations (object relations theory). These shifts in emphasis have resulted in four different and distinct submodels (drive theory, structural theory, object relations theory, self theory) or perspectives for understanding a person.

Drive theory refers to Freud's earliest stages of theory construction in which he was primarily interested in identifying the basic instincts (Freud, 1923/1961). Despite changes in his theory of instincts over time, in his latest writings he settled upon two instincts: libido and aggression. Current writers tend not to use the term *instinct*, but instead evoke terms such as *wishes, desires, urges, needs,* and others. Although different words are used, this model focuses on the motivational aspect of behavior.

From his initial interest in drive identification, Freud's work shifted to an emphasis on understanding those processes that controlled and regulated the drives (Freud, 1923/1961). He began to outline the characteristics, synthesis, and functions of the ego with particular emphasis on the defensive function. This change in theoretical emphasis ushered in the structural model and eventuated in Freud's formulations regarding the tripartite (ego, superego, id) structure of the personality.

A recent advance in psychoanalytic theory has been the elaboration of an object relations model. Basic to this perspective is the recognition of the complex, yet defining, interactions among early formative interpersonal relationships, the quality of internal psychological structures, and the nature of ongoing interpersonal relations including the ways they are internalized and become part of the personality. Core psychoanalytic concepts, which had been understood in exclusively intrapsychic terms such as *defense* and *thought processes,* have been reconceptualized so as to take into account their interpersonal implications.

In a series of major publications, Kohut (1977, 1978) laid the conceptual groundwork for a comprehensive psychoanalytic psychology of the self. Before Kohut, the concept of self had occupied a relatively peripheral role for psychoanalytic thinkers; however, in conceptualizing the self as a superordinate concept, outlining the various dimensions of the self, and emphasizing self-experiences, Kohut elevated the concept to the status of a full submodel.

It is important to bear in mind that most psychoanalysts and psychodynamic therapists do not adhere exclusively to one specific perspective, but instead make conceptual use of all four.

In concert with this evolution in theory has been movement away from an experience-distant metapsychology couched in a mechanistic natural-science framework of impersonal structures, forces, and energies to a more experience-near clinical theory concerned primarily with experiences and subjective meanings.

With this changing emphasis in theory have also come new conceptualizations of psychopathology. The older model of psychopathology—based on drive theory and structural theory—stressed impulses pressing for discharge, defenses evoked, and the interplay between the two that resulted in conflict, increased anxiety, and symptom formation. From object relations theory and self psychology has come an alternative conceptualization, a "developmental arrest" or "structural deficit" model, which highlights impairments in the personality structure itself as a consequence of faulty development.

Implicit in these differing models of psychopathology are also different ways of thinking about the treatment process. Theories of treatment rooted in the earlier conflict model stressed interpretation and insight, with therapy seen as a unique type of education and the therapeutic relationship as a special laboratory for exploring and experiencing the critical dynamic configurations as they emerged in the transference. In this classical treatment model, the analyst pays particular attention to the resistances and transference reactions and relies on the patient's free associations as the major means of communication. The core intervention is interpretation, which consists of confrontation, clarification, interpretation, and working through (Greenson, 1967). The analyst maintains a somewhat detached position and adheres to a policy of neutrality.

In contrast, as Michaels (1983) has noted, conceptualizations of treatment based on later models of psychopathology "emphasize the psychological substrata and nutriments necessary for growth and development, with therapy being construed as a special kind of parenting, the interpretive process as a model of growth promoting interaction, and the therapeutic relationship as a substitute for the nuclear family as a matrix for individuation and growth" (p. 5). Representative of this newer perspective is Modell's (1978) extension of Winnicott's (1960) concept of the "holding environment" to the treatment situation, Cohen and Sherwood's (1991) evocative and helpful notion of "standing still," and the importance Kohut (1977) attached to "empathic failures."

In addition, there has been a strong tendency to cast older and basic concepts in a more contemporary mold. For example, regression, in its broadest sense, as Ornstein and Ornstein (1980) noted, involves "a return to, or a revival of genetically earlier modes of thought, behavior, and object relations" (p. 12). Regression in treatment, within the drive and structural submodels, has meant the unfolding of the patient's psychopathology in treatment. Although retaining these earlier meanings, theorists from a self-psychology perspective have highlighted a second aspect of regression—its restorative function. Herein, regression is conceptualized as also implying a state in which, through conflict resolution or belated structure building, arrested development may again proceed.

As an eclectic psychoanalyst, I make use of theoretical concepts, dynamic formulations, and technical recommendations issuing from each of the four submodels. I do this with the recognition that the models are complimentary and that my guiding intent is to understand the patient and assist that individual to get well.

1. In being constant and reliable, placing the patient's needs above one's own, accepting what is offensive and obnoxious, judiciously setting

limits, attempting to clarify what for the patient is confusing and bewildering, and enabling the patient to feel understood, one is not only applying good therapeutic techniques, but for some patients, one is also providing symbolic equivalents of parent-child relationship elements.

2. Understanding the patient—typically based on a theory of personality and psychopathology that is related to, but independent of, the treatment—precedes action and furnishes the basis for interventions.

3. Treatment consists of several distinguishable types and levels of relationships, including transference and countertransference reactions, which can and are used to promote the treatment and achieve therapeutic goals.

4. The therapist's major therapeutic tool is his or her empathy. Following upon Kohut (1959/1978), I view empathy as a mode of relating, an aspect of the therapeutic action of treatment, and as an information gathering activity—a way of coming to know another as it were.

5. Interventions are most useful when they are pitched at a level as close to the patient's experience as possible and couched in the patient's language. Stepping into, and making use of, the patient's metaphors is helpful. For example, during his final session an analytic patient repeatedly referred to a valued radio from childhood that served as his lifeline to the news of the outside world and the creative imagery of the inside world. Typically, his analyst ended sessions by saying, "Our time is up." This final hour, instead, he sensitively moved into the metaphor and said, "Signing off."

6. For patient and therapist alike, time should be regarded as a valuable ally. A therapist conveys this in any number of ways, including a readiness to be steady and empathetically present without being intrusive or problem solving in response to the patient's sense of urgency.

7. An important goal of treatment as well as a means to other hoped-for outcomes is self-understanding rooted in a self-reflective attitude.

8. It is my experience that treatment has an unfolding quality. All my treatment cases share a common structure of having a beginning, a middle, and an ending; however, each case has its own unique dynamics which unfold as treatment deepens and progresses.

THE THERAPISTS' SKILLS AND ATTRIBUTES

To do psychoanalytic work requires a number of capacities and skills together with a specific set of attitudes. Greenson (1967) emphasizes two in particular—the capacity to understand the unconscious and the ability to communicate to the patient.

By understanding the unconscious, Greenson is referring to the ability to translate the patient's conscious thoughts, affects, fantasies, urges, and behaviors into their unconscious antecedents. As he puts it, the analyst or therapist "must listen to the obvious melody but also hear the hidden (unconscious) themes in the 'left hand,' the counterpoint" (p. 365).

To hear the music—the unconscious, not just the words—is no mean achievement. It requires a knowledge of psychoanalytic theory, intuition. Greenson (1967) draws a distinction between empathy and intuition, viewing the former as the capacity to experience and share another's feelings and desires and the latter as related to ideas. This distinction also implies a split in function in which the therapist simultaneously experiences with the patient (empathy) and observes the patient's offerings (intuition).

The second capacity Greenson highlights involves the ability to communicate with the patient. Here, the therapist must translate understandings couched in his or her own vocabulary into the very language of the patient's. As well, the therapist needs to decide what to tell the patient, when to tell it, and how to tell it. In itself, the ability to communicate helpfully and effectively assumes various other capacities including empathy, sound judgment, the ability to listen, interest in people, and skill in the use of silence.

In addition to the two capacities Greenson highlights and the requisite subskills, psychoanalytic treatment requires that the therapist also be able to tolerate not knowing, confusion, ambiguity, and aloneness; have available a sense of humor; and have attained a strong sense of professional identity.

Professional identity, in part, consists of ethical standards and one's theoretical orientation. There is another component, however, that extends beyond ethical guidelines and cuts across theoretical persuasions. What I am referring to here is professional identity as reflected in one's attitude toward and approach to patients. Psychoanalytic work, as I see it, is based upon a humanistic-clinical attitude.

By *humanistic,* I mean the humanness of the therapist as expressed in his or her compassion, concern, and therapeutic intent toward the patient. This involves the continuous awareness that the individuals who seek our help are in pain and are suffering. Our task is to understand the nature of their difficulties and to assist them in getting well. One attempts to do this with an appreciation and respect for the patient's separateness and a concern for the patient's self-esteem, self-regard, and dignity.

With respect to the clinical component of this attitude, this first includes a stance of receptive openness. The term "analytic neutrality" has been incorrectly taken to mean abstinence and deprivation. Rather, the concept has to do with an "even hovering attention," an openness to the patient with a striving to understand, not judge.

A second aspect of a clinical attitude involves one's willingness and capacity to accord each session full importance. One is emotionally available, present and unhindered by internal or external distractions. The final element is the therapist's meaning-seeking orientation. I am referring here to one's unwavering pursuit of meaning, understanding, and truth.

THE CASE OF SANDRA

From a psychoanalytic perspective, *DSM-IV* presents serious limitations. Like its more immediate predecessors, almost total emphasis is accorded that which is observable and can be described, with little attention paid to underlying and more invisible structures, dynamics, and meanings. As one consequence, such an approach cannot conceptualize individuals who present marked contradictions between external and internal spheres of functioning.

In addition, each *DSM* edition has made use of a categorical schema rather than a dimensional or contextual one. By definition, different types of psychopathology are viewed as discrete and discontinuous, and the distinction between normalcy and pathology is considered as one of kind, not as one of degree. The attempt to negotiate this by assigning dual or multiple diagnoses with the implied premise that each diagnosis signifies a distinct disturbance is antithetical to the psychoanalytic clinician who views various external expressions (e.g., symptoms, complaints, etc.) as arising from a common internal source, what McWilliams (1998) refers to as the "same overall sickness of the soul" (p. 199).

Because of these difficulties, together with the consideration that the *DSM* schema does little to inform a more dynamic form of treatment, I use an alternative diagnostic scheme, one proposed by Kernberg (1970). Kernberg's diagnostic scheme involves assessing patients along two relatively independent dimensions. The first dimension consists of a descriptive characterlogical diagnosis in terms of character structure. Representative and commonly encounted character structures would include the hysterical character, the obsessive compulsive character, the depressive character, the masochistic character, the infantile personality, the narcissistic personality, the schizoid personality, and the paranoid personality. For a fuller description of these particular character structures and a comprehensive discussion of the concept of character refer to Lerner (1998).

Recognizing that a descriptive characterlogical diagnosis is necessary but not sufficient, Kernberg (1970) outlined a second dimension. Referred to as "levels of personality organization," this dimension involves a systematic appraisal of underlying psychological structures. The specific structures assessed include level of instinctual development, signs of ego weakness, defenses, quality of internalized object relations, level of superego development, and ego identity. Each of these structures is placed on a three-level continuum, ranging from higher level to intermediate level to lower level.

In keeping with psychoanalytic practice and with my own style of working, I will slightly depart from the editors' proposed outline and begin with the case conceptualization.

Assessment, Conceptualization, and Treatment Planning

Case Conceptualization

From a symptomatic perspective, most striking is the nature and extent of the patient's anxiety and her way of dealing with it. Her anxiety is chronic, unremitting, diffuse, and free-floating. Ever present, it imposes severe restrictions on her daily life. In addition to various psychophysiological expressions, her anxiety is manifest in a constant state of apprehension and fear, in thought content that is dominated by an assortment of worries, and in the recurring fear that she will be intruded upon by an unknown assailant.

Although her family home was in fact broken into when she was a teenager, I understand this specific apprehension as an externalization of the internal threat of her conscious state being intruded upon by primary process expressions, including primitive urges, affects, and fantasies and the accompanying loss of reality. This is to say, it is my hunch that one core fear underlying her pervasive anxiety is the fear of "going crazy" and becoming like the psychotic mother of her childhood.

Accompanying the anxiety is marked avoidance, numerous phobias, and a regime of rituals all designed to lower the anxiety and allow her to function in the world. Although these behaviors permit her to function, they clearly do not totally bind her anxiety. In addition, her external world has become remarkably restrictive.

In the assessment provided, I was also impressed with the nature of the patent's object relations (interpersonal relations) and the way in which she treats those individuals closest to her. She is painfully aware of her intense anxiety and fear of aloneness; however, she seems unaware of her impact on others. More specifically, through her symptoms she exerts tremendous control over her objects (individuals). For example, when her boyfriend leaves early, she finds herself unable to shower. And when her boss expresses anger, she dreamed of a man stabbing her and her parents. Attuning to the latent rather than overt meaning, I view each incident as also reflecting either the intense anger or resentment the patient feels when she is unable to control one or the other. In the first instance, her reaction to her boyfriend's leaving is to relinquish a self-caring function with the implied message that he is to blame. In the second instance, the anger toward her boss is reversed in her dream so that rather than her wishing to injure and kill him, it is instead she herself who is the passive and wounded party. Viewed from this perspective—her symptoms as a way of controlling her objects—it is my impression that pervasive fears of separation are driving the need for such control.

Interpersonally, the patient is described as emotionally aloof, superficial, and dependent. Further to the issue of her need to control her objects, I view the patient not as relating herself to others in a dependent way, but rather in a narcissistic way. By this I mean that she does not regard others as separate and distinct, but rather as extensions of her self who are to provide functions she internally cannot provide for herself. These specific functions include a sense of security, safety, protection, and well-being. In addition, she is unable to calm and soothe herself; hence, she looks to others for self-soothing as well.

Her need for a sense of security and well-being and her desire to be soothed are legitimate; however, that she cannot provide these self-sustaining functions for herself implies a significantly disturbed early mother-child relationship together with failures in internalization. One can but imagine the experiences with, and impact of, a paranoid schizophrenic mother. What we do know is that her mother not only failed to provide a sense of safety and well-being, but to the contrary filled the patient with her own anxieties and sense of the world as fearsome and dangerous. Then too, it is from this relationship that the patient emerged with a basic sense of distrust of others.

Other and later aspects of the patient's childhood are also troubling and of concern. Repeated themes include abandonment and threats of abandonment, instability, betrayal, disillusionment, sexual molestation, and not being listened to.

Because of the nature and severity of the patient's symptoms—in particular, the pervasiveness of her anxiety and the degree to which it controls and rules her life; the narcissistic quality of her relationships including her need to control her objects; and the developmentally early level of struggles (i.e., fear of madness, fear of separation, distrust of others, etc.)—she is continually attempting to negotiate; I consider the patient more disturbed and injured than is implied in her *DSM-IV* diagnosis of specific phobia and generalized anxiety disorder.

The above diagnosis is essentially descriptive and rests solely on presentation of symptoms. In terms of Kernberg's (1970) model, what is missing is a consideration of structural and dynamic factors. Were one to consider these variables, one might conclude that beyond her disabling symptoms the patient also presents a damaged personality as evidenced by severe ego weaknesses (i.e., poor anxiety tolerance), primitive defenses (projective identification, denial), and impaired object relations.

Despite the significant level of impairment, the patient also demonstrates several capacities that can be mobilized in treatment. Specifically, she functions relatively effectively with structure, historically has stood up for herself, and on her job reveals determination, stick-to-itiveness, and commitment. Also, although effected in a narcissistic way, she has shown the ability to constructively make use of others. Finally, the patient is in pain and is suffering, and these are powerful motives for continuing in treatment.

Assessment

As indicated earlier, I do not view the patient's debilitating and pervasive anxiety as an isolated symptom. Rather, I conceive of her anxiety as both a part of and an expression of a primitive personality organization with a number of structural impairments. The furnished material hints at the nature of several of these impairments; however, it does not address them directly nor does it attend to others. For example, in the service of attempting to calm and regulate her anxiety, one sees clearly how the patient acts upon her external world. Less clear are the internal processes, the defenses, that are employed to contain the anxiety.

Because of the lack of attention to structural and dynamic concerns, I would ask that the patient be psychologically tested in which she is administered a battery of tests including the WAIS-III, Rorschach, and TAT. Based on Rapaport's (1950) concept of "levels of structure," a test battery, as opposed to any one test, allows the examiner to observe an individual in a variety of situations that differ in their relative degree of structure. For instance, we are familiar with those patients who function smoothly and efficiently on the WAIS-III yet experience serious difficulties, including regressive responses, on the less structured Rorschach test. Noting the quality of an individual's reaction to different levels of external structure often has important diagnostic and treatment implications.

From such an assessment, I would hope to obtain a clearer sense of the patient's defensive structure, coherence of self, capacity of object constancy, and the effects of lesser degrees of external structure on her thinking and functioning. Also, if the examiner were able to pinpoint especially troublesome dynamic areas, identify narcissistic vulnerabilities, and outline potential treatment pitfalls, that too would be especially helpful. Finally, recognizing that any case conceptualization is tentative and amenable to change, an external assessment would assist in supporting, refuting, and refining several of my preliminary hypotheses.

Findings from the psychological testing would be integrated with my own clinical impressions to assist in structuring the treatment. With specific reference to this case, such findings would help determine how structured the treatment itself should be, frequency of sessions, and how out-of-session events like phone calls and requests for extra sessions should be handled.

Therapeutic Goals

Although the distinction is somewhat artificial, as noted in the case conceptualization, I consider the patient's difficulties as arising from structural impairment rather than from higher level structural conflict. Therefore, the overall goal is one of structure building so as to promote individuation and growth.

Previously, I indicated that the impaired structures in this patient are those that would afford her a sense of safety, security, protection, and well-being. Because she is unable to effect these functions intrapsychically, others are relied upon to provide them for her. A prime goal of treatment, then, is to repair the faulty structures that underlie her lack of sense of well-being and also interfere with her capacity to soothe herself.

Intimately related to these impairments is her failure to have fully completed the separation-individuation process. Mahler, Pine, and Bergmann (1975) carefully outlined the specific stages of this developmental process. Separation, according to these authors, begins with the infant's differentiating himself or herself from the mother. This is then followed by a stage, characterized by forms of locomotion, in which the infant becomes so absorbed in his or her own autonomous functioning that mother is virtually excluded. Increasingly recognizing the greater independence and distance, the child then redirects his or her main attention back to mother. This stage, referred to as rapproachment, is characterized by constant shifts in the child between the need for closeness and the desire for distance. With the completion of rapproachment the child moves into the final stages of feeling the beginnings of a sense of self and of constancy of the object. It is the development of a sense of self and of object constancy that ultimately affords and guarantees full and lasting separation.

One senses that Sandra's psychic survival depends upon the availability of her objects. This dependence extends well beyond residing in her adoptive parents' home, occasionally sleeping in their bedroom, and refusing to shower when her boyfriend is away. She experiences her objects as her lifeline. This basic level of relatedness, in terms of Mahler's theory, clearly implies an arressment in the separation process. Another prime goal, therefore, paraphrasing Michaels (1983), involves therapy as a matrix for completing separation and individuation.

A third goal, one consistent with the two previous ones, relates to the nature of the patient's anxiety. From the furnished material, it is my impression that the patient suffers from a particular form of anxiety referred to in the psychoanalytic literature as "annihilation anxiety" (Hurvich, 1989). As its name suggests, annihilation anxiety refers to an individual's subjective fear of impending psychic or physical destruction. It finds expression in fears of being overwhelmed, of loss of control, of fading away, and of being destroyed.

A core aspect of annihilation anxiety is traumatic anxiety (Freud, 1926/1959), a form that floods and overwhelms the individual. Traumatic anxiety heralds the reemergence of a traumatic situation, conceptualized by Freud as "a recognized, remembered, expected situation of helplessness" (Freud, 1926/1959, p. 166). It is useful to distinguish annihilation anxiety from the signal variety. Signal anxiety is a complex development achievement in which anxiety is experienced and expressed in a greatly attenuated form. It is based on the capacity for anticipation and adaptively alerts the individual to specific and realistic dangers. Because annihilation anxiety can come to be anticipated and its affective component tamed, this represents another prime goal of treatment.

It is important to bear in mind that although the treatment goals were discussed separately, they are inextricably intertwined. Progress toward one necessarily will involve movement toward the others. For example, the shift from annihilation anxiety to signal anxiety also implies a shift from a disrupted personality to a functional one.

Timeline for Therapy

A core feature of this patient's pathology is her not having attained object constancy. The concept refers to the child's capacity to remain attached to the mother even in her physical absence, when there is no instinctual need of her, or even when the child is angry with her. Constancy is fully established when the child can evoke a comforting inner image of the mother in her physical absence. Such an image continues throughout life, comforting the adult much as the actual mother had comforted the young child. As a consequence of this failure, subsequent development achievements, including the capacity for mature attachments, the ability to tolerate aloneness, and a sense of continuity of self over time are all severely compromised.

Patients who have not achieved object constancy, who have not internalized the comforting mother of childhood, require a treatment framework that takes into account their struggle in forming attachments, ongoing fear of abandonment, difficulty in modulating affects, and most important, distrust of subsequent caregivers. Therefore, I would need to see the patient at least once a week but preferably twice a week. My sessions typically last 50 minutes.

I envision a long-term treatment, meaning years; however, I cannot speculate as to its precise length. When patients ask me this question, almost always at the onset of treatment, I point out that our concern should be with beginning not with ending. I also point out that because it took them a lifetime to get to this particular point, they should not expect instantaneous change.

The Therapeutic Relationship

The Therapeutic Bond

From a psychoanalytic perspective, the therapeutic bond—indeed the entire treatment—rests on the establishment of a "treatment frame." Like earlier terms such as the "analytic situation" and the "contract," the treatment frame refers to the structural conditions that provide the framework for treatment to occur. The frame commonly consists of the place where sessions will be held, the frequency and length of sessions, the agreed upon fee, the way in which missed appointments will be handled, and how the participants are to refer to each other (e.g., by last name, first name, title). In addition, as part of the frame, roles, although subject to distortion, are relatively prescribed and confidentiality is safeguarded.

The frame serves several functions. While allowing for the emergence of certain psychic phenomena, at the same time it provides a containment of their expression. Furthermore, its stability and permanence distinguish, spacially and temporally, the inside from the outside, regulate the physical and psychical attitudes of the two participants, and permit the appearance and observation of transference reactions.

Whereas the frame defines the therapeutic space, treatment itself is a relational experience that consists of a multiplicity of different relationships. Greenson (1967) has identified and distinguished three of these relationships, all of which occur simultaneously in any treatment: the real relationship, the working alliance, and the transference. The real relationship refers to the real relationship between patient and therapist. It is real in both senses of being undistorted and genuine. The working alliance, as the term implies, involves the patient's capacity to work purposefully with the therapist in the therapeutic situation.

The concept of transference is highly complex and has been used loosely to refer to a variety of interpersonal phenomena. Authors have used the concept to describe an individual's general interpersonal expectations, an individual's tendency to engage in certain types of interactions, and an individual's replacing a current figure (the therapist) with one from the past. Despite differences in usage, transference phenomena in general share common characteristics: They involve repetitions, they are resistant to change, and they are defenses against memory, although they indirectly lead in that direction.

With the patient we are considering, I would expect that establishing a working alliance would be particularly difficult. An alliance presupposes that the patient has the ego strength to maintain a split between his or her experiencing self and observing self. As such, the alliance involves the level of mutuality and cooperativeness between the patient's and the therapist's observing selves. I see little evidence that the patient has the capacity to effect this split at this time.

Different from transference, projective identification is another type of interpersonal transaction that is often experienced with patient who have not achieved object constancy and is to be expected with this patient. The term was coined by Melanie Klein to describe a developmental and defensive process in which "parts of the self and internal object are split off and projected into the external object, which then becomes possessed by, controlled, and identified with the projected parts" (Segal, 1973, p. 27). Bion (1956/1967) extended the concept by using the metaphor of the container and the contained. Underlying this metaphor is the image of an infant emptying its bad contents into the mother, who accepts the unwanted projection, contains it, and alters it in such a way as to permit its reintrojection by the infant. For Bion, "projective identification is an interpersonal process in which one finds oneself being manipulated so as to be playing a part, no matter how difficult to recognize, in somebody else's fantasy. In the interpersonal setting, the person projectively identifying engages in an unconscious fantasy of ejecting an unwanted or endangered aspect of himself and of depositing that part of himself in a controlled way" (Ogden, 1983, p. 232).

Implicit in projective identification, then, are the following elements: the presence of an unconscious fantasy, pressure on the other to experience himself or herself in a way congruent with the unconscious fantasy, the defensive aspects of ridding oneself of unwanted parts, and the attempt to control the external object. More current writers (Lerner, 1998) have drawn attention to the nonverbal communicative aspects of projective identification.

Roles in the Therapeutic Relationships

Because of the unfolding nature of psychoanalytic treatment and that each case is remarkably unique, it is difficult to conceptualize the treatment in terms of roles. Nonetheless, I will try to outline several basic principles.

Overall, the therapist is responsible for establishing and maintaining the therapeutic frame, safeguarding the patient's confidentiality and welfare, placing the patient's interest above his or her own, and within ethical guidelines, conducting the treatment in such a way as to assist the patient in getting well. This further means that the therapist recognizes his or her own limitations, including intense and interfering countertransference reactions, and must be prepared to seek consultation or refer the patient elsewhere if needed.

Reciprocally, the patient is responsible for both adhering to the treatment frame, and, more generally, for his or her behavior. I recognize that the issue of general responsibility is complex, contentious, and subject to a number of factors; nonetheless, the notion of an individual's being held accountable for his or her actions and thoughts is necessary and basic to this model of treatment.

More specific roles or functions, such as a more active involvement versus a more passive involvement (listening) or level of directedness versus nondirectedness, are based upon a respect for the patient's separateness, an awareness of the patient's needs and capacities, and a sense of what is necessary to further the treatment and meet therapeutic goals. For example, a remarkably timid, socially awkward, shy young woman acknowledged she could not begin a session and asked me if I would. I agreed to her request. Yet I do not offer instructions and seldom engage in problem solving, preferring instead to understand and explore, and respond to the frequently asked question of "what should I do?" with, "why do anything?"

Ideally, treatment is a collaborative effort; however, it is often a goal one moves toward rather than a given. The capacity to engage in treatment and to do the work of treatment (e.g., openness, self-reflection, etc.) varies from person to person, and, in my experience, develops as therapy progresses. Indeed, an important assessment question involves the patient's capacity to think psychologically and to envision a role for himself or herself in treatment.

As to the patient being discussed here, based upon her work history, rigidity, and tendency to behave ritualistically, I believe she will comply with and adhere to the treatment frame. At the same time, her pervasive anxiety, inability to trust or entrust, and lack of object constancy all suggest that during the beginning phase, she will have difficulty involving herself in her treatment in an invested and emotional way. This will need to be taken into account in terms of how the treatment is fashioned and conceptualized.

Treatment Implementation and Outcome

Techniques and Methods of Working

As indicated previously, patients who present with significant structural impairments require a treatment different from traditional analysis, one that places greater emphasis on the therapeutic milieu and views the therapeutic relationship as a metaphorical type of re-parenting. An example of this relatively new look, and one especially well suited for this patient, is Modell's (1978) conceptualization of treatment as a "holding environment."

Extending Winnicott's (1960) concept of maternal holding and Bion's (1956/1967) metaphor of the container and the contained to the treatment situation, Modell (1978) suggests that "the analytic setting and the analytic work itself leads to the development of an actual and current object relationship which is itself the source of dependent gratification, and the field in which early developmental conflicts can be recapitulated" (p. 494).

To create a holding environment, the therapist need not introduce new techniques or procedures, but rather carefully follow traditional therapeutic practices. For example, in being steady and reliable, placing the patient's needs above one's own, remaining empathically attuned to the patient's concerns, and doing what one believes to be in the patient's best interest—like the "good enough mother"—one is symbolically holding the patent.

A patient, not unlike the one under discussion here, felt compelled to attend every session regardless of her own physical health or the weather. Recognizing that the patient herself was unable to cancel appointments when the weather was especially nasty and driving hazardous, I would call her to cancel and reschedule as part of tending to her best interests.

In accepting what is offensive and obnoxious, judiciously setting limits, and quietly sitting still in response to the patient's intense affectivity and demand for action, the therapist is performing another function symbolically equivalent to the ideal parent-child relationship: containing the patient.

In addition to holding and containing the patient, the holding environment also involves the therapist's empathically listening to the patient. Through his or her empathy, the therapist assists the patient in sorting through what feels confusing and bewildering while conveying to the patient a sense of understanding. Sitting still, listening, and responding empathically does something else too. Mindful that these more disturbed patients tend to engage in projective identification, these quieter activities permit the therapist to take in the patient's projections, metabolize them, and give them back to the patient in a form devoid of its intense affects that can then be understood and digested.

With patents such as the one being considered, establishing the holding environment constitutes the opening phase of treatment. Once established, the holding environment continues; however, it is during the opening period that it is the focus of therapeutic action. Although interpretive work is done during this period, it needs to be done carefully and empathically. For instance, if interpretations do not touch on the patient's conscious experience or are experienced but felt as painful, they are either quickly dismissed or experienced as cruel and interrupting intrusions.

Empathy, particularly at this stage but in other stages too, is the therapist's major therapeutic tool. However, regardless of the therapist's alertness and sensitivity, there will be empathic failures in style and in content. Because such failures recapitulate previous experiences with earlier caregivers, it is crucial that they be recognized and fully understood.

The holding environment serves several purposes. It provides a background of safety and security that then allows the patient to invest more fully in the treatment, as manifest in the patient's increasing openness, spontaneity, and ventureness. As in Modell's (1978) term, an "object relationship," it enables the patient to relate to the therapist in a way different from how he or she related to the caregivers of childhood. These patients typically describe themselves and are seen by others as distrustful; however, to be more accurate, I believe that their struggles and apprehensions relate more directly to their fear of entrusting themselves to others.

As the therapeutic action of the holding environment takes hold and there is a greater degree of affective relatedness between therapist and patient, slowly but increasingly the therapist can then make greater use of the traditional analytic techniques of interpreting resistances and transference reactions. Even at this point, the therapist is still guided by his or her own empathy and is ever alert to empathic failures.

Medical and Nutritional Issues

At a time when biological psychiatry holds sway, one must be especially careful and thoughtful regarding the role of medication. Too readily, patients and physicians alike look to medication as a magical solution. Except for patients who are psychotic and individuals in acute distress, my bias is against medication. As I see it, medication is directed exclusively at symptoms and does little to affect underlying causes; may counteract a patient's sense of having control over, and responsibility for, his or her own behavior; and conveys the message that change can be immediate, effortless, and magical.

Medication can be antitherapeutic too. For instance, feelings of sadness and grief in response to loss are not only appropriate, but for some individuals may be an indication of therapeutic and developmental progress. To medicate a patient at that point is to deny him or her the opportunity to live through a feeling. As well, it unnecessarily interrupts the mourning process.

Although my bias is against the use of medication, I am not rigidly or completely opposed. For example, if a patient is not benefiting from psychotherapy, then clearly other alternatives, including medication, should be considered. Then too, we are all familiar with those patients who are amenable to psychotherapy only when they are taking medication.

With this current patient, I would begin treatment without medication. If, however, her level of anxiety reached the point that she could not tolerate or make use of the treatment situation, then I would refer her for a medication-related consultation. If, too, treatment appeared to be of little help, then at that time I would also seek a consultation.

Potential Pitfalls

There are several pitfalls, problems, or resistances to be anticipated with this patient. As described, she did not seek help on her own, but rather was encouraged by her boyfriend who was concerned with the toll it was taking on her life. Perhaps, he was concerned with the toll it was taking on his life as well. In any event, this suggests to me that even as uncomfortable as her anxiety might be and even as restricted as her life is, her condition is more ego-syntonic than ego-dystonic. That is, it has become her familiar way of being in the world. To put is somewhat differently, despite the complaints her anxiety has become a long-term companion. In addition and as noted previously, it has also become her means of exercising inordinate control over her objects. Given that she has organized her life and the lives of others around the anxiety, it will be a difficult symptom for her to relinquish. In addition to the secondary gains, I feel that coupled with the control of others is an unspoken and probably unrecognized sense of omnipotence. Therefore, and quite paradoxically, to give up the symptom is also to relent on the sense of omnipotence.

It is my sense that the patient will come to treatment more in body than in spirit. What will appear as cooperation will in fact be closer to compliance. Recognizing her basic fear of entrusting herself to another, that which is most important and intimate will be maintained in privacy. It is my experience with this type of defense (i.e., compliance) that one continue to empathize with her pain and suffering with the expectation that as she feels the safety of the holding environment, it will enable her to increasingly become more genuinely open.

As noted, the patient relates herself to others as if they are her psychic lifeline. Apart from the others' capacity to provide safety or security, there is little else in the relationship that seems to matter. Rather than immediately looking to her therapist to meet these needs and in keeping with her being described as emotionally aloof, there will be a period of affective nonrelatedness. This, too, will constitute an important resistance.

Finally, because of her tendency to avoid, and need to control, others, there is a likelihood that as she begins to experience relief from her anxiety, she will consider prematurely leaving therapy. Little evidence has been provided to indicate that this patient is psychologically minded or psychologically aware. Therefore, I question whether she will be interested or willing to push beyond her symptoms and look at underlying causes. I have found this to be of issue in other patients bearing this diagnosis and presenting as does this patient.

Termination and Relapse Prevention

Treatment from a psychoanalytic perspective, regardless of length, has an implicit structure consisting of a beginning, a middle, and an end. Although these phases flow seamlessly into each other, they are distinct and have their own requirements, tasks, and points of emphasis. For example, the beginning stage has as its objectives defining the treatment frame, clarifying misconceptions regarding therapy, and establishing a working alliance.

The ending phase, as the term implies, involves bringing the treatment to a close. The phase actually has two separate parts. The initial part consists of the patient and therapist together deciding to terminate and then setting a specific date. Although subject to variation, termination is typically spread over several months. Once the date is set, one then enters the second part, doing the work of terminating.

Although the idea of terminating provokes a vast array of feelings, including relief, regret, satisfaction, gratitude, disappointment, like death more than anything else, it represents and stirs feelings of loss. It is in the nature of loss that a current and immediate loss will rekindle memories and feelings associated with earlier losses (Lerner, 1990). To paraphrase Dylan Thomas, after the first loss there is no other. Therefore, whereas the task of this period is to end treatment, the experience is one of loss and mourning.

In order to mourn, one must see clearly what it is that has been lost. In "Mourning and Melancholia," Freud (1917/1957) put it this way: "He knows whom he has lost but not what he has lost in him" (p. 245). He went on to observe that "in mourning it is the world which has become poor and empty; in melancholia it is the ego itself" (p. 246).

To know clearly whom and what one has lost depends upon a full inner representation of the lost object (Lerner, 1990). Patients who have not achieved a level of object constancy are therefore unable to truly mourn. The depressive affect they do experience is similar to Freud's description of melancholia, in that the felt loss is of aspects of the self and not of the object.

If, during the earlier phases of treatment, the patient we have been discussing does achieve a level of object constancy, then the termination phase will include reviewing the significant losses in her life such as the loss of her natural father and of her mother who is schizophrenic. Other related issues including disappointment, disillusionment, and abandonment will occupy center stage. Although each of these themes will have arisen during the course of her treatment, they commonly reemerge in the termination phase and with a renewed sense of urgency.

The term *relapse prevention* has little meaning to me; however, I do encourage the patient to return for additional sessions in the event of a relapse or if he or she is unable to work out a problem. It is important throughout treatment that the therapeutic frame be adhered to and that the therapist maintain his or her professional posture. Changing or relaxing either will make it more difficult and uncomfortable for the patient to return posttermination.

Mechanisms of Change

With more intact patients in which conflict rather than deficit is the difficulty, insight and self-understanding gained through interpretation is considered the major vehicle of change. By contrast, with less intact patients in which structural impairment poses the problem, it is my impression that internalization constitutes the therapeutic action of change.

Beginning with Freud, the concept of internalization has occupied a prominent position in the psychoanalytic literature. Based on different strands in Freud's writings, it has been discussed from various vantage points, including the importance of inadequate or distorted internalizations in psychopathology, the function of internalizing mechanisms as defenses, and the role of internalization in growth and development including its place in the treatment process.

In his 1923 article "The Ego and the Id," Freud used the term *introjection* to account for the process by which external experiences are transformed and re-created on the terrain of inner experience (Freud, 1923/1961). In his discussion of superego development, he explained how the guiding, restraining, and punishing functions originally imposed on children by their parents in time become part of the child and are experienced not as other-regulators, but as self-regulators.

Authors subsequent to Freud replaced the term with "internalization" and viewed introjection as one type of internalization. Representative of this refinement is Kernberg (1976), who distinguished between introjection and identification but saw both as subordinate aspects of internalization. For Kernberg, identification, unlike introjection, implies a firm separation between self representations and object representations and presupposes an actual relationship in which the individual experiences himself or herself as the subject interacting with another person.

For psychoanalysts, the internalizing process—the transforming of outer experiences to inner experience—occurs in the context of an object relationship. Prompting the process is the affective relatedness (i.e., love, hate, respect, fear, etc.) between the participants. Included in the internalization is not just the personhood of the other and the nature of the relationship, but also roles, functions, and attitudes. For instance, with internalization the individual is progressively able to do for himself or herself what others previously had done for him or her. Or, as Cohen and Sherwood (1991) pointed out, when a child internalizes his or her mother, he or she also internalizes the sense of being (or of not being) seen, defined, and validated.

Because internalization involves transforming functions, attitudes, and an entire array of external events, it is, as Loewald (1962) reminded us, structure building. This is also to say that psychic structures are based on and modified by internalized object relations. This view of internalization as a mediating process for growth, development, and change is also highly consistent with Piaget's theory of cognitive development. Both emphasize the progressive internalization and structuring of external environmental experiences, and both focus on the continuous growth, reorganization, and revision of existing internal structures.

Further to internalization, all psychoanalytically oriented therapists point to a very specific type of internalization. Each sets as a treatment goal the patient's internalizing of the therapist's way of working. This is to say, each hopes by the completion of treatment that the patient is not only more self-aware, but has also internalized a method of approaching and thinking about his or her struggles. It is in this context—the patient's transforming the therapist's introspective, reflective, meaning-seeking attitude into his or her own—that Freud spoke of treatment as interminable.

CONCLUSION

There always has been an intimate relationship between psychoanalytic theory and practice. Clinical data obtained in the laboratory of the clinician's consulting room has served to forge modifications and changes in theory, which in turn have influenced practice. In response to a changing clinical population, emphasis has shifted from conceptualizations of structural conflict to conceptualizations of structural impairment. In concert with these shifts, later models of treatment have drawn attention to psychological nutriments inherent in the treatment situation that promote growth and development.

Although diagnosed as specific phobia and general anxiety disorder, looking at and beyond her symptoms, the patient being considered here shows evidence of reasonably severe disturbances. Her anxiety, which phenomenologically has the quality of annihilation anxiety, is chronic and pervasive; she seemingly has not achieved object constancy, seeks to control her objects, and relies on others to provide basic psychological functions she cannot provide for herself.

Several treatment goals were outlined in which structure building and repair was emphasized. It is assumed that focusing on the underlying structures will not only afford symptom relief, but will also facilitate psychological development.

In keeping with the nature of her difficulties, the holding and containing aspects of treatment were emphasized. If and as the patient attains object constancy and achieves a more consolidated sense of self, treatment will take on a more traditional quality. Without diminishing the importance of self-understanding and the therapeutic action of empathy, internalization is suggested as the major agent of change.

REFERENCES

Bion, W. (1967). Development of schizophrenic thought. In W. Bion (Ed.), *Second thoughts* (pp. 36–42). New York: Aronson. (Original work published in 1956)

Cohen, C., & Sherwood, V. (1991). *Becoming a constant object in psychotherapy with the borderline patient.* New York: Aronson.

Freud, S. (1957). Mourning and melancholia. In J. Strachey (Ed. and Trans.), *The standard edition of the complete psychological works of Sigmund Freud* (Vol. 14, pp. 237–260). London: Hogarth Press. (Original work published 1917)

Freud, S. (1959). Inhibitions, symptoms, and anxiety. In J. Strachey (Ed. and Trans.), *The standard edition of the complete psychological works of Sigmund Freud* (Vol. 20, pp. 87–172). London: Hogarth Press. (Original work published 1926)

Freud, S. (1961). The ego and the id. In J. Strachey (Ed. and Trans.), *The standard edition of the complete psychological works of Sigmund Freud* (Vol. 19, pp. 12–59). London: Hogarth Press. (Original work published 1923)

Greenson, R. (1967). *The technique and practice of psychoanalysis.* New York: International Universities Press.

Hurvich, M. (1989). Traumatic moment, basic dangers, and annihilation anxiety. *Psychoanalytic Psychology, 6,* 309–323.

Kernberg, O. (1970). A psychoanalytic classification of character pathology. *Journal of the American Psychoanalytic Association, 18,* 800–822.

Kernberg, O. (1976). *Object relations theory and clinical psychoanalysis.* New York: Aronson.

Kohut, H. (1977). *The restoration of the self.* New York: International Universities Press.

Kohut, H. (1978). Introspection, empathy, and psychoanalysis. In P. Ornstein (Ed.), *The search for the self, Vol. 1* (pp. 205–232). Madison, CT: International Universities Press. (Original work published in 1959)

Lerner, P. (1990). The treatment of early object loss: The need to search. *Psychoanalytic Psychology, 7,* 79–90.

Lerner, P. (1998). *Psychoanalytic perspectives on the Rorschach.* Hillsdale, NJ: The Analytic Press.

Loewald, H. (1962). Internalization, separation, mourning and the superego. *Psychoanalytic Quarterly, 31,* 483–504.

Mahler, M., Pine, F., & Bergmann, A. (1975). *The psychological birth of the human infant.* New York: Basic Books.

McWilliams, N. (1998). Relationship, subjectivity, and inference in diagnosis. In J. Barron (Ed.), *Making diagnosis meaningful* (pp. 197–226). Washington, DC: American Psychological Association.

Michaels, R. (1983). Plenary address. Presented at the symposium *Distortions of Personality Development and Their Management,* Toronto, Ontario.

Modell, A. (1978). The conceptualization of the therapeutic action of psychoanalysis: The action of the holding environment. *Bulletin of the Menninger Clinic, 42,* 493–504.

Ogden, T. (1983). The concept of internal object relations. *International Journal of Psychoanalysis, 64,* 227–243.

Ornstein, P., & Ornstein, A. (1980). Self psychology and the process of regression. Paper presented at the meeting of the Toronto Psychoanalytic Society, Toronto, Ontario.

Rapaport, D. (1950). The theoretical implications of diagnostic testing procedures. *Congres International de Psychiatric, 2,* 241–271.

Segal, H. (1973). *Introduction to the work of Melanie Klein.* London: Hogarth Press.

Winnicott, D. (1960). The theory of the parent-infant relationship. *International Journal of Psychoanalysis, 41,* 385–395.

13

Psychopharmacological Treatment

Agnieszka Popiel, Lynn Montgomery, and Robert A. DiTomasso

TREATMENT MODEL

From the earliest of times people have attempted to find chemical ways to eliminate the distressing symptoms of anxiety. For example, Sir Richard Blackmore recommended the usage of "Pacific Medicines" such as opium in 1795: "First as it calms and soothes the Disorders and Perturbations of the animal Spirits which then lulled and charmed by the soporiferous Drug, cease their Tumults and settle into a state of Tranquility" (Hunter & Macalpine, 1963). The early civilizations of China, India, the Mediterranean, and the Middle East employed a number of plants and minerals for remedial and preventative purposes.

While the need for substances to quell the disturbing symptoms of anxiety evolved, consideration was also given to the adaptive role of fear in human survival. The protective role of the normal physiological fear response serves to warn an individual about danger and mobilizes the individual to act or to escape by increasing autonomic sympathetic nervous system activity. This mechanism is the same in acutely pathological anxiety; however, the response is disproportional to the threatening stimulus, is of longer duration, and ultimately impairs the ability to lead a normal life. This state of arousal is manifested by changes, usually increases, in blood pressure and heart rate, dry mouth, and an erratic respiratory rate.

Based on the present state of knowledge, this response is mainly connected with three substances: noradrenaline, serotonin (5 hydroxy-tryptamine), and GABA (gamma-aminobutyric acid). Noradrenaline and serotonin can be considered excitatory transmitters. GABA is an inhibitory substance, which has a modulating effect on other neuro-transmitter systems in the brain. Some forms of severe anxiety, commonly found in panic episodes and in anxious depressive states, are most likely to be associated with enhanced noradrenergic release. The anxiolytic effect results from the reduction of serotonergic transmission, especially in the raphe region. Although the mechanisms related to escape-safety behavior are understood, the mechanisms underlying anxiety disorders are still largely unknown. The application of the biochemical model involves the use of different classes of psychotropic drugs in treating anxiety that modify serotonergic and noradrenergic transmission such as with antidepressants and agonists of GABA receptors, like the benzodiazepines. Medications that do not belong to these groups exert their effect through the modification of one of the three substances (noradrenaline, serotonin, and GABA).

The 19th century actually marked the beginning of the era of psychopharmacology. At that point, the most commonly used substances in the treatment of anxiety and sleep disturbances were barbiturates, bromides, paraldehyde, glutethimide meprobamate, methaqualone, and methyprylon. Their narrow therapeutic index, or basic value in treating anxiety, their high abuse potential, and potential for lethality in overdose led to their gradual disappearance. Today, benzodiazepines and other newer agents have largely replaced these older substances.

The psychopharmacological treatment model is fairly straightforward and simple although the technical details and biochemical pathway are not. This model presupposes that neurological or neurochemical pathways are either malfunctioning or maladaptive. For example, if the brain of the patient is not producing enough, or the specific kind, of neurotransmitters, then that patient's behavior, mood, perception, or cognition will be adversely affected. If a therapeutic chemical agent is prescribed and ingested and makes its ways into the correct area in the nervous system, then the right neurotransmitter is either mimicked, stimulated, or bypassed in some beneficial way. Sometimes the wrong neurochemicals or damaged neuropathways are blocked from causing difficulties.

The decision to prescribe medication is ideally based upon scientific data supporting the efficacy of the medication for a specific disorder. Ideally, in this model the medication will normalize the abnormality, balance the imbalance, stabilize the instability, or enhance an otherwise exiting insufficiency. Of course, this is a very simplistic conceptualization of somewhat complicated, interlocking mechanisms. In the case of a patient with an anxiety disorder, the approach would be to relieve abnormal symptoms, most of which are abnormal expressions of normal physiology. Ideally, this would be achieved with minimal or no unwanted side effects, such as sedation or diminished libido. The patient is then left mechanically intact and free from unnecessary distractions to get about the business of life, free to make ordinary choices for good or ill. Several different medications are available today for treating the patient with an anxiety disorder.

Benzodiazepines

Benzodiazepines are the agonists of the benzodiazepine receptors. An agonist is a "drug or chemical that mimics the effects of a naturally occurring substance (such as a hormone or transmitter) or of another chemical; for example, beta-adrenergic agonist medications mimic epinephrine and produce relaxation of bronchial (lung) muscles to treat asthma" (Preston, O'Neal, & Talaga, 1997; Shader & Greenblatt, 1993). They stimulate GABA-ergic transmission, which has an inhibitory result on the CNS. All of the substances in this group differ according to their pharmacokinetics, that is, the way they are absorbed, metabolized, and eliminated. They may also differ in their pharmacodynamics, that is, the affinity of the drug to certain subtypes of receptors in the brain. These factors influence the different clinical properties and responses, whether anxiolytic, anticonvulsant, or hypnotic; the half-life, and the possibility of accumulation in the body system.

In and of themselves benzodiazepines are relatively safe drugs. An overdose of benzodiazepines usually leads to somnolence. However, when combined with alcohol, the inhibitory influence on the respiratory center may lead to death. Over the years, there have been numerous studies confirming the efficacy of the benzodiazepines group in the treatment of generalized anxiety disorder (Leonard, 1998). For example in a recent study, approximately 35% of patients with GAD achieved marked benefit from a trial of a benzodiazepine, and 40% of patients achieved moderate relief (Leonard, 1998). Patients usually respond to benzodiazepine treatment within the first week. Tolerance usually develops to the sedative and psychomotor effects of the benzodiazepines, but few data support tolerance to the antianxiety effect. In some cases, the response to treatment can be 6 weeks, but there are no data that prolonging the period or increasing the dose will lead to improvement in response (Leonard, 1998).

Antidepressants

The biological concept of anxiety is not limited to the GABA transmission that is influenced by benzodiazepines. The anxiolytic effect of the drugs used in the treatment of depression has been described since the 1960s. Antidepressants effectively treat anxiety and comorbid anxiety-depression (Feighner, 1999). This group of drugs is especially connected with the noradrenergic and the serotonin systems. Classic tricyclic antidepressants were first synthesized in the late 1950s. The most popular tricyclics are amitriptyline, imipramine, nortriptyline, clomipramine, and doxepine. The second generation of antidepressants includes the SSRIs (selective serotonin reuptake inhibitors), alpha-2 adrenoreceptor antagonists, noradrenaline reuptake inhibitors, and serotonin reuptake enhancers. To date, the research that has supported the efficacy of tricyclic antidepressants in the treatment of anxiety has examined doxepine, imipramine, and clomipramine. Tricyclic antidepressants have an advantage over benzodiazepines in that they do not cause dependency. Their rather narrow therapeutic index, however, quite often creates adverse effects and the dosing regime makes their use quite limited. The most common side effects connected with these drugs are anticholinergic effects including dry mouth, blurred vision, as well as alpha-adrenergic activity (orthostatic hypotension, sedation, slowing of cardiac conduction, and weight gain). They also lower the seizure threshold.

Selective serotonin reuptake inhibitors (SSRIs), which have been proven to have antianxiety effects include Paxil (paroxetine), Luvox (fluvoxamine), and Celexa (citalopram) (Allgulander, Cloninger, Przybeck, & Brandt, 1998; Rocca, Fonzo, Scotta, Zanalda, & Ravissa, 1997). They are associated with fewer side effects, fewer interactions with other drugs, lower toxicity when overdosed, and a more favorable dosing regime (usually once a day). Their side effects are connected with the activation of serotonin peripheral receptors and include nausea, headache, restlessness, and sexual dysfunction. Serzone (nefazodone), belonging to the group of "modified SSRIs," has an additional anxiolytic effect due to its action on 5HT2 receptors.

Alpha-2 adrenoreceptor antagonists facilitate the release of noradrenaline. Their side effects include sedation, postural hypotension, dry mouth, and nausea. Noradrenaline reuptake inhibitors include Effexor (venlafaxine), which is the best examined drug of this group that has an anxiolytic effect. Its efficacy has been demonstrated in a number of research studies (Davidson et al., 1999; Gelenberg et al., 2000; Rickels et al., 2000; Sheehan, 1999). Its side effects include nausea (early in therapy), headache, sleep disturbance, dizziness, sexual dysfunction, and an elevation in supine diastolic blood pressure.

Buspirone

Buspar (buspirone) is not related to the benzodiazepines. Its mechanism of action is probably through the 5HT1A serotonin receptor. It acts also on dopamine receptor (D2), and its metabolite has an affinity to alpha-2 adrenoreceptors. The mechanism of action seems to be the result of more complex interactions of buspirone itself and its metabolites, but still has been not well examined. It does not cause muscle relaxation as do the benzodiazepines. It acts slowly (usually after 2 to 4 weeks) when compared to Valium (diazepam) but does not give the side effects characteristic of benzodiazepines. It also does not have the negative interaction with alcohol or dependence effects. Its efficacy in GAD has been demonstrated in many studies and is comparable to the efficacy of benzodiazepines (Lader & Scott, 1998; Roerig, 1999; Sramek et al., 1999). Side effects of buspirone include dizziness, nausea, and headache.

Several other miscellaneous compounds have been used to treat various symptoms of anxiety, including adrenergic antagonists, hydroxyzine, ondansetron, and some antipsychotics (Ballenger, 1999; Bazire, 2000; El-Khayat & Baldwin, 1998). Currently, the Food and Drug Administration (FDA) has approved three classes of medication for the treatment of GAD (Roerig, 1999), each with a different mechanism of action, side effects profile, and abuse potential.

THE THERAPIST'S SKILLS AND ATTRIBUTES

The person responsible for pharmacotherapy, ideally, should be a psychiatrist or a general practitioner. The personal attribute most essential for successful pharmacotherapy is the ability to create a secure base for the patient. The doctor's verbal and nonverbal communication should express the idea that anxiety is a nonlethal, although chronic condition, which can be treated successfully with medication, psychotherapy or, more likely, some combination of both modalities.

In order to be effective, the pharmacotherapist must be able to gather and decipher information, some of which he or she may directly observe, but most of which must be gathered in conversation, usually in a dialogue with the patient or those close to the patient. The pharmacotherapist will be most effective as a coinvestigator with the patient, looking together at what's happening in the patient's body and mind. It is most profitable to be able to collaborate in the examination of symptoms, creating for the patient a sense of mutual discovery in an open-minded inquisitive way. An effective therapist takes the stance of partnership, reassuring the patient when necessary, advising and recommending, but always from a position of respect.

The therapist or physician must be able to communicate at the level of understanding of the patient. Rapport is essential for compliance and for open communication. Rarely are medications perfect. Feedback from the patient is therefore essential. Having positive feelings about the therapist is necessary for the sustained and sometimes long-term relationship of trust in which medications are initiated, monitored, adjusted, changed, and discontinued. In this state of rapport an understanding of the psychiatric condition as well as the potential benefits and limitations of the medication are openly discussed.

In the case of Sandra, her precise prescription regime would be especially important. A very focused medication-education component would be critical. In this manner the pharmacotherapist would present, describe, and discuss in detail the rules for taking the medication(s) and the expectations regarding the various effects of the medication(s). All this information would serve to help to limit her anxiety. Given the potential for addiction, in prescribing benzodiazepines emphasis on the dosing regime would also be necessary. Obviously, the pharmacotherapist would need to have extensive, accurate, and up-to-date knowledge of pharmacotherapy.

The contact with Sandra would be structured and mainly informative. She would need to receive very focused information concerning the realistic goals of the drug treatment, the expected direct effects of the drug, the approximate time of the onset of the drug action, and its side effects. If she were treated with antidepressive drugs or buspirone, information about the time of action should not raise her expectations (and anxiety) for an immediate effect. Given her basic excessive-worry style, the information shared with Sandra about side effects would not be downplayed or exaggerated.

The influence of anxiety in exacerbating her somatic symptoms should also be explained. At all times, Sandra would be given complete information. It is only with that information that she will then be able to offer informed consent to the pharmacotherapy.

THE CASE OF SANDRA

Assessment, Conceptualization, and Treatment Planning

Assessment

Sandra does not presently take any medication and does not suffer from medical illness, other than an allergy. As the baseline for the treatment of Sandra's symptoms of anxiety, the physician should order basic blood tests to assess her electrolyte level and thyroid hormones, and an EKG. This would help to rule out some of the most frequent possible somatic reasons, which might manifest themselves as anxiety-like symptoms. A complete medical examination would also be in order. During the medical examination, attention would be paid to habits concerning Sandra's caffeine use and sleep hygiene, which may be contributory to her anxious state.

Sandra presents with two diagnoses: specific phobia and generalized anxiety disorder. The treatment for specific phobia is psychotherapy. The possible treatments for generalized anxiety disorder, however, depend on the nature and extent of the symptoms. From the case presentation, we have deduced that Sandra views her world as dangerous. She has a general lack of trust in people, in large part conditioned and determined by conclusions she has drawn from confronting danger as a child. Her fear response is heightened, and physiologically she responds with muscle tension, palpitations, a pounding heart, an accelerated heart rate, sweating, trembling, and shakiness. These responses are sympathetic-autonomic responses to danger and are designed to mobilize her to flee or survive attack. Her psychic response is one of worry, apprehensiveness, and lack of trust.

Further psychiatric assessment should include an attempt to distinguish the level of anxiety she experiences when not acutely present to perceived threat. If possible, information regarding other close blood relatives should be obtained to enrich the understanding of her biological tendencies. Apart from a thorough psychiatric interview, no other assessment instruments are necessary. Of course, periodic reassessment with the Beck Anxiety Inventory may be a useful "objective" tool, although the patient's satisfaction is generally unparalleled by written testing.

Therapeutic Goals

The pharmacotherapy of anxiety disorders is focused on symptomatic improvement rather than cure. Sandra presents anxiety on emotional (fear), cognitive (worry, mistrust) and biological levels (anxious arousal, muscle tension, shakiness, and sleep disturbances). An immediate goal of her treatment would be a small decrement in her level of anxiety as well as the improvement of her sleep pattern. It would be extremely important for Sandra, whose life is now governed by her anxiety, to experience a decrease in her symptoms. This improvement would allow her some measure of control and relief from her anxiety. Given her use of avoidance as a coping strategy, it would be therapeutic and ultimately beneficial to show her, as powerfully as possible, that controlling her anxiety symptoms is a possibility. Because of her attitude of mistrust, important factors worthy of consideration would be her statements regarding the probability of negative outcome with psychiatric treatment (her mother's unfavorable course of chronic psychosis with numerous hospitalizations), and her coming to treatment at the behest of her boyfriend (rather than as a function of her own decision). Establishing the therapeutic alliance may be difficult and problematic in this instance.

There are limits to pharmacotherapy in the treatment of anxiety, especially when considering the long-term outcome. One short-term goal would involve engaging Sandra into therapy by showing her the possibilities of decreasing the symptoms of arousal. By doing so, Sandra would likely experience enhanced motivation to participate and continue treatment. Her participation would, ideally, form the basis of Sandra's psychotherapy, which would help her to gain a new way of coping and thinking (Fisher & Durham, 1999).

Sandra's treatment should be a combination of psychotherapy and psychopharmacology, with the use of medication to assist in her growth and development, not as a substitute for it. She may have brain physiology that will forever need chemical mediation, but her world view must be altered in order for her to have a satisfying and fulfilling life. On the other hand, it is most likely that her physiology will begin to normalize as she experiences the world differently. Psychopharmacology plays a supporting role in this case. The treatment goal of combined therapy should be a fully functioning human being with an opportunity for ongoing unobstructed growth and development. This patient could be helped immediately with medication to sleep better and reduce her hyperarousal. Intrapsychic symptoms of worry may also be diminished by medication.

Moreover, the patient would also be able to experience rapid relief from muscle tension and other autonomic symptoms, such as palpitations and sweating. Irritability would be expected to diminish, and overall the patient should feel freed from her physiological burden. She would then be able to face the risks she perceives with fewer unwanted body sensations, thus enabling the therapeutic process to proceed with less resistance.

Timeline for Pharmacotherapy

There are no standards concerning the overall length of pharmacotherapy in the treatment of anxiety. However, there are some factors to consider when determining this time, such as the addictive potential of benzodiazepines. The possibility for addiction translates into making the pharmacotherapy as short a treatment as possible. The long onset of action found in other groups, such as antidepressants and buspirone, would lead us to expect the first signs of improvement after at least 2 weeks of treatment.

The timeline for Sandra, then, should be flexible. This would also apply to the frequency of the pharmacotherapy monitoring sessions. At the beginning of treatment, we would suggest seeing the patient 2 to 3 times a week. After the first diagnostic interview lasting 1 hour, the next sessions would be shorter, approximately 30 minutes. If everything was progressing well up to that point, seeing her every 3 to 4 weeks for about 30 minutes for a period of approximately 6 months would be appropriate.

Case Conceptualization

From a psychiatric standpoint, Sandra is a patient with an euthymic mood, but in a hyperaroused state with phobic and anxiety-related symptoms. These symptoms are primarily due to a nervous system and perceptual system overly conditioned to danger with subsequent avoidant behavior. She was trained in the past to be untrusting and suspicious. She has been unable to complete developmental milestones and make the transition into adulthood with the ability to form functional bonds and affiliations. Although she does not meet the criteria for obsessive-compulsive personality she is obsessive in response to her anxiety and fears. This obsessiveness, although socially disabling, can be used to her advantage, by driving her to "prove herself" as evidenced by her successful career. In spite of her difficulties, Sandra has been able to maintain a relationship with a boyfriend for 5 years.

Clearly, the boyfriend may be an asset to her treatment. He prompted her to seek treatment and may be a useful source of information, feedback, and support for treatment. Sandra is resourceful and has managed two careers, one professional, and one in creating a world to manage her symptoms. Her intelligence is therefore a potential strength. Her suffering is also a strength as this will help motivate her to recover.

Sandra's symptoms present in three main areas: motor tension, automatic hyperactivity, and hyperarousal, which underlie the feelings of anxiety, worry, and avoidance behavior. Her positive or negative ideas regarding medication will come from her preconceived ideas, what she has read, or from friends and family members. The subjective experience of feeling relief will be helpful in increasing her motivation. The duration of treatment is individualized. Sandra may need some medication for a few weeks or she may require some medication for years. This issue must be determined in ongoing dialogues between the physician and Sandra, the therapist and Sandra, and, one hopes, the physician and the therapist. This may even include dialogue with her boyfriend. Initially, Sandra and the psychiatrist should see each other more frequently. In the beginning, twice a month would seem like a reasonable amount of time to determine efficacy of treatment for the first 2 to 3 months. After the initial period, medication follow-up can be less frequent, going from monthly to bimonthly. This plan assumes, of course, a stable ongoing therapeutic process and adequate communication with the parties involved (patient, therapist, and physician).

The Therapeutic Relationship

The Therapeutic Bond

In order to be effective, the psychiatrist must be credible as an authority, but warm enough in the relationship for the patient to be willing to try the recommended treatment. Ideally, the patient is loyal enough to the physician to be compliant, but not to a degree that the patient feels obligated to continue a treatment that is not working.

The physician must be in a position to make recommendations based on the physician's knowledge, information, and wisdom. As a medication consultant, the physician must manage transference and countertransference, even making use of positive transference to aid compliance. The key stance is to use what works, promoting the medical and nonmedical aspects of treatment. The patient's confidence that the physician is working *with* the patient rather than working *on* her is paramount.

Roles in the Therapeutic Relationship

The role of the physician (psychiatrist) is that of an expert advisor, not an all-knowing father or mother. To be most effective, particularly when the treatment configuration is patient-therapist-physician, the physician acts as a consultant, like a wise uncle or aunt whose recommendations are worthy of consideration. The role of the patient or the patient's advocate is to make a rational informed choice, weighing the risks and benefits of treatment. When there is a menu of possible medical approaches, the physician should be candid about his or her recommendations and reasons. The patient and physician are partners in finding those treatments that are optimal for that patient.

In pharmacotherapy it would be essential that Sandra trust the physician's knowledge, experience, and competence. As an expert, the pharmacotherapist would provide information and set the rules for the administration of the treatment. With Sandra, as with many anxious patients, both too much information (e.g., sharing doubts) and lack of necessary information (the drug effects, side effects, onset of action) could be expected to increase her anxiety.

Treatment Implementation and Outcome

Techniques and Methods of Working

The work of the psychiatrist acting as physician and psychopharmacologist is in *dialogue.* Collaboration with therapists, family members, and significant others should always be an option, depending on the specific patient's case. The patient may be asked to track symptoms by keeping a journal or charting different levels of response to treatment. If not part of the psychotherapist's expertise, the physician may also instruct the patient in relaxation techniques and other methods of managing emotionality. The physician also is a partner with the psychotherapist and as such should expect both feedback about the patient and the therapist's support of the patient in communicating with the physician. For this patient, the boyfriend is a valuable source of support and information and should be included when possible in office visits.

In initiating Sandra's treatment, the therapeutic alliance is no less important than it is in psychotherapy, and for the same reasons. It is, in fact, crucial in motivating others. Sandra did not experience a great deal of understanding and support in her life. Moreover, her only experience with mental health professionals was due to her mother's disease. It is important for her to start the process of therapy with the sense of safety and of being understood.

She would need to receive an explanation of the somatic and psychic symptoms of anxiety, its chronic yet nonlethal nature, and the role of anxiety as a coping mechanism. An explanation would include two of three different ways that we could proceed in treating her anxiety disorder. Research studies show that all treatments appear to be beneficial, but the best results can be obtained by combined treatment. Pharmacological therapy would be beneficial for symptomatic improvement; psychological therapy for changing the patient's way of coping, her view of herself and the world, and whatever is essential for long term functioning.

The treatment protocol would be based on several presumptions. First, the patient has had the symptoms of anxiety for several years. Second, she presents with many features of arousal and autonomic system activation, as well as worry and apprehension. Third, anxiety is a chronic condition. In approximately two-thirds of treated patients a decrease of symptoms and better control over anxiety can be achieved, as opposed to the total disappearance of symptoms (Fisher & Durham, 1999; Roerig, 1999). Finally, psychotherapy is the method of proven efficacy in the treatment of GAD. Given all this, we would recommend that she be involved in both pharmacotherapy and psychotherapy (Uhlenhuth, Balter, Ban, & Yang, 1999).

Specific medicines that may be used to treat Sandra are appropriate to discuss at this time. Current treatment choices include SSRIs, venlafaxine, benzodiazepines (Xanax, Ativan, Klonopin, Valium), buspirone (Buspar), and at times, antihistaminic medications such as Vistaril.

With Sandra, the psychiatrist would likely begin by starting with an SSRI or venlafaxine, either of which will potentially be useful for the psychic symptoms, particularly worry. Benzodiazepines may also be of use temporarily or on an as-needed basis. Considering the chronic and nonemergent nature of Sandra's condition, the psychiatrist should start with only an SSRI or venlafaxine. This medication may take a few weeks to be effective, but this approach may help avoid some pitfalls.

As with any medication, the specific therapeutic effects are variable with any given patient. Because this patient is new to any psychotropic medication, each new trial should be observed carefully and documented for beneficial effects and unwanted side effects. Nutritional issues are also important and extend beyond food to include caffeine and alcohol consumption.

Pharmacotherapy would be our first choice because the long history of the patient's symptoms suggests that she may need longer pharmacotherapy. This suggests the administration of drugs that can be used safely for longer period of time, such as antidepressants. The severity of her symptoms, the negative impact of her present functioning, and the need for enhancing Sandra's motivation to treatment would support the decision of also prescribing benzodiazepines in the first stage of therapy before the onset of action of antidepressants.

One drug that we would strongly consider is extended-release venlafaxine. This is an antidepressant drug approved by the FDA for the treatment of generalized anxiety disorder. The dose of 75 mgs has been proven to be a safe and effective treatment for both the psychic and somatic symptoms associated with GAD in short- and long-term (6 months) treatment (Davidson et al., 1999; Gelenberg et al., 2000; Rickles et al., 2000; Sheenan, 1999). The recommended starting dose is 37.5 mgs once a day for 4 days, then usually 75 mgs/day is efficient.

Improvements in Sandra's symptoms of anxiety and arousal, irritability, and difficulties in falling asleep usually will take place in the second week of treatment. This information should be clearly explained to her because this is also the rationale for the short-term use of benzodiazepines.

In Sandra's case the goal for benzodiazepines would be to decrease her somatic symptoms of anxiety such as the reported muscle tension, "feeling on edge," palpitations, pounding heart, trembling, shakiness, and difficulty in falling asleep. Such an effect at the onset of the treatment can be expected to improve her motivation and future compliance. Sandra's anxiety lasts most of the time during the day and is exacerbated by certain situations. Our recommendation would be to use one of the benzodiazepines of long duration, for example Tranxene (clorazepate), starting from a dose of 5 mg (up to 60 mg) once a day in the evening. Benzodiazepines of long duration also have a lower addictive potential. The discontinuation of the use of benzodiazepines should take place gradually after 2 weeks of treatment. At this point, we would expect that Sandra will begin to experience the effects of venlafaxine. There are no data on interactions between venlafaxine and benzodiazepines that could have a negative impact on her. She should be informed about the structure of the treatment, possible side effects, the need to keep within the prescribed dose and time of the treatment, and any influence on her reaction time. The effects on one's reaction time when driving or the use of machinery are very important.

Medical and Nutritional Issues

Sandra has already had a medical examination by her family physician. This may not have included a thyroid profile or EKG, which may uncover treatable medical problems such as hypo- or hyperthyroidism. An EKG may reveal arrhythmias that may intensify anxious responses or warn against the use of certain types of medication, for example, tricyclic antidepressant medication. Routine medical and gynecological examinations are appropriate. She also has upper respiratory problems related to allergies, which may cause difficulty breathing, and this may increase her anxiety. Furthermore, certain types of medication, bronchodilators, and decongestants may themselves contribute to hyperarousal and make her symptoms of anxiety worse. The psychiatrist should be aware of any and all prescribed or over-the-counter medications that the patient is taking, including "nutriceuticals" and nontraditional remedies. Many over-the-counter products may contain stimulants such as caffeine or ephedrine, which may also exacerbate anxiety.

With a patient who is anxious it is important to note how much coffee, tea, cola, or chocolate is consumed and the reaction to alcohol, even in moderate amounts. Anxiety may be increased when blood glucose drops after delays in eating or as a result of the body's overly compensating for high carbohydrate, sugary meals. Generally, drops in blood sugar can be prevented in the normal patient by eating meals with adequate protein-rich foods at frequent intervals. Exercise may also be an important variable and should be explored with Sandra, as this may be a source of stress relief and has many benefits to health and well-being.

Potential Pitfalls

There are a number of pitfalls to be aware of in this case, including establishing the roles of psychotherapist, physician, and patient. Resistances exist in any therapy, and pharmacotherapy is no exception. The psychiatrist must avoid "splitting" or "rescuing" the patient from what may be difficult memories and emotional states that arise in the course of therapy. One reason to minimize the use of benzodiazepines is that these medications may sometimes be used to escape difficult therapeutic work that needs to be accomplished. As noted previously, these medications are also addictive. Of course, sedation is sometimes needed, but that needs to be coordinated with the psychotherapist. Sometimes symptoms are initially made worse with medication. Careful encouragement and support of the patient throughout the beginning of treatment may help prevent aborting a potentially beneficial treatment. The patient may resist medication, seeing a lessening of her hypervigilance as a threat and feeling that she's letting her guard down to potential threats. The necessary cognitive restructuring may not yet be in place and this issue should also be discussed with the therapist when and if this resistance occurs. Sandra may also have a secondary gain of seeking attention or protecting a point of view. With Sandra, being dogmatic or forceful is likely to allow her to "reenact" her earlier victimization, making compliance and therapy more difficult. One special consideration to be taken into account in women of child-bearing age is the possibility of pregnancy. This issue needs must be handled at the beginning of treatment, given the potential risk to a fetus. In pharmacotherapy treatment, planning for birth control and pregnancy are important. These scenarios should be addressed before starting medication, including when and if to stop medication as well as delineating what the psychological and hormonal effects of pregnancy are likely to be.

Difficulties in pharmacotherapy may also arise because of side effects, lack of effect, lack of patient compliance and need for discontinuation (e.g., because of pregnancy). The most common side effects of venlafaxine include anorexia, dry mouth, dizziness, constipation, somnolence, sweating, tremor, nausea, and sexual dysfunction; they occur, however, in only 2% to 5% of treated patients. The possibility and likelihood of side effects should be explained to Sandra at the beginning of treatment.

That side effects occur rarely and usually only at the beginning of the treatment should also be explained.

Adverse effects in short-term treatment with benzodiazepines are usually not severe. Sedation, psychomotor impairment, occasional ante-retrograde amnesia (impairment of the acquisition of new memory) and, very rarely, paradoxical excitement may occur.

The lack of effect of the first-choice treatment or a need for discontinuation due to the side effects of venlafaxine can be a reason for choosing the second-choice drug, buspirone, a nonbenzodiazepine anxiolytic. The choice would be based on the proven efficacy of buspirone in the treatment of anxiety. Its sedative, antianxiety, and muscle relaxant properties could be beneficial for Sandra, but usually the onset of action is slow (2 to 4 weeks) with the effective dose of 30 mg, administered twice or three times daily (Sramek et al., 1999). The advantages of buspirone are that there is a lower incidence of dependence than with benzodiazepines, no effects upon withdrawal, and less cognitive and memory impairment. The third choice of medication for Sandra would be an antidepressant, probably one of the SSRIs such as paroxetine, with similar expectations and regimens as with the first-choice drug. Lack of compliance with any prescribed medication may be associated with side effects.

Termination and Relapse Prevention

The length of treatment for Sandra is unpredictable, and because of the chronic nature of her illness may last for years. The decision of when and if medication is to be stopped necessitates considering how long the symptoms have been in remission, what personal and occupational responsibilities are at risk should symptoms reemerge, what if any medical complications of continuing medications exist (for example, risk to pregnancy), and what the risks are versus the benefits in stopping treatment. For the physician, periodic follow-up with patients after medication has been stopped is routine and may serve as a reinforcement to patients that they have indeed recovered. Termination is termination of a treatment, not of the relationship. The psychiatrist should have an open-door policy for other potential problems or symptoms that reemerge. Medications may be stopped rapidly or over a long period of time, depending on the type of medication, the reliability of the patient, and the level of comfort the patient has. With a patient who has had a chronic condition and she is now symptom free, the common wisdom is to taper and stop slowly, observing for reemergent symptoms, and to continue to reassure the patient throughout that period.

Mechanisms of Change

Sandra will change when she constructs a less hostile world view. With a more positive world view, she will experience more pleasurable and less painful affective states. She will then be more comfortable in her body and mind, allowing her to achieve more of her potential in life, without the blocking effect of fear and worry. This helps set in motion a positive feedback loop of action-success-more action-more success.

CONCLUSION

Sandra will change if the world she experiences changes. This includes the world she experiences within and the world she experiences without. Medicines can help reduce the interference or intrapersonal "noise," thus allowing the patient to hear and attend to the matters of life and growth with less unnecessary obstruction and with the possibility of a fulfilled and happy life.

REFERENCES

Allgulander, C., Cloninger, C. R., Przybeck, T. R., & Brandt, L. (1998). Changes on the temperament and character inventory after paroxetine treatment in volunteers with generalized anxiety disorder. *Psychopharmacology Bulletin, 34,* 165–166.

Ballenger, J. C. (1999). Current treatments of the anxiety disorders in adults. *Biological Psychiatry, 46,* 1579–1594.

Bazire, S. (2000). *Psychotropic Drug Directory 2000.* Quay Books: Exeter.

Davidson, J. R., DuPont, R. L., Hedges, D., & Haskins, J. T. (1999). Efficacy, safety, and tolerability of venlafaxine extended release and buspirone in outpatients with generalized anxiety disorder. *Journal of Clinical Psychiatry, 60,* 528–535.

El-Khayat, R., & Baldwin, D. S. (1998). Antipsychotic drugs for non-psychotic patients: Assessment of the benefit/risk ratio in generalized anxiety disorder. *Journal of Psychopharmacology, 12,* 323–329.

Feighner, J. P. (1999). Overview of antidepressants currently used to treat anxiety disorders. *Journal of Clinical Psychiatry, 60,* 18–22.

Fisher, P. L., & Durham, R. C. (1999). Recovery rates in GAD following psychological therapy: An analysis clinically significant change in the STAI-T across outcome studies since 1900. *Psychological Medicine, 29*, 1425–1434.

Gelenberg, A. J., Lydiard, R. B., Rudolph, R. L., Aguiar, L., Haskins, J. T., & Salinas, E. (2000). Efficacy of venlafaxine extended-release capsules in nondepressed outpatients with generalized anxiety disorder: A 6-month randomized controlled trial. *Journal of the American Medical Association, 283*, 3082–3088.

Hunter, R., & Macalpine, I. (1963). *Three hundred years of psychiatry 1535–1860*. Oxford University Press: London.

Lader, M., & Scott, J. C. (1998). A multicentre, double-blind comparison of hydroxyzine, buspirone and placebo in patients with generalized anxiety disorder. *Psychopharmacology, 139*, 402–406.

Leonard, B. E. (1998). *Fundamentals of psychopharmacology (2nd ed.)*. Chichester: Wiley.

Preston, J. D., O'Neal, J. H., & Talaga, M. C. (1998). *Consumer's guide to psychiatric drugs*. New Harbinger Publications: Oakland.

Rickels, K., Pollack, M. H., Sheehan, D. V., & Haskins, J. T. (2000). Efficacy of extended-release venlafaxine in nondepressed outpatients with generalized anxiety disorder. *American Journal of Psychiatry, 157*, 968–974.

Rocca, P., Fonzo, V., Scotta, M., Zanalda, E., & Ravizza, L. (1997). Paroxetine efficacy in the treatment of generalized anxiety disorder. *Acta Psychiatrica Scandinavica, 95*, 444–450.

Roering, J. L. (1999). Diagnosis and Management of Generalized Anxiety Disorder. *Journal of the American Pharmaceutical Association, 39*, 811–821.

Shader, R. I., & Greenblatt, D. J. (1993). Use of benzodiazepines in anxiety disorders. *New England Journal of Medicine, 328*, 1398–1405.

Sheehan, D. V. (1999). Venlafaxine extended release (XR) in the treatment of generalized anxiety disorder. *Journal of Clinical Psychiatry, 60*, 23–28.

Sramek, J. J., Hong, W. W., Hamid, S., Nape, B., & Cutler, N. R. (1999). Meta-analysis of the safety and tolerability of two dose regimens of buspirone in patients with persistent anxiety. *Depression & Anxiety, 9*, 131–134.

Uhlenhuth, E. H., Balter, M. B., Ban T. A., & Yang, K. (1999). International study of expert judgment on therapeutic use of benzodiazepines and other psychotherapeutic medications: VI. Trends in recommendations for the pharmacotherapy of anxiety disorders, 1992–1997. *Depression & Anxiety, 9*, 107–116.

14

Comparison of Treatment Approaches

Robert A. DiTomasso and Elizabeth A. Gosch

The goal of this chapter is to provide the reader with a comprehensive overview of both the essential similarities and critical distinguishing features of the theoretical approaches presented in the preceding pages. We have been fortunate in being able to assemble a group of very experienced clinicians who practice within the framework of their own identified theoretical orientation. We specifically sought practicing clinicians who strongly identify with a major theoretical orientation and treat patients within their professed theoretical scheme. In so doing, our hope is that these clinicians have elucidated the distinguishing aspects of their craft in assessing and treating a patient with anxiety from the various theoretical perspectives represented herein. Of equal import, existing similarities between these approaches will also be apparent. Moreover, our goal is to provide the reader with a real world flavor, or ecologically valid view, about what may actually transpire in the mind of the clinician in approaching a particular patient and how this information is translated into what may happen in the treatment room. In this manner, the reader has the opportunity to peek inside the theoretical workings of the clinician's mind who is digesting, seeking, and weighing the clinical information presented; why it is or is not important and what aspects of it are most significant; how it is interpreted and synthesized; and what methods are utilized in forming a conceptualization, treatment goals, and a plan of action.

As clinicians ourselves, we suspect the old notions that *therapy is only as good as the assessment upon which it is based* and *good therapy is good therapy* are never more apparent than in the words of the contributors to this volume. Unlike their novice counterparts, experienced therapists of different theoretical persuasions may be expected to attend to what most experienced therapists would consider important. Although the manner in which the problems, thoughts, feelings, and behaviors of the patient are construed and interpreted may be distinct—as well perhaps as the weighing of their importance—we expect that qualified therapists will generally concur about what should be addressed in the assessment and treatment of patients. On the other hand, it will be interesting to see on what points clinicians of differing orientations will diverge. In other words, the similarities may be just as important as the differences noted. We believe that no single therapeutic orientation to date has accounted for all of the variance in the assessment and conceptualization and treatment of anxiety disorders. What clinicians who are operating from differing orientations may learn from one another will only serve to help patients who have anxiety problems in the future. In this spirit, the information presented in Appendix A and our analysis of these approaches in the treatment of Sandra are presented, and the defining characteristics of each of the major psychotherapy models are presented, including the following cognitive-behavioral therapy (CBT), problem-solving therapy (PST), acceptance and commitment therapy (ACT), contextual family therapy (CFT), Adlerian therapy (AT), context-centered therapy (CCT), interpersonal psychotherapy (IPT), person-centered therapy (PCT), supportive-expressive therapy (SET), psychodynamic psychotherapy (PP), and psychopharmacological treatments.

THE THERAPISTS' SKILLS AND ATTRIBUTES

A comparison of the ideal therapists' skills and attributes across the theoretical approaches reveals interesting and important similarities. These commonalities underscore the critical importance of the therapeutic alliance and the ability of the therapist to establish a therapeutic relationship. We are reminded here that psychotherapy is a social psychological process, whereby the capacity of the helper to positively influence the one who is being helped is in part a function of the relationship that ensues between them.

Not surprisingly, the requisite and specific skill mix espoused by proponents of a particular approach is inherently defined by each respective theory. In other words, the required important skills are in large part defined by what is deemed necessary to occur during the course of the therapeutic encounter in order to promote change. Competencies in specific techniques are clearly derived from each theory. These proposed therapeutic strategies are congruent with the models from which they are derived and are intertwined with the expected role of the therapist. In all instances except one (PCT), specific techniques are used to effect change.

ASSESSMENT

In almost all instances described in this text, the contributors sought formal assessment information from the patient. The nature, type, and specificity of information and the method used to obtain it are dimensions along which differences are noted. All approaches, however, rely upon assessment information obtained during the course of clinical interviewing. Of course, the specific information sought relates to the content that is deemed most relevant to each approach, an example of the theoretical consistency within each model. In addition, some contributors (CBT, PST, ACT, PP) utilize formalized assessment instruments derived from their theoretical position. Others (CCT, PCT) do not use assessment instruments at all. Still others (CFT, AT) use strategies designed to elicit useful information from patients. Examples here include genograms (CFT) and early recollections (AT). Only two approaches (SET, PP) rely upon the use of projective techniques.

THERAPEUTIC GOALS

Each of the contributors identified therapeutic goals for treatment. In some instances (CBT, PST, CCT, IPT, SET) these goals are carefully and clearly specified and focus upon learning skills and reducing distressing symptoms. In only one instance (PST), the goals were actually divided intro short-term instrumental goals and long-term goals. Other approaches (CCT, AT, PCT, PP) described more global goals and sought to promote insight or self-understanding.

TIMELINE

Although the duration of therapy was addressed by all contributors, only some identified the length of sessions. Cognitive-behavioral-oriented therapists predicted more time-limited, weekly treatment complemented by booster sessions, if necessary, with therapy ranging anywhere from a minimum of 8 (CBT) to a maximum of 24 sessions (ACT). Two of these approaches (CBT, PST) recommended 90-minute sessions. Interpersonal therapy was also time-limited ranging from 12 to 16 weeks; context-centered therapy, ten sessions or less. However, and perhaps the most unusual, context-centered therapy sessions were reported to last from as little as 10 minutes to as much as 3 hours. Session frequency was dictated by patient problems and tasks to be addressed (ACT, CCT). In one instance (CCT), sessions could occur on several consecutive days or not occur over the course of a month. In one instance (PCT), weekly 50-minute sessions were recommended but duration was left unspecified and dependent upon the patient. Psychoanalytic therapy was recommended preferably twice a week for 50 minutes over the course of years. Finally, supportive-expressive therapy represented the standard 50-minute session in both open-ended (months to years) and time-limited (6 months to 2 years) formats.

CASE CONCEPTUALIZATION

From the standpoint of case conceptualization, most of the approaches emphasized the deleterious effects of early negative experiences related to abandonment and trauma, mistrust, and the problem of maintaining the role of avoidance in the patient's life. In three models (CBT, PST, CCT), the role of biological predispositions or reactivity were noted. Also, the view of the world as a dangerous place where one could encounter harm was stressed by three of the contributors (CBT, ACT, AT). Finally, dependency upon others to achieve security, safety, and protection is evidenced in several approaches (CBT, PST, AT, PCT, SET, PP).

TECHNIQUES AND INTERVENTIONS

In the models discussed in this volume, the psychotherapeutic techniques and interventions are specifically related and directed toward the presumed nature of the patient's problems. For example, the cognitive- and behavioral-oriented therapies emphasize, among other things, the use of psychoeducation, cognitive restructuring strategies, relaxation therapies, and homework, the latter as a means of generalizing treatment beyond the therapy session. Other models (CFT, AT, IPT, SET) emphasize the importance of the patient's relationship patterns. One model (PCT) relies exclusively upon the therapist's interpersonal attributes to foster a communicated and perceived sense of caring, warmth, acceptance, and empathic understanding in the patient's quest for self-exploration and self-acceptance.

TERMINATION AND RELAPSE PREVENTION

The process of terminating therapy, usually and understandably considered a critical issue, is addressed by every model. Essentially, all models appear to incorporate mechanisms designed to attribute treatment success to the patient. Specific means of accomplishing this important task include the following: reinforcing the notion that the success of therapy is due to the patient (CBT, PST, ACT, IPT) or those participating in therapy (CFT); tapering sessions over time (CBT, PST, ACT); recognizing that as the patient improves she will come less often (CCT); and discussing and reviewing therapy and the growth attained by the patient (AT, SET).

Specific efforts at relapse prevention by discussing anticipated obstacles and plans to address them are particularly characteristic of cognitive behavioral models (CBT, PST). However, the majority of the theoretical approaches leave the door open to the patient for future booster or follow-up sessions, when needed.

MECHANISMS OF CHANGE

The specific mechanisms to which change in psychotherapy is attributed may depend upon a number of factors. The theoretical assumptions of a given model, how problems are presumed to develop, the roles and functions of the psychotherapist, and the techniques, strategies, and interventions developed and implemented to resolve problems appear to play a major role. Each model in this volume displays a consistency across each of these domains, which is theoretically congruent within itself. The manner in which assumptions, concepts, and principles of a model are operationalized is directly related to its parent theory. A theoretical model, then, guides the thoughts, feelings, beliefs, assumptions, and behaviors of the therapist practicing within it. A review of the mechanisms of change across the models contained in this volume clearly displays a remarkable internal consistency. Except perhaps for the therapist-patient relationship, each model dictates and prescribes certain and often unique ways of conceptualizing, assessing, and treating anxiety. Even when the contributors speak about similar or perhaps identical phenomena, different terms may be used to describe it. Not unexpectedly, each model attributes change mechanisms to its own unique explanation. Common factors across all psychotherapies and factors that are specific to a given therapy may combine in ways that help experienced clinicians help patients who are anxious to improve. When psychotherapists challenge cognitive distortions, expose anxious patients to what they fear, teach problem-solving skills, increase self-acceptance, change dysfunctional relationships, foster insight and a sense of belonging, facilitate effective interpersonal interactions, and promote self-exploration and self-understanding, change may occur. The final common pathways across all these therapies are alterations in the ways patients think, believe, feel, act, react, and relate.

CONCLUSION

In this volume we have sought to present a comprehensive overview of the treatment of a patient who is anxious from a variety of theoretical perspectives. We presented a case example that reflects the characteristics of a patient with an anxiety disorder, which is commonly seen in clinical practice today. By utilizing as contributors experienced clinicians from several popular psychotherapeutic models who profess to practice from a single theoretical orientation, our hope was to present the reader with an appreciation of how clinicians within each model approach, conceptualize, plan, and implement treatment of a patient with anxiety disorder. It is hoped that by allowing the reader to figuratively "sit in and watch" these master therapists at work, we have whet the reader's appetite for understanding the manner in which various psychotherapies evolve in clinical practice with patients who are anxious. At best, if we can assume that in actual practice prototypical clinicians actually do what they say they do, then we have elucidated the common and distinctive features of these models. Otherwise, we have presented an ideal that clinicians of each theoretical perspective can seek to emulate. For those readers interested in integrative approaches to psychotherapy, the preceding chapters, taken as a whole, provide a vast, enriched landscape from which they may harvest. Also, perhaps budding clinicians in search of an orientation will find an approach that meets their professional needs. At the very least, we have attempted to provide a thorough comparison of selected available treatments for anxiety. By carefully explicating the similarities and differences between these approaches, we may stimulate a process of further understanding critical concepts and constructs that may offer important implications for assisting our understanding about the nature and treatment of anxiety.

Appendix

<table>
<tr><td></td><td>*Treatment Model*</td></tr>
<tr><td>Cognitive-
Behavioral</td><td>Individuals are subject to laws of operant and classical conditioning. Problems develop from faulty learning, inadequate learning, and distorted interpretation of events—an interaction of cognition, affect, and behavior. Mowrer's two-factor theory is used to explain development of anxiety disorders, i.e., acquired by classical conditioning and maintained by operant contingencies. Each component (cognitive, behavioral, and physical) is targeted; exposure, extinction, reinforcement of alternative responses and challenging and replacing erroneous beliefs with rational beliefs are used to solve problems.</td></tr>
<tr><td>Problem-
Solving</td><td>Patient problems are idiographic—what constitutes a problem for one individual is defined individually by the person experiencing the problem. Problem-solving deficits in the form of ineffective coping responses are what lead to distress and maladaptive psychological and physical responses. Distress develops from the reciprocal interacting relationships among stressful life events, negative mood states, and problem-solving and coping deficits. Patients need to learn a formal, systematic, and rational approach to the personal, interpersonal, and objective/impersonal problems they confront and to initiate self-directed purposeful action designed to change the nature of the problem, reactions, or both.</td></tr>
<tr><td>Acceptance and
Commitment</td><td>A contextual-behavioral psychotherapy approach that views psychopathology as a frequent side effect of</td></tr>
</table>

normal human language processes. People use language arbitrarily to relate events and transform the stimulus functions of one event based on the other, leading to higher thinking processes but also to "symptoms." ACT interventions aim to undermine experiential avoidance, deliteralize language representations, teach acceptance and willingness, and help clients behave in accord with chosen values.

Context-
Centered

Words and symbols (language) determine how people experience themselves and their world and how they relate to one another. Language constrains and motivates actions. People's choices are linguistically grounded. Problems are seen as high-cost operants. Through orthogonal interactions, therapy helps make lower-cost solutions available to clients.

Contextual
Family

The unification of the totality of one's relationships and the ethics and loyalties inherent within those relationships are the central foci of CFT. Rooted in the work of Ivan Boszormenyi-Nagy, this multigenerational systemic family approach to treatment attends to four primary dimensions: facts, psychology, transactions, and relational ethics.

Adlerian

A person is a holistic, self-consistent unity striving toward a subjectively conceived sense of significance and security within a social-interpersonal field; a person's lifestyle goal is a person's unique way of striving for significance, security, completeness, and a sense of power and efficacy; most psychopathology results from discouragement (i.e., lacking confidence and seeking to avoid life's demands); distortions in lifestyle beliefs and goals and development of symptoms results in nonconscious strategies designed to avoid situations that one believes will reveal to the world one's feelings of inadequateness and worthlessness.

Interpersonal

Originally developed as a treatment for depression, IPT is based on a diathesis-stress model of illness, viewing mental disorders as resulting from a combination of biology, life stressors, interpersonal relationships, and personality. IPT is designed to alleviate symptoms by specifically focusing upon the client's current stressors in interpersonal relationships as well as the stress response associated with those relationships. One of the following interpersonal problem areas is targeted for intervention: (a) grief or complicated bereavement, (b) interpersonal role disputes, (c) role transitions, and (d) interpersonal deficits.

Person-Centered

People have desire and capacity to self-actualize; internal guiding system of an individual is skewed by external judgments and capacity to self-actualize; incongruence between real and ideal self is root of psychopathology; goal is to provide necessary and sufficient conditions for psychological growth; therapeutic relationship is based on respect and valuing of person, his or her thoughts, perceptions, and ability to grow; therapeutic conditions of unconditional positive regard, empathy, and congruence are offered by therapist, and client experiences feeling of incongruence and identifies same dynamic in daily interactions; important for client to express feelings in an accepting environment where conditions of worth are not placed on person.

Supportive-Expressive

Grounded in principles of psychodynamic change through which individuals come to a greater understanding of their behavior, particularly with respect to insight into their interpersonal relationship patterns. Core conflictual relationship themes (CCRTs) are examined as a refined understanding of individual's central relational need (wish) from others, typical responses from others (RO), and the resulting response from the individual (RS).

Psychodynamic

Four conceptual submodels often utilized by practitioners: drive, structural, self psychology, and object relations theory. Drive theory emphasizes the interplay between basic, instinctual impulses pressing for discharge and the evocation of defenses, which causes intrapsychic conflict leading to anxiety symptoms. Structural theory focuses on the control and regulation of drives through the id, ego, and superego. Self psychology and object relations theory emphasizes early formative relationships, quality of internal psychological structures, and the nature of ongoing interpersonal relationships in treatment.

Pharmacological

Heightened autonomic sympathetic nervous system activity is disproportional to the threatening stimuli, lasts longer, and impairs the ability of an individual to lead a normal life. According to the present state of knowledge, this heightened arousal is connected mainly with three substances: noradrenaline, serotonin (5 hydroxytryptamine), and GABA (gamma amino butyric acid). The present biochemical model calls for the use of different classes of psychotropic medications in the treatment of anxiety, which modify serotonergic and noradrenergic transmission or agonists of GABA receptors.

The Therapist's Skills and Attributes

Cognitive-Behavioral

Ability to engender trust, think logically, express empathy, foster collaboration, question one's actions, and demonstrate competence. Depending on problem, therapeutic relationship may take on more or less import; therapist may use reaction to patient in formulating case conceptualization and therapist may disclose how CBT has been personally helpful. Thorough grounding in cognitive-behavioral conceptualization and implementation of cognitive behavioral techniques. Interpersonally skilled and able to provide a collaborative focus, therapist is active, directive teacher, guide, and collaborator.

Problem-Solving

Therapist must possess warmth, genuineness, empathy, positive regard, and ability to establish rapport/collaboration. Therapist must have sound clinical decision-making skills and convey knowledge of clinical research that supports therapy. Ability to identify patient's patterns in the therapeutic relationship (sample of the patient's reactions, behaviors, and feelings). Competencies with techniques from cognitive-behavioral models including imagery, Socratic questioning, role-playing, and exposure are important. As a problem solver, therapist seeks out all facts about patient, considers possible interventions, makes effective treatment decisions, monitors progress through time-series assessment, and adjusts therapy plan as necessary. Therapist prescribes a collaborative therapeutic treatment alliance. Therapist is expert in problem solving; patient is expert in his or her own personal experiences.

Acceptance and Commitment

ACT therapists adopt a posture of radical acceptance of private experiences, compassionately accepting no reason-giving from clients in the context of a warm, nonjudgmental, direct, and honest therapeutic relationship. Therapists' understanding of ACT strategies at a deep, functional level is aided by therapists' using ACT techniques on their problems. Therapists benefit from the ability to track verbal events at multiple levels and to intervene in the function of the behavior.

Context-Centered

Therapists able to identify client's rhetoric for clues about unexamined assumptions and linguistic evasions (half-truths, exaggerations, circular assumptions, disclaimed actions). Therapeutic attitude is direct, friendly, efficient, straightforward, and compassionate as therapist questions the linguistic usage of the client. Promoting orthogonal interactions, therapists are able to demonstrate how clients are imprisoned by their own belief systems and "club" allegiances.

Contextual Family

The CFT therapist needs to understand the power inherent in relationships, networks, and systems. As a catalyst and choreographer, the therapist needs to be able to identify loyalties and reoccurring themes in the family, while helping move the client toward patterns of increasingly positive connectedness with others. Therapists benefit from having dealt with their own family history and issues, as well as training in contextual therapy, multigenerational psychodynamics, and developmental stages.

Adlerian	Ability to enter client's world and maintain a therapeutic relationship based on mutual respect; most significant is the ability to model for patient and stimulate the expression of social interest; therapist seeks to understand patient's lifestyle (private meaning or logic) free of one's own biases; relationship is characterized by cooperation, social equality, social interest, respect, ability to encourage and stimulate courage to be imperfect; receive didactic therapy to increase awareness of one's own lifestyle and its impact in conducting therapy.
Interpersonal	The IPT therapist should receive specialized IPT training. Acting to instill hope, the therapist plays an active, educative role (e.g., explicitly asserts that disorder is treatable, provides diagnostic clarification) but does not provide direct advice or reassurance. Focusing on present interpersonal functioning as opposed to intrapsychic or cognitive/behavioral realm, the therapist acts as a warm, nonjudgmental advocate for the client.
Person-Centered	Ability to offer and have person perceive unconditional positive regard, empathy, and genuineness; to possess patience and trust in person's ability to grow; therapist must have a deep, conscious level of self-acceptance upon which to draw; therapist is fully aware of feelings and thoughts person evokes in him or her; relationship is promoted through necessary and sufficient conditions, not techniques; therapist is most effective when therapist has had chance to know/accept himself or herself under the guided hand of an experienced clinician.
Supportive-Expressive	Attention to the various elements of the therapeutic relationship: building of a positive therapeutic alliance (i.e., facilitating an atmosphere of trust, collaboration, respect, and responsiveness), becoming empathically involved through listening and understanding and patience. Therapist is active in eliciting specific and detailed interpersonal interactions between the patient and other individuals in the present

                    and past. Therapists are active in setting clear, agreed-
                    upon goals that are frequently revisited.

Psychodynamic   The therapist maintains a stance of acceptance, re-
                    spect, concern, limit-setting, and analytic neutrality
                    (attentiveness) with the patient. Tolerant of ambiguity
                    and confusion, the therapist balances empathizing
                    with the patient's experience and observing the pa-
                    tient's thoughts, feelings, impulses, and behaviors.
                    The therapist must have the ability to translate con-
                    scious material into unconscious antecedents and
                    communicate this meaning effectively to the client.

Pharmacolog-   A physician, ideally a psychiatrist, with extensive, accu-
ical   rate, and up-to-date knowledge of pharmacotherapy
                    who communicates that anxiety is a condition that can
                    be successfully treated. The well-structured contact
                    between physician and patient would be designed to
                    provide patient with information about his or her
                    condition and treatment through a focused, detailed
                    medication-education program.

                    Assessment

Cognitive-   Administer Anxiety Disorders Interview Schedule-
Behavioral   Revised and Penn State Worry Questionnaire; patient
                    self-monitoring of the content, frequency, severity,
                    and context of a variety of Sandra's symptoms; con-
                    sider Sandra's biological propensity for schizophrenia
                    and role of modeling from her mother (world is a
                    dangerous place necessitating self-protection) and di-
                    rect experience (past abuse and presence of intruder
                    in home).

Problem-   Administer the Social Problem Solving Inventory
Solving   (measure of coping skills) before and at the end of
                    therapy. Various methods used to define problem,
                    identify etiological and functionally related factors
                    related to problem, establish therapy goals, and iden-
                    tify obstacles to treatment. Within biopsychosocial
                    framework, collect patient data using an empirically

based, multimodal (interpersonal, intrapersonal, and environmental), multimethod (observations, interview, and physiological), multiformat (self, other) approach to identify well-defined causal variables. Monitor Sandra's moods, identify antecedents and consequences, frequency of symptoms, somatic arousal, depressive symptoms, coping history, current records of coping (thoughts, feelings, emotions, behaviors), strengths, and adaptive skills.

Acceptance and Commitment	Specific assessment information includes the function of client's current and historical symptoms, cognitive fusion, experiential avoidance, control strategies, emotional control and historical factors, verbal story that supports avoidance behaviors, and values assessment. Acceptance and Action Questionnaire assesses experiential avoidance. Daily self-monitoring of the intensity of negative feeling, the intensity of trying not to feel that emotion, and the workability of client's life approach that day.
Context-Centered	No specific tools. Therapist assesses linguistic rhetoric of the client for inaccuracies, inconsistencies, circular logic, disclaimed actions, etc.
Contextual Family	Multigenerational family background information regarding patterns of relating, connectedness, abuse, trauma, support, abandonment, denial, parenting, etc. A genogram provides a pictorial map of multigenerational family patterns. The authors also call for further diagnostic symptom clarification and a psychiatric pharmacotherapy consultation.
Adlerian	Collect six to eight early recollections (subjective reconstruction of past events) at outset of therapy; family constellation interview (early subjective experiences of family system) that help to provide information about circumstances within which client's personal beliefs, meanings, and behavior patterns developed. Examine Sandra's relationship to her father and how abuse by brothers contributed to her lack of trust.

Interpersonal	Use of formal diagnostic assessment, mood/diagnostic rating instruments, psychiatric history, and the Interpersonal Inventory. The authors suggest using the MCMI-III, Trauma Symptom Inventory, and projective assessment techniques. Assessment would clarify the nature of Sandra's interactions with important individuals in her life, including type of contact, recurrent interpersonal patterns, each person's interpersonal expectations, satisfying and unsatisfying aspects of relationships, communication styles, and the ways Sandra would like to change the relationships.
Person-Centered	Assessment tools are not used for these reasons: person is healthy enough to provide own history; therapist is not put in role of judge or in position of power; diagnostic labels take away from the person of the client. Specific information sought by therapist: Sandra's level of self-acceptance; if she understands self-acceptance and its importance for healthy ego development; how Sandra's mother's condition makes her feel about herself; how information was stored or symbolized; how Sandra introjects values into understanding of herself; how Sandra is re-creating relationships with family with her boss; and her relationships with her loved ones.
Supportive-Expressive	Developmental history, current presenting symptoms, precipitating events, medical problems, and *DSM-IV* diagnoses. Psychodiagnostic testing can include projective measures from which finer distinctions of a patient's psychology can be enunciated. Additional information from Sandra's history: others in her relational network, past and present intimate relationships and close friends, previous treatment experiences. Sandra's ideas regarding the nature of her symptoms and what contributes or maintains their presence.
Psychodynamic	Cognitive and projective instruments (e.g., WAIS-III, Rorschach, TAT) to elucidate Sandra's structural dynamics, character structure, and level of personality organization. The structures assessed include level of

instinctual development, signs of ego weakness, defenses, quality of internalized object relationship, superego development, and ego identity.

Pharmacological · Complete medical evaluation and blood tests.

Therapeutic Goals

Cognitive-Behavioral · Learn skills to reduce fear of being alone (which will generalize to other problems); reduce worry; sleep with less difficulty; increase social sphere and sense of connection to others; accept and resolve anger/guilt related to her family.

Problem-Solving · Identify ultimate outcomes (desired by client) and instrumental outcomes (cognitive, behavioral, emotional, social, and environmental changes) judged necessary in order to achieve ultimate outcome. Short-term goals: Help Sandra change to positive problem orientation (problems are seen as normal, expected, challenging, solvable by self); recognize relationship between thoughts, feelings and behaviors; self-monitor thinking and emotions; engage in more productive, rational thinking and expectations; adopt a more adaptive core belief system; learn new ways to think about past events, new ways of coping with negative emotions, and new ways of controlling impact of her past on her future; increased reliance on rational problem-solving skills. Long-term goals: Decrease fear of harm, somatic anxiety symptoms, daily rituals and obsessive behavior, avoidant behavior, helplessness and powerlessness, guilt and anger (resolve past experiences with family), dependency; improve or increase relationship quality, sense of trust in others, coping skills, sense of control over problems, self-sufficiency, quality of life, and future functioning.

Acceptance and Commitment · Encourage cognitive defusion and experiential acceptance so that Sandra can abandon the agenda of regulating her private events (avoidance) and engage in behaviors that align with her values in the presence of difficult private events. In concert, accept herself, her inner experience (including pain), and her history.

Context-
Centered

Discussion of the therapist-client contract leads to establishing goals. Aim not to cure or change personality traits but to initiate a specialized form of dialogue that will lead to change in linguistic inaccuracies, impasses, and assumptions/beliefs which in turn will lighten Sandra's life burdens and interpersonal impasses. Assist Sandra to accept herself nonjudgmentally, step back and observe her own processes at work, and embrace an adult role.

Contextual
Family

Assist Sandra to develop a more individually differentiated life, to distance herself in a healthy way from her family and her reliance on her boyfriend. Clarification of her birth parent's role regarding her identity and the reenactment of abandonment in her foster family. Lessening guilt or shame from past molestations and family betrayal.

Adlerian

Encourage hope for change; gain insight into Sandra's lifestyle; help her understand how she strives for significance and security in world; understand how the experience of being victimized and betrayed as child influenced her development of her current views of self, others, and world; understand how her lifestyle conclusions were appropriate during childhood but presently exaggerate dangers; understand how her emotions move her toward a goal of safeguarding; increase involvement with others to foster sense of belonging.

Interpersonal

The therapist would work with Sandra to ameliorate interpersonal role disputes or interpersonal deficits. If focusing on the interpersonal role dispute, IPT would seek to understand the dispute fully, choose a plan of action, and bring about an acceptable resolution by modifying expectation or problematic communication style. If focusing on interpersonal deficits, a primary therapeutic goal would be for Sandra to recognize the association between problematic social skills and the maintenance of her anxiety/social isolation, while seeking to reduce Sandra's social isolation and encourage the development of new relationships.

Person-
Centered

Increase Sandra's self-acceptance; become a fully functioning self-reliant adult; reconstruct personality, not simply symptom reduction or external behavioral control; form new connections and symbolizations based on what Sandra internally values based on life experiences and not introjected values; think for herself and have thoughts congruent with organismic valuing system; identify her own natural inclinations about situations that cause her the most incongruence.

Supportive-
Expressive

Identify symptoms in an interpersonal context; discuss and agree on specific, achievable goals. Increase understanding of pervasive anxiety, fear of personal injury/attack, avoidance of perceived danger situations, how they relate to CCRT and begin to exert a sense of control over their expression. Reduce anxiety and worry, fear of her surroundings, avoidance of typical daily activities and need to obsessively rely on a rigid timetable to manage her anxiety. Experience relationships as reliable, safe and worthy of trust. Experience deeper, more affective connections and autonomy in relationships.

Psychodynamic

An overarching goal for Sandra is self-understanding rooted in self-reflection. Emphasize structural repair and building versus high level structural conflict resolution; promote individuation, growth, and the ability to soothe herself.

Pharmacolog-
ical

Decrease motor tension, hyperarousal, and avoidance behavior.

Timeline for Therapy

Cognitive-
Behavioral

Time-limited treatment with 90-minute sessions occurring one time a week (sometimes twice a week) for 10 to 15 weeks.

Problem- Solving	Once a week for 90-minute sessions; given complexity of developmental and learning history, a high level of family/significant other involvement may necessitate more than the typical 8 to 12 sessions.
Acceptance and Commitment	Session frequency dictated by Sandra's situation. Typically, 16 to 24 sessions with additional and booster sessions as needed.
Context- Centered	Sessions are scheduled when there are specific tasks to accomplish. Sometimes sessions may occur several days in a row or not for a month at a time. Sessions last from 10 minutes to 3 hours as the time is a function of the job at hand. Usually meet for 10 sessions or less.
Contextual Family	A minimum of 3 to 6 months of treatment during which Sandra would attend sessions weekly or possibly biweekly. Some sessions would be longer than 1 hour, especially when more than one person is in attendance or important issues need to be addressed.
Adlerian	Ask if Sandra would prefer to meet once or twice a week at outset; therapy would last 28 to 36 months.
Interpersonal	Designed as a time-limited therapy, IPT would involve Sandra's attending weekly psychotherapy sessions for 12 to 16 weeks.
Person- Centered	Weekly 50-minute sessions; varies according to Sandra's level of comfort, intelligence, and awareness of feelings.
Supportive- Expressive	Dependent upon Sandra's goals. Therapy can be open-ended (TO) or time-limited (TL). TL therapy typically involves a planned treatment of 6 to 24 sessions with TO running from months to years. Weekly sessions (usually 50 minutes each), in some cases twice weekly or biweekly, depending on Sandra's acuity, therapy phase, and therapist's judgment.
Psychodynamic	One or preferably two sessions per week, for 50 minutes, over a period of years.
Pharmacological	Flexible timeline. Initially, Sandra would be seen two to three times a week then every 3 to 4 weeks for 30-minute sessions over 6 months.

Case Conceptualization

Cognitive-Behavioral	Focus upon etiological and maintaining variables; early experience and her biological predisposition play key roles; early trauma and her biological mother have led to development of danger schema and anxiety is maintained through avoidance.
Problem-Solving	Synthesis of previously collected biopsychosocial information and functional analysis reveals that Sandra exhibits difficulties in cognitive, affective, behavioral, physical/biological, and social/interpersonal areas. These difficulties have been shaped by negative life events related to trust and she developed maladaptive schemas about herself, her self-worth, and others. Her problems were learned at an early age and have been reinforced throughout her life. Her anxiety and avoidances have been reinforced and maintained by her family and boyfriend.
Acceptance and Commitment	Sandra has an experiential avoidance disorder. She engages in costly and ultimately ineffective coping strategies (e.g., avoidance, suppression, perfectionism, achievement, workaholism, self-attack, ruminative worry, and interpersonal distancing) in her attempts to avoid pain and produce an outward appearance of success. She has not learned to accept and love herself, with her pain, and is trying to drive perfect performances out of herself in vain attempts to make herself feel better.
Context-Centered	Sandra is struggling to maintain an adult façade within the infantilizing effects of a hyperreactive biochemistry. She is a prisoner of *primitive survival mechanisms* as opposed to having a pathological mental health condition. Her experience of anxiety is not a reified state but a concept, a subjective report of distress, and not an "affliction." She may misunderstand and despise her own coping needs especially if others have pathologized her behavior.
Contextual Family	Parentified and with few deep emotional attachments, Sandra's ruminations may act as cognitive avoidance

of her own lack of a true self. Sandra's basic male-female role concepts are split in an all-or-nothing fashion, contributing to feelings of distrust, loneliness, and fear of others. On a positive note, her hypervigilance also demonstrates her desire to protect herself.

Adlerian

Subjective perception of experience in early childhood is basis upon which one's lifestyle beliefs and goals are based. Sandra's image of life and the world are hostile, dangerous, and scary; image of self is vulnerable, victimized, and in danger when alone; image of others is untrustworthy, critical, unfair, and hurtful; her goal is to protect herself from situations she believes will cause her harm; fear and anxiety are protective mechanisms for maintaining safety.

Interpersonal

The authors identify Sandra's numerous strengths (e.g., capable, professionally successful, young) and suggest that Sandra may have PTSD with notable detachment, disconnectedness, and possible depersonalization. Interpersonal role disputes and interpersonal deficits appear the predominant interpersonal stressors with which Sandra struggles.

Person-Centered

Anxiety and fearfulness are based on early abandonment by mother and father; dependent on others to manage her fears; seeks mother's level of approval and acceptance despite being an adult who no longer needs to rely on adults to guide her; poorly formed sense of self based on distorted introjections and low self-efficacy; broken trust is at core of Sandra's psychopathology.

Supportive-Expressive

Sandra's CCRT: (Wish) To be safe and protected, to trust, depend upon others; to be appreciated and valued; (Response of Other) Abuse, punishment, abandonment; disinterest; (Response of Self) Feeling anxious, angry, fearful, alone, and disconnected. Relationship patterns have an integral role in generating and escalating Sandra's symptom patterns, which she has generalized to the world. Her personality style is dependent; she depends upon others to protect her from a terrifying world yet cannot become too close for fear of the emotional connection. Sandra presents many features of an individual with a chronic, post-traumatic adjustment to a trauma. For Sandra, the world is a threatening place, and much of the stimuli present are potential threats to be avoided.

Psychodynamic	Sandra suffers from unremitting, diffuse, and free-floating annihilation anxiety in which she fears conscious expression of unconscious primary process urges, thoughts, fantasies, and the accompanying loss of reality (core fear of going crazy). She exhibits a pervasive fear of separation and a driving need to control external objects (e.g., her boyfriend) whom she utilizes to provide security, safety, and well-being. Damaged personality structure evidenced by severe ego weakness, use of primitive defenses (denial, projective identification), and impaired object relations. She demonstrates strengths in her ability to function effectively with structure and make constructive use of others.
Pharmacological	Sandra's difficulties include motor tension, autonomic hyperactivity, and hyperarousal. These problems exacerbate her feelings of anxiety, worry, and avoidance behavior.

Techniques and Methods of Working

Cognitive-Behavioral	Functional assessment used to develop treatment plan; target one problem for treatment with assumption it will lead to improvement in other problems; use treatment package for specific disorder that has been shown to be effective. For Sandra, exposure is treatment of choice; obtain physical consultation with physician and assess caffeine intake; review protocols for treatment of specific phobia and generalized anxiety disorder. Specific techniques: psychoeducation, coping strategies, cognitive restructuring, progressive

	muscle relaxation, breathing retraining, confrontation (exposure) of fears in hierarchical fashion; and homework.

Problem-Solving

Techniques include tasks specific to stage of treatment: problem definition and formulation, generating alternatives, decision-making, solution implementation and verification, and homework. Other techniques include cognitive restructuring, exposure, covert desensitization, behavioral exercises, role-playing, relaxation, and diaphragmatic breathing.

Acceptance and Commitment

Specific techniques such as metaphor, paradox, exercises, homework, and confusion to break up existing structural linkages created by verbal language. Using these techniques, the therapist would find examples in Sandra's life that illustrate how strategies of control and avoidance are the problem, not Sandra herself. The six domains of treatment include creative hopelessness, control as the problem, self as context/defusion and deliteralization, experiential willingness, choices and values, and commitment to action and change.

Context-Centered

Promote orthogonal interactions that cause Sandra to examine gaps in logic, assumptions, inaccuracies, inconsistencies, circular logic, disclaimed actions, etc. Help Sandra trade a familiar viewpoint for a novel one by making the new perspective's payoff seem worthwhile. Engage in projects and exercises that (a) demonstrate how Sandra's choices operate, (b) help her practice acceptance, detachment, and commitment, and (c) make new declarations for herself.

Contextual Family

Help family members develop the ability to nonjudgmentally hear, understand, and acknowledge each person's perspective or construction of meaning. Expanding the context of relating to include the dimension of "meaning" allows new insights to be gained through multigenerational understanding and multidimensional enlightenment. The authors also advocate some individually focused interventions such as EMDR for dealing with trauma.

Adlerian	Develop alliance by rapport, encouraging collaboration, understanding subjective world of patient; model expression of social interest; investigate dynamics by gaining understanding of lifestyle through interpreting early recollections and family constellation; therapist seeks to understand client's movement and goals in early and current relationships, including therapy relationship; develop insight by exploring metaphoric expression of interpretation of beliefs and purposes of client's behaviors; stimulate change; understand and deal with resistance.
Interpersonal	A combination of IPT and pharmacotherapy while Sandra monitors her symptoms over time through self-report inventories like the Beck Anxiety Inventory. Promotion of the "sick role" and diagnostic clarification while addressing negative and positive aspects of important relationships with an emphasis on solving problems. Communication analysis and role-play to address interpersonal deficits.
Person-Centered	Therapist is caring listener and client is courageous explorer; therapist creates atmosphere of acceptance and permission for Sandra to express her emotional turmoil; therapist is active listener, empathizing with Sandra as they embark on journey of self-exploration with client as a fellow traveler and participant; therapist is not the expert as this is disingenuous and creates distance between therapist and Sandra—the antithesis of mechanism of change; move at Sandra's pace doing all to support and enhance client's level of self-acceptance.
Supportive-Expressive	The therapist must persistently present as trustworthy and reliable and communicate genuine concern and attentiveness through listening and empathic responding. The therapeutic relationship is collaborative. Language is important; including the terms "we" or "let's" (let us) highlights the collaborative nature of the treatment. Sandra's role is to be open with their thoughts and feelings. Therapist will help solve problems through listening and understanding, not

giving advice, and assists patients in making them aware of aspects of their emotional life of which they may not have been aware. Patients are educated about the role of the unconscious and relationship patterns. The therapist should communicate that change is difficult and that things may worsen before they improve. Encourage discussion of negative feelings about the treatment or therapist. Therapist must be active in elucidating the CCRT though typically is not directive.

Psychodynamic   Creating a holding and containing environment in which Sandra can experience and resolve early developmental conflicts. Empathetic listening will help Sandra sort through what feels confusing, while conveying a sense of understanding. Therapist takes in Sandra's projections, metabolizes them, and gives them back to her in a form that can be understood. As affective relatedness grows between the therapist and Sandra, the therapist makes greater use of interpreting resistances and transference reactions. Recognizing and understanding of empathetic failures is also of crucial importance because these failures recapitulate previous experiences with earlier caregivers.

Pharmacolog-   Establishing a good therapeutic alliance is critical.
ical   Pharmacotherapy education, including the nature of anxiety symptoms and medication treatment options. Advocate a combination of pharmacotherapy and psychological therapy for optimal treatment response. Possible recommended medications include extended-release venlafaxine (Effexor XR), a long acting benzodiazepine such as Clorazepate, buspirone, or possibly a selective serotonin reuptake inhibitor such as sertraline (Zoloft).

Potential Pitfalls

Cognitive-   Improvement may change patient's relationships;
Behavioral   nonadherence to treatment possibly due to fear, lack of confidence in therapy, lack of support from others, heavy demands of time necessary for treatment; onset

of relaxation-induced anxiety; dissociation or numbing during exposure, which prevents the experience of fear; becoming overwhelmed with fear; feelings of frustration, anger, or shame. To ameliorate: address reasons for nonadherence; address reasons for the relaxation-induced anxiety, drop this component, or use alternative relaxation procedures; modify the exposure procedure.

Problem-Solving	Viewing problem-solving therapy as skills-training alone and not as psychotherapy. Presenting treatment in a mechanistic, generic, and superficial manner and minimizing patient's feelings. With Sandra, failure to address trust and safety issues, validate her feelings, consider impact of therapy on others in her life, and her possible dependence on therapy and therapist.
Acceptance and Commitment	Sandra's tendency to intellectualize may lead the therapist to "tell ACT stories" that fit her case without Sandra's experiencing acceptance directly. Because of her dependence on others and her tendency to intellectualize, Sandra may wish to justify and evaluate her choices, leading to cognitive entanglement. Sandra may want to maintain a story in which she is a victim. Although she may have been a victim in the past, she may have difficulty understanding her role in maintaining this story in her current life.
Context-Centered	Sandra's decision to pursue treatment may be motivated by her wish to appease her boyfriend rather than her own intentionality. Recommend that Sandra claim therapy as her own personal choice and as an example of her own responsible behavior.
Contextual Family	The inclusion of multiple treatment participants may increase the chances for negative dynamics to be enacted. Disorders of personality or refusal to accept needed medication may compromise the treatment. The possibility of uncovered traumas emerging for Sandra or other participants can affect the treatment.
Adlerian	Sandra doesn't feel able to successfully prevent intrusion and abuse from others. She may resist directive

interventions designed to decrease her anxiety because she maintains these symptoms as a way of keeping safe. Reframing her symptoms as coping strategies changes her relationship to these symptoms and may enable her to experience change.

Interpersonal   The evolution of her symptoms into comorbid major depressive disorder, PTSD, or psychotic disorder. Sandra's struggles with dependency, inability to trust, avoidance, and superficiality may impact upon her ability to form a collaborative relationship with the therapist. Her past experience with invalidation may impact upon her ability to tolerate distress or success in treatment.

Person-Centered   Sandra may have difficulty making connection with therapist; Sandra may have difficulty accepting conditions therapist offers and may resist assuming responsibility for her life.

Supportive-Expressive   Developing a trusting therapeutic relationship may be initially difficult; prospects that the therapy would be potentially even more distressing than symptoms. Avoidance of painful issues may manifest in psychotherapy in patient's obsessive and avoidant style. When symptom change occurs, relationships will change as will how others view her. Change in relationships may precipitate other than supportive responses from others.

Psychodynamic   The long-term nature of her anxiety symptoms has become Sandra's way of being in the world and her means of exercising control over others. In addition to these secondary gains there is an unspoken and unrecognized sense of omnipotence. To give up the symptom is to relinquish the secondary gains and sense of omnipotence, which may be difficult for Sandra. Fears of entrusting herself to others may lead her to keep private what is most important and intimate. She may not be interested in looking beyond her symptoms to underlying causes and may consider prematurely leaving therapy once she experiences some relief from anxiety.

Pharmacological	Physical dependence on medication, intolerable side-effects of medication, and relapse following cessation of medication. Sandra's difficulty with trust may impinge upon her ability to communicate with her physician or follow the prescribed medication regime.

Inclusion of Others in Treatment

Cognitive-Behavioral	Significant others may be used as coaches, reminding patient and encouraging her to practice.
Problem-Solving	Sandra's parents and boyfriend.
Acceptance and Commitment	Experiential exercises may include other individuals.
Context-Centered	May include family and friends in the sessions or projects/exercises.
Contextual Family	The therapy includes relevant family and friends with adequate preparation of the client.
Adlerian	Depending on the type of problem, couple or family therapy may be utilized. A psychiatric referral to assess the need for medication to control anxiety or depression may be considered. Sandra would be encouraged to consider a referral to a molestation support group.
Interpersonal	If the IPT therapist is not a physician, the therapist would collaborate with a psychiatrist or physician to provide medication management.
Person-Centered	Invite boyfriend; refer to physician if relevant issues arise.
Supportive-Expressive	Including family members in the treatment process—either in joint sessions or via information gathering in person or by phone—is not contraindicated. Helpful to observe interactions between Sandra and significant others as a way of increasing understanding of the CCRT and the therapeutic relationship.
Psychodynamic	No other individuals were mentioned by author but pharmacotherapy was to be considered as needed.

| Pharmacological | Involvement of others was not mentioned by authors. |

Termination and Relapse Prevention

| Cognitive-Behavioral | During termination, assess Sandra's view of progress; attribute success to her rather than to therapist's efforts; find others with whom she can discuss practice, discuss issue of dependence; stretch out sessions. To prevent relapse: discuss future obstacles; prepare her for dealing with eventualities and temporary setback; conduct formal practice if anxiety increases; use booster sessions as needed. |

| Problem-Solving | At termination of therapy Sandra may fear independence. Therapist should communicate confidence in Sandra's coping ability. To prevent relapse therapist should work with Sandra in anticipating difficulties and future obstacles, generate options, make plans if anticipated problems arise, and taper last few sessions. If her anxiety increases, schedule follow-up booster sessions, being careful not to communicate a lack of confidence in Sandra. Provide her with handouts, work sheets, and copies of completed homework assignments for future use. |

| Acceptance and Commitment | Termination is a gradual process of tapering over time, based on a collaborative sense that the process of living is now ahead for Sandra. However, Sandra is never "cured" or "failed/relapsed," as ACT views living as an ongoing process. Booster sessions may be helpful; Sandra may come back periodically over several years. |

| Context-Centered | Views termination as an artificial punctuation that creates more problems than it solves. As Sandra's life improves, she will naturally come in less often. If problems occur, she may come back for additional sessions. |

| Contextual Family | Termination of the therapeutic relationship is seen as difficult and needs to be addressed with all participants. It may be helpful to have a session scheduled after an extended period following the "official" ter- |

mination. Therapist seeks to frame termination as an accomplishment and reinforce the positive accomplishments of all participants. Systemic relational networks put into place with mobilization of needed professionals following treatment.

Adlerian

Review of therapist's and Sandra's perspectives about therapeutic work. Assessment of present level of social interest expressed in work, love, and friendship. Discussion of possible symptom reoccurrence with suggestion that the intensity may be diminished. Sandra able to return for additional therapy if needed in the future.

Interpersonal

Issues pertaining to termination, such as mourning the end of treatment and bolstering Sandra's sense of competence, would be addressed in the final 2 to 4 sessions of treatment. If Sandra requires further treatment, a new treatment contract emphasizing a different treatment focus could be developed or she could be referred for treatment to another mental health professional.

Person-Centered

Discuss growth Sandra has experienced through therapy; reinforce her internal valuing system and level of congruence achieved thus far; client decides when she is ready to terminate. Sandra will discuss what she can do to prevent herself from relapsing into old habits and behaviors; relapse is not a major issue in person-centered work, as once Sandra accepts herself and once her behavior is congruent with her thoughts and feelings and her internal evaluation system, there is no pressure to revert back to old patterns which are no longer valued.

Supportive-Expressive

Termination facilitates a review of the entire treatment process, endeavors to assist Sandra in maintaining the gains made in treatment, and works toward helping the patient understand separation. Symptoms may arise again at termination; helping Sandra understand their meaning in the context of the therapeutic relationship and separation aids in closure. Sandra would not be dissuaded from contacting the therapist after termination to inform the therapist of progress or to seek further treatment if required.

Psychodynamic   Sandra and therapist decide together when to terminate. The termination process occurs over several months, during which time Sandra would explore a variety of issues including the experience of loss. Memories and feelings associated with earlier losses would be reviewed with accompanying issues of disappointment, disillusionment, and abandonment. Sandra can return for additional sessions as needed. Maintenance of professional posture and therapeutic frame is important.

Pharmacolog-   Patients develop tolerance and a physical dependence
ical   to many medications, particularly benzodiazepines. Gradual tapering of medication over time minimizes withdrawal and relapse effects. After pharmacotherapy termination, two to three follow-up visits would occur to monitor symptom reoccurrence.

Mechanisms of Change

Cognitive-   Breaking erroneous or maladaptive associations; fears
Behavioral   have likely been maintained by avoidance. Through exposure, the associations between avoidance and anxiety reduction would be broken: Sandra learns new information—that being alone is not necessarily dangerous, learns an increased sense of control over environment particularly over potentially threatening events. Through exposure and psychoeducation, Sandra's erroneous beliefs are challenged and replaced with more realistic beliefs.

Problem-   Improvement in problem-solving skills, coping, and
Solving   anxiety management will improve her sense of control, problem-solving self-efficacy, proactive coping, decreased avoidance, increased trust, and increased pleasure in prosocial activities. Changes in thoughts, feelings, behaviors, and coping will lead to improve-

ment in her relationships, daily functioning, and quality of life.

Acceptance and Commitment
: Increase in acceptance skills; reduction in believability of negative self-evaluation, worrisome thoughts, and anxious constructions; increase in emotional openness and experiential acceptance; display of new and valued behaviors; significant reduction in phobic avoidances; and improved relationships.

Context-Centered
: Orthogonal interactions between Sandra and the therapist will help Sandra break out of self-perpetuating linguistic structures/belief systems, negotiate role conflicts, tap underutilized resources, and contemplate new ways of being. Calling attention to the framework of assumptions that dictates how relationships develop and how symptoms are experienced creates positive change. Acceptance, detachment, and commitment serve to recontextualize symptoms, leading symptoms to decrease.

Contextual Family
: Participants identify those aspects of their relationships that they have felt to be false and exploitive. Concurrently, a multigenerational dialogue of open questioning, answering, and understanding leads to change in individual and relational functioning. Understanding each person's justice system and ledger of merits, receiving relational dispensation for past perceived injustices, reworking of injured relationships, and uncovering negative aspects of invisible loyalty help lead to the abandonment of long-standing imbalanced roles in relationships.

Adlerian
: A therapeutic relationship characterized by cooperation, mutual respect, and the experience of being deeply understood stimulates hope and encouragement. Develop insight and awareness of her lifestyle and symptom purposes. Understand how childhood experiences shape current conclusions about self, life, others, symptoms, and safety behaviors. Reframe symptoms and resistances. Education about how people function. Increase expression of social interest.

Interpersonal
Promotion of the sick role, use of the interpersonal inventory, and identification of Sandra's social isolation (lack of meaningful relationships). Establishment of a treatment contract as well as interventions such as communication analysis and role-playing will instill hope for symptom reduction. The therapist's adherence to boundaries and attention to Sandra's dependency, avoidance, and inability to trust will offer her a chance to feel validated as well as to tolerate distress and success.

Person-Centered
Development of an internal evaluation system. Decrease in incongruence between real and ideal self. Increase in self-acceptance.

Supportive-Expressive
Patients gain understanding into symptoms and into their relationships with important people in their life. By attending to the emotional insights, an understanding of their relational world (with conflicting wishes, expected responses from others, and typical symptom patterns) can be gained. The use of the current therapeutic relationship facilitates this process through an understanding of transference and assisting the patient in exercising more adaptive ways of relating. Change is also facilitated by the patient's experiencing the therapist as a supportive ally. The therapeutic alliance is crucial to therapy as the patient encounters in the present successive manifestations of difficult, anachronistic relationships from the past. At termination, acknowledging feelings that emerge provides an opportunity to negotiate separation and reinforce gains.

Psychodynamic
With patients for whom conflict rather than deficit is the difficulty, insight and self-understanding gained through interpretation is a major vehicle of change. For Sandra, who appears to suffer from structural impairment, internalization (transforming outer experiences to inner experiences) would constitute the therapeutic action of change. The affective relatedness, nature of the relationship, roles, functions,

and attitudes between therapist and patient serve to prompt the process of internalization for the patient.

Pharmacological

Different classes of psychotropic medications modify serotonergic and noradrenergic transmission—such as antidepressants (selective serotonin reuptake inhibitors, alpha-2 adrenoreceptor antagonists), buspirone, and agonists of GABA receptors like the benzodiazepines. Decreasing symptoms of arousal through medication may provide a basis from which Sandra could learn new ways of thinking, experiencing, and coping.

Index

Springer Publishing Company

Brief But Comprehensive Psychotherapy: *The Multimodal Way*

Arnold A. Lazarus, PhD, ABPP

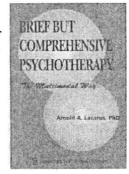

"...substantially advances the practice of short-term psychotherapy. Dr. Lazarus distills his many years of experience as a master clinician and teacher and outlines the fundamentals of multimodal therapy in an exciting and readable fashion. I highly recommend this volume to everybody in the mental health field, from students to advanced psychotherapists."
—**Aaron T. Beck,** Univ. Professor Emeritus
University of Pennsylvania

The current healthcare environment has created a need for short-term and cost-effective forms of psychotherapy, emphasizing efficiency and efficacy. The central message is "don't waste time." But how can one be so brief and also comprehensive?

Using his traditional acronym — BASIC ID — Dr. Lazarus stresses the assessment of seven dimensions of a client's personality: behavior, affect, sensation, imagery, cognition, interpersonal relationships, and the need for drugs. Featuring distinctive assessment procedures and therapeutic recommendations, this volume enhances the skills and clinical repertoires of every therapist.

Contents:
• Let's Cut to the Chase
• Elucidating the Main Rationale
• What is the Multimodal Way?
• Theories and Techniques
• Multimodal Assessment Procedures: Bridging and Tracking
• Multimodal Assessment Procedures: Second-Order Basic ID and Structural Profiles
• Some Elements of Effective Brevity
• Activity and Serendipity
• Two Specific Applications: Sexual Desire Disorders and Dysthymia
• Couples Therapy
• Some Common Time Wasters

Springer Series on Behavior Therapy and Behavioral Medicine
1997   192 pp   0-8261-9640-3   hard

536 Broadway, New York, NY 10012• (212) 431-4370 • Fax (212) 941-7842
Order Toll-Free: (877) 687-7476 • *www.springerpub.com*

Springer Publishing Company

Empirically Supported Cognitive Therapies
Current and Future Applications

William J. Lyddon, PhD
John V. Jones, Jr., PhD, LPC, NCC, ACT, Editors

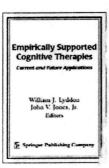

In the spirit of disseminating some of the most recent research on empirically supported treatments, this volume brings together distinguished practitioners and researchers in the field who use a cognitive model as the basis of their research and practice.

Cognitive techniques for common clinical problems such as depression, bipolar I disorder, phobias, panic disorder, obsessive compulsive disorders, post traumatic stress disorders, and eating disorders are described in clinical detail. Newer applications for anger management and antisocial behavior in children and adolescents are also reviewed. Illustrative case examples are integral to each discussion.

Including recent trends, current limitations, and new directions and developments, this text offers a fundamental knowledge base for students and practitioners alike.

Contents:

2001   272pp   0-8261-2299-X   hard

536 Broadway, New York, NY 10012 • Telephone: 212-431-4370
Fax: 212-941-7842 • Order Toll-Free: 877-687-7476
Order On-line: www.springerpub.com